Springer Series in

Series Editors
Peter Bickel, CA, USA
Peter Diggle, Lancaster, UK
Stephen E. Fienberg, Pittsburgh, PA, USA
Ursula Gather, Dortmund, Germany
Ingram Olkin, Stanford, CA, USA
Scott Zeger, Baltimore, MD, USA

More information about this series at
http://www.springer.com/series/692

Peter Müller • Fernando Andrés Quintana • Alejandro Jara • Tim Hanson

Bayesian Nonparametric Data Analysis

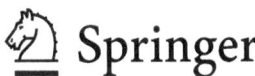 Springer

Peter Müller
Department of Mathematics
University of Texas at Austin
Austin, TX
USA

Fernando Andrés Quintana
Departamento de Estadística
Pontificia Universidad Católica
Santiago, Chile

Alejandro Jara
Departamento de Estadística
Pontificia Universidad Católica
Santiago, Chile

Tim Hanson
Department of Statistics
University of South Carolina
Columbia, SC
USA

ISSN 0172-7397   ISSN 2197-568X   (electronic)
Springer Series in Statistics
ISBN 978-3-319-18967-3   ISBN 978-3-319-18968-0   (eBook)
DOI 10.1007/978-3-319-18968-0

Library of Congress Control Number: 2015943065

Springer Cham Heidelberg New York Dordrecht London
© Springer International Publishing Switzerland 2015
This work is subject to copyright. All rights are reserved by the Publisher, whether the whole or part of the material is concerned, specifically the rights of translation, reprinting, reuse of illustrations, recitation, broadcasting, reproduction on microfilms or in any other physical way, and transmission or information storage and retrieval, electronic adaptation, computer software, or by similar or dissimilar methodology now known or hereafter developed.
The use of general descriptive names, registered names, trademarks, service marks, etc. in this publication does not imply, even in the absence of a specific statement, that such names are exempt from the relevant protective laws and regulations and therefore free for general use.
The publisher, the authors and the editors are safe to assume that the advice and information in this book are believed to be true and accurate at the date of publication. Neither the publisher nor the authors or the editors give a warranty, express or implied, with respect to the material contained herein or for any errors or omissions that may have been made.

Printed on acid-free paper

Springer International Publishing AG Switzerland is part of Springer Science+Business Media (www.springer.com)

Preface

In this book, we review nonparametric Bayesian methods and models. The organization of the book follows a data analysis perspective. Rather than focusing on specific models, chapters are organized by traditional data analysis problems. For each problem, we introduce suitable nonparametric Bayesian models and show how they are used to implement inference in the given data analysis problem. In selecting specific nonparametric models, we favor simpler and traditional models over specialized ones. The organization by inferential problem leads to some repetition in the discussion of specific models when the same nonparametric prior is used in different contexts.

Historically, Bayesian nonparametrics and indeed Bayesian statistics in general remained largely theoretical except for very simple models. The "discovery" and subsequent widespread use of Markov chain Monte Carlo and other Monte Carlo methods in the 1990s has made Bayesian nonparametric models an attractive and computationally viable possibility only in the last 20 years. Thus, a review of Bayesian nonparametric data analysis would be incomplete without a discussion of posterior simulation methods. We include pointers to available software, in particular public domain R packages. R code for some of the examples is available at a software page for the book at

https://www.ma.utexas.edu/users/pmueller/bnp/.

In the text, references to the software page are labeled as "**Software note**."

Chapter 1 introduces the framework for nonparametric and semiparametric inference and discusses the distinction between Bayesian and classical nonparametric inference. Chapters 2 and 3 start with a discussion of density estimation problems. Density estimation is one of the simplest statistical inference problems, and has traditionally been a popular application for nonparametric Bayesian methods. The emphasis is on the Dirichlet process, Polya trees, and related models. Chapter 4 is about nonparametric regression, including nonparametric priors on residual distributions, nonparametric mean functions, and fully nonparametric regression. The latter is also known as density regression. Chapter 5 introduces methods for categorical data, including contingency tables for multivariate categorical data and methods specifically for ordinal data. Chapter 6 discusses applications to survival

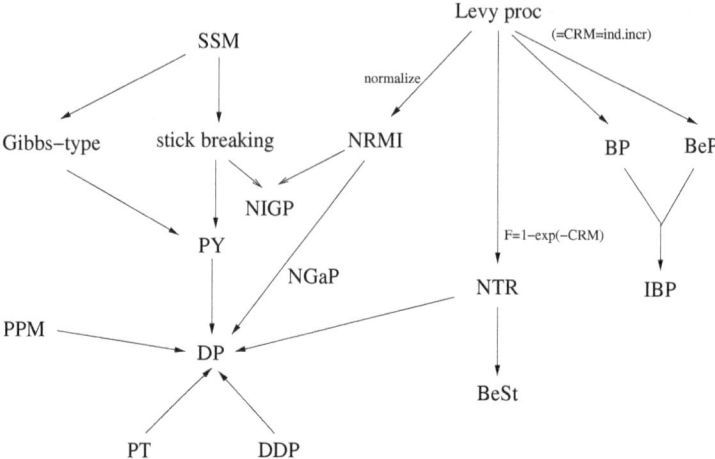

Fig. 1 Overview of some popular Bayesian nonparametric models for random probability measures. An *arrow* from model M1 to model M2 indicates that M2 is a special case of M1. For the case of NRMI and NTR, the *arrow* indicates that the descendant model is defined through a transformation of the CRM. Notice the central role of the Dirichlet process (DP) model

analysis. Probability models for a hazard function and random probability models for event times are a traditional use of nonparametric Bayesian methods. Perhaps this is the case because for event times it is natural to focus on details of the unknown distribution, beyond just the mean. Chapter 7 considers the use of random probability models in hierarchical models. Nonparametric priors for random effects distributions are some of the most successful and widespread applications of nonparametric Bayesian inference. In Chap. 8, we discuss models for random clustering and for feature allocation problems. Finally, in Chap. 9, we conclude with a brief discussion of some more problems. In the Appendix, we include a brief introduction to DPpackage, a public domain R package that implements inference for many of the models that are discussed in this book.

Figure 1 gives an idea of how popular nonparametric Bayesian models relate to each other. The Dirichlet process (DP), Polya tree (PT), Pitman Yor process (PY), normalized random measures (NRMI), and stick-breaking priors are discussed as priors for random probability measures in Chaps. 2 and 3. The dependent DP (DDP) is used to define a fully nonparametric regression model in Chap. 4, and then also features again in Chap. 6 for survival regression, and again in Chap. 7 to define a prior for a family of dependent random probability measures. Neutral to the right (NTR) processes come up in Chap. 6. The product partition model (PPM) and Gibbs-type priors are introduced as priors for random partitions, that is, cluster arrangement, in Chap. 8. The Indian buffet process (IBP) is introduced as a feature allocation model, also in Chap. 8.

The selection and focus is necessarily tainted by subjective choices and preferences. Finally, we recognize that the outlined classification of data analysis problems is arbitrary. Meaningful alternative organizations could have focused on the probability models, or on application areas.

Austin, TX, USA Peter Müller
Santiago, Chile Fernando Andrés Quintana
Santiago, Chile Alejandro Jara
Columbia, SC, USA Tim Hanson

Acronyms

We use the following acronyms. When applicable we list a corresponding section number in parentheses. We omit acronyms that are only used within specific examples.

AH	Accelerated hazards (Sect. 6.2.4)
AFT	Accelerated failure time (Sect. 6.2.2)
ANOVA DDP	DDP with AN(C)OVA model on $\{m_{hx},\ x \in X\}$ (Sect. 4.4.2)
BART	Bayesian additive regression trees (Sect. 4.3.4)
BNP	Bayesian nonparametric (model, inference)
CALGB	Cancer and Leukemia Group B
CART	Classification and regression tree (Sect. 4.3.4)
c.d.f.	Cumulative distribution function
CI	Credible interval
CPO	Conditional predictive ordinate (Chap. 9)
CRM	Completely random measure (Sect. 3.5.2)
CSDP	Centrally standardized Dirichlet process (Sect. 5.2.1)
DDP	Dependent Dirichlet process (Sect. 4.4.1)
DP_K	Finite Dirichlet process (Sect. 2.4.6)
DPM	Dirichlet process mixture (Sect. 2.2)
DPT	Dependent Polya tree (Sect. 4.4.3)
DP	Dirichlet process (Sect. 2.1)
FFNN	Feed-forward neural network (Sect. 4.3.1)
FPT	Finite Polya tree (Sect. 3.2.2)
GLM	Generalized linear model (Sect. 5.2.)
GLMM	Generalized linear mixed model (Sect. 5.2.2)
GP	Gaussian process (Sect. 4.3.3)
HDPM	Hierarchical Dirichlet process mixture (Sect. 7.3.1)
IBP	Indian buffet process (Sect. 8.5.2)
LDTFP	Linear dependent tail-free process (Sect. 4.4.3)
LPML	Log pseudo marginal likelihood (Chap. 9)
MAD	MAP-based asymptotic derivation

MAP	Maximum a posterior estimate
MCMC	Markov chain Monte Carlo (posterior simulation)
m.l.e.	Maximum likelihood estimator
MPT	Mixture of Polya tree (Sect. 3.2.1)
NRMI	Normalized random measure with independent increments (Sect. 3.5.2)
NTR	Neutral to the right (Sect. 6.1.1)
p.d.f.	Probability density function
PD	Pharmacodynamics (Sect. 7.2)
PH	Proportional hazards (Sect. 6.2.1)
PK	Pharmacokinetics (Sect. 7.2)
PO	Proportional odds (Sect. 6.2.3)
PPM	Product partition model (Sect. 8.3)
PPMx	Product partition model with regression on covariates (Sect. 8.4.1)
PT	Polya tree (Sect. 3.1)
PY	Pitman-Yor process (Sect. 2.5.2)
SSM	Species sampling model (Sect. 2.5.2)
TF	Tail free (Sect. 2.5.1)
WBC	White blood cell counts
WDDP	Weight dependent Dirichlet process (Sect. 4.4.4).

We use the following notational conventions. *Probability measures:* We use $p(\cdot)$ to generically indicate probability measures. The use of the arguments in $p(\cdot)$ or the context clarifies which probability measure is meant. Only when needed we use subindices, such as $p_X(\cdot)$, or introduce specific names, such as $q(\cdot)$. We use $\pi(\cdot)$ to indicate (upper level) prior probability models, usually BNP priors on a random probability measure, for example, $\pi(G)$ for a random probability measure G. When the use is clear from the context, we use $p(\cdot)$, etc. to also refer to the p.d.f, and introduce separate notation only when we wish to highlight something. We use $f_\theta(\cdot)$ for kernels and $f_G(\cdot) = \int f_\theta(\cdot) \, dG(\theta)$ for a mixture. We use notation like $\text{Be}(\epsilon \mid a, b)$ to indicate that the random variable ϵ follows a $\text{Be}(a, b)$ distribution. *Variables:* We use y_i for observed outcomes, x_i for known covariates, boldface ($\boldsymbol{y}$) for vectors, and uppercase symbols (A), or boldface uppercase ($\boldsymbol{C}$) when needed for distinction or emphasis, for matrices. *Clusters:* Many models include a notion of clusters. We use $\star$ to mark quantities that are cluster-specific, such as $\boldsymbol{y}_j^\star$, $\theta_j^\star$, etc.

Contents

1	**Introduction**		1
	References		5
2	**Density Estimation: DP Models**		7
	2.1	Dirichlet Process	7
		2.1.1 Definition	7
		2.1.2 Posterior and Marginal Distributions	9
	2.2	Dirichlet Process Mixture	11
		2.2.1 The DPM Model	11
		2.2.2 Mixture of DPM	15
	2.3	Clustering Under the DPM	15
	2.4	Posterior Simulation for DPM Models	16
		2.4.1 Conjugate DPM Models	17
		2.4.2 Updating Hyper-Parameters	19
		2.4.3 Non-Conjugate DPM Models	20
		2.4.4 Neal's Algorithm 8	22
		2.4.5 Slice Sampler	23
		2.4.6 Finite DP	25
	2.5	Generalizations of the Dirichlet Processes	26
		2.5.1 Tail-Free Processes	26
		2.5.2 Species Sampling Models (SSM)	27
		2.5.3 Generalized Dirichlet Processes	28
	References		29
3	**Density Estimation: Models Beyond the DP**		33
	3.1	Polya Trees	33
		3.1.1 Definition	33
		3.1.2 Prior Centering	35
		3.1.3 Posterior Updating and Marginal Model	37
	3.2	Variations of the Polya Tree Processes	39
		3.2.1 Mixture of Polya Trees	39
		3.2.2 Partially Specified Polya Trees	41

	3.3	Posterior Simulation for Polya Tree Models	41
		3.3.1 FTP and i.i.d. Sampling	41
		3.3.2 PT and MPT Prior Under i.i.d. Sampling	42
		3.3.3 Posterior Inference for Non-Conjugate Models	45
	3.4	A Comparison of DP Versus PT Models	46
	3.5	NRMI	48
		3.5.1 Other Generalizations of the DP Prior	48
		3.5.2 Mixture of NRMI	49
	References		49

4 Regression ... 51
- 4.1 Bayesian Nonparametric Regression ... 51
- 4.2 Nonparametric Residual Distribution ... 52
- 4.3 Nonparametric Mean Function ... 54
  - 4.3.1 Basis Expansions ... 54
  - 4.3.2 B-Splines ... 59
  - 4.3.3 Gaussian Process Priors ... 62
  - 4.3.4 Regression Trees ... 63
- 4.4 Fully Nonparametric Regression ... 64
  - 4.4.1 Priors on Families of Random Probability Measures ... 65
  - 4.4.2 ANOVA DDP and LDDP ... 67
  - 4.4.3 Dependent PT Prior ... 70
  - 4.4.4 Conditional Regression ... 72
- References ... 74

5 Categorical Data ... 77
- 5.1 Categorical Responses Without Covariates ... 77
  - 5.1.1 Binomial Responses ... 77
  - 5.1.2 Categorical Responses ... 80
  - 5.1.3 Multivariate Ordinal Data ... 83
- 5.2 Categorical Responses with Covariates ... 86
  - 5.2.1 Nonparametric Link Function: A Semiparametric GLM ... 87
  - 5.2.2 Models for Latent Scores ... 90
  - 5.2.3 Nonparametric Random Effects Model ... 92
  - 5.2.4 Multivariate Ordinal Regression ... 95
- 5.3 ROC Curve Estimation ... 96
- References ... 99

6 Survival Analysis ... 101
- 6.1 Distribution Estimation for Event Times ... 101
  - 6.1.1 Neutral to the Right Processes ... 102
  - 6.1.2 Dependent Increments Models ... 103
- 6.2 Semiparametric Survival Regression ... 104
  - 6.2.1 Proportional Hazards ... 105
  - 6.2.2 Accelerated Failure Time ... 107

	6.2.3	Proportional Odds	108
	6.2.4	Other Semiparametric Models and Extensions	109
6.3	Fully Nonparametric Survival Regression		110
	6.3.1	Extensions of the AFT model	110
	6.3.2	ANCOVA-DDP: Linear Dependent DP Mixture	110
	6.3.3	Linear Dependent Tail-Free Process (LDTFP)	113
6.4	More Examples		114
	6.4.1	Example 17: Breast Retraction Data	114
	6.4.2	Example 8 (ctd.): Breast Cancer Trial	116
	6.4.3	Example 18: Lung Cancer Data	118
References			121

7 Hierarchical Models ... 125

7.1	Nonparametric Random Effects Distributions		125
7.2	Population PK/PD Models		129
7.3	Hierarchical Models of RPMs		132
	7.3.1	Finite Mixtures of Random Probability Measures	132
	7.3.2	Dependent Random Probability Measures	136
	7.3.3	Classification	138
7.4	Hierarchical, Nested and Enriched DP		139
References			141

8 Clustering and Feature Allocation ... 145

8.1	Random Partitions and Feature Allocations		145
8.2	Polya Urn and Model Based Clustering		147
8.3	Product Partition Models (PPMs)		150
	8.3.1	Definition	150
	8.3.2	Posterior Simulation	152
8.4	Clustering and Regression		155
	8.4.1	The PPMx Model	155
	8.4.2	PPMx with Variable Selection	158
	8.4.3	Example 26: A PPMx Model for Outlier Detection	160
8.5	Feature Allocation Models		164
	8.5.1	Feature Allocation	164
	8.5.2	Indian Buffet Process	165
	8.5.3	Approximate Posterior Inference with MAD Bayes	168
8.6	Nested Clustering Models		170
References			173

9 Other Inference Problems and Conclusion ... 175
References ... 178

A	**DPpackage**		179
	A.1 Overview		180
	A.2 An Example		182
		A.2.1 The Models	182
		A.2.2 Example 29: Simulated Data	184
	References		188

Index 191

Chapter 1
Introduction

Abstract We introduce the setup of nonparametric and semiparametric Bayesian models and inference.

Statistical problems are described using probability models. That is, data are envisioned as realizations of a collection of random variables $y_1, \ldots, y_n$, where y_i itself could be a vector of random variables corresponding to data that are collected on the i-th experimental unit in a sample of n units from some population of interest. A common assumption is that the y_i are drawn independently from some underlying probability distribution G. The statistical problem begins when there exists uncertainty about G. Let g denote the probability density function (p.d.f.) of G. A statistical model arises when g is known to be a member g_θ from a family $\mathcal{G} = \{g_\theta : \theta \in \Theta\}$, labeled by a set of parameters θ from an index set Θ.

Models that are described through a vector θ of a finite number of, typically, real values are referred to as finite-dimensional or *parametric models*. Parametric models can be described as $\mathcal{G} = \{g_\theta : \boldsymbol{\theta} \in \boldsymbol{\Theta} \subset \mathbb{R}^p\}$. The aim of the analysis is then to use the observed sample to report a plausible value for $\boldsymbol{\theta}$, or at least to determine a subset of $\boldsymbol{\Theta}$ which plausibly contains $\boldsymbol{\theta}$. In many situations, however, constraining inference to a specific parametric form may limit the scope and type of inferences that can be drawn from such models. Therefore, we would like to relax parametric assumptions to allow greater modeling flexibility and robustness against mis-specification of a parametric statistical model. In these cases, we may want to consider models where the class of densities is so large that it can no longer be indexed by a finite dimensional parameter $\boldsymbol{\theta}$, and we therefore require parameters $\boldsymbol{\theta}$ in an infinite dimensional space.

Example 1 (Density Estimation) Consider a simple random sample $y_i \mid G \overset{iid}{\sim} G$, $i = 1, \ldots, n$, from some unknown distribution G. One could now proceed by restricting G to a normal location family, say $\mathcal{G} = \{N(\theta, 1) : \theta \subset \mathbb{R}\}$. Figure 1.1a shows the resulting inference conditional on an assumed random sample $y_1, \ldots, y_n$. Naturally, inference about the unknown G is restricted to the assumed normal location family and does not allow for multi-modality or skewness. In contrast, a nonparametric model would proceed with a prior probability model π for the unknown distribution G. For example, later we will introduce the Dirichlet process mixture prior for G.

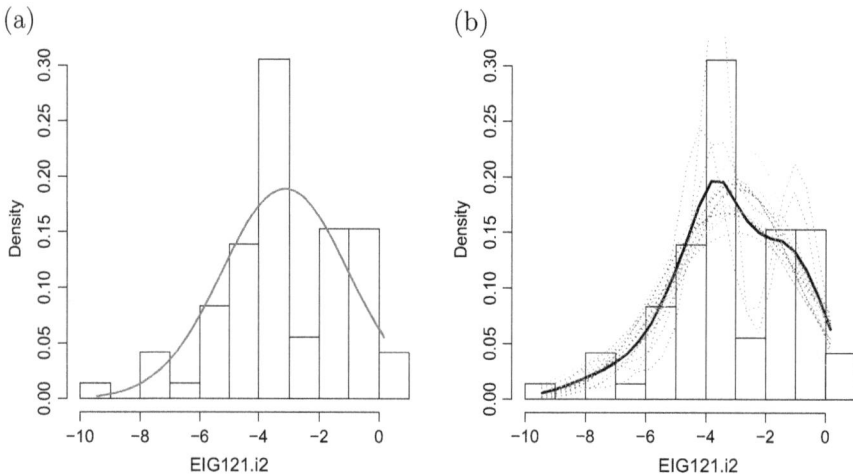

Fig. 1.1 Example 1. Inference on the unknown distribution G under a parametric model (panel **a**) and nonparametric model (panel **b**). The histogram of the observed data is also displayed. The *dotted lines* in panel (**b**) correspond to posterior draws

Figure 1.1b contrasts the parametric inference with the flexible BNP inference under a Dirichlet process mixture prior.

In Example 1 the unknown, infinite dimensional, parameter is the distribution G itself. Another example of an infinite-dimensional parameter space is the space of continuous functions defined on the real line, $\mathcal{S} = \{m(z) : z \in \mathbb{R}, m(\cdot) \text{ is a continuous function}\}$. This could arise, for example, in a regression model with unknown mean function $m(z)$. Models with infinite-dimensional parameters are referred to as *nonparametric models* (Ghosh and Ramamoorthi 2003; Tsiatis 2006). In some other cases, it is useful to write the infinite-dimensional parameter θ as (θ_1, θ_2), where θ_1 is a q-dimensional parameter and θ_2 is an infinite-dimensional parameter. These models are referred to as *semiparametric models* because both a parametric component θ_1 and a nonparametric component θ_2 describe the model (see e.g., Tsiatis 2006). As an example of a semiparametric model, consider the proportional hazards model that is commonly used in modeling a survival time T as a function of a vector of covariates z. The model was first introduced by Cox (1972). Let

$$\lambda(t \mid z) = \lim_{h \to 0} \left\{ \frac{p(t \leq T < t + h \mid T \geq t, z)}{h} \right\} \tag{1.1}$$

denote the conditional hazard rate, conditional on some covariates z. The proportional hazards model assumes

$$\lambda(t \mid z) = \lambda_0(t) \exp(z'\boldsymbol{\beta}). \tag{1.2}$$

where $\lambda_0(\cdot)$ is the underlying or baseline hazard function and $\boldsymbol{\beta}$ is a q-dimensional vector of regression coefficients. In the classical semiparametric version of the model, the underlying hazard function is left unspecified. Since this function can be any positive function in t, subject to some regularity conditions, it is an infinite-dimensional parameter. The parameters $\boldsymbol{\theta} = (\boldsymbol{\beta}, \lambda_0)$ completely characterize the data generating mechanism. In fact, the density f_T of the survival time T is related to the hazard function through

$$f_T(t \mid z) = \lambda_0(t) \exp(z'\boldsymbol{\beta}) \exp\left\{-\exp(z'\boldsymbol{\beta}) \int_0^t \lambda_0(u) du\right\}.$$

The parameters of interest can be written as $\boldsymbol{\theta}_1 = \boldsymbol{\beta}$ and $\boldsymbol{\theta}_2 = \lambda_0$, where $\boldsymbol{\theta} = (\boldsymbol{\theta}_1, \boldsymbol{\theta}_2) \in \Theta = \mathbb{R}^q \times \mathcal{S}$ and $\mathcal{S}$ is the infinite-dimensional space of all nonnegative functions on $\mathbb{R}^+$ with infinite integral over $[0, \infty)$.

Example 2 (Oral Cancer) We use a dataset from Klein and Moeschberger (2003, Sect. 1.11). The data report survival times for 80 patients with cancers of the mouth. Samples are recorded as aneuploid (abnormal number of chromosomes) versus diploid (two copies of each chromosome) tumors. We define $z_i \in \{0, 1\}$ as an indicator for aneuploid tumors and carry out inference under model (1.2) with a BNP prior on λ_0. Figure 1.2 shows the estimated hazard curves under $z = 0$ and

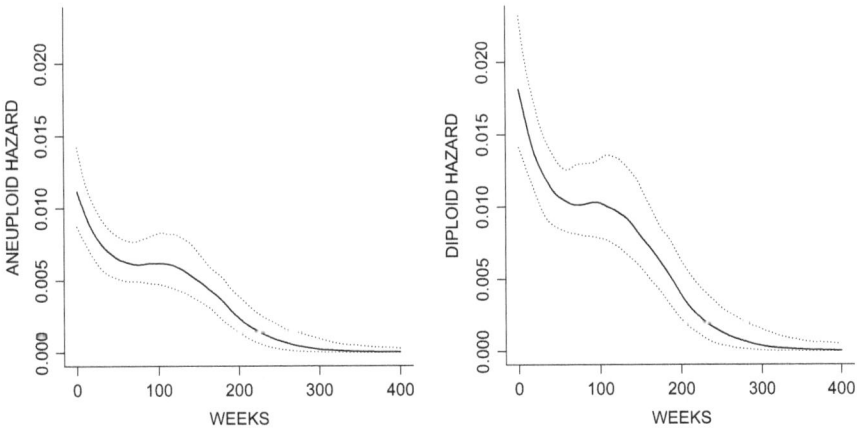

Fig. 1.2 Example 2. Hazard curves for aneuploid and diploid groups under the proportional hazard model with point-wise 50% CIs

$z = 1$. The prior on $\log\{\lambda_0(\cdot)\}$ is a penalized B-spline, fit through the R package R2BayesX.

To proceed with Bayesian inference in a nonparametric model we need to complete the probability model with a prior on the infinite-dimensional parameter. Such priors are known as Bayesian nonparametric (BNP) priors. We take this as a definition of BNP models. That is, we define BNP priors as probability models for infinite-dimensional parameters and refer to the entire inference model as a BNP model. This highlights the similarities and distinctions of Bayesian versus classical nonparametric inference. Under both BNP and classical nonparametric approaches an infinite-dimensional parameter characterizes the family of sampling probability models. The major difference between Bayesian and classical nonparametrics is that Bayesian inference completes the model with a prior on the infinite-dimensional parameter (random probability measure, regression function, etc.). As a result, inference includes a full probabilistic description of all relevant uncertainties. Classical nonparametrics, on the other hand, treats infinite-dimensional parameters as nuisance parameters and derives procedures where they are left unspecified to make inferences on finite-dimensional parameters of interest.

Infinite-dimensional parameters of interest are usually functions. Functions of common interest include probability distributions, or conditional trends, e.g. mean or median regression functions. Consideration of probability distributions requires the definition of probability measures on a collection of distribution functions. Such probability measures are generically referred to as random probability measures.

While our main focus is on data analysis and how to build models in some important special cases, it is important to know that there is a solid body of theory supporting the use of nonparametric models. In the upcoming discussion we will briefly state some of the important results and the particular effect they have on models. But we stop short of an exhaustive list of BNP prior models. An excellent recent review of a large number of BNP models appears in Phadia (2013). See also Figure 1.1 in Phadia (2013), which is an interesting variation of Fig. 1 in the preface of the current text. Other recent discussions of BNP priors include Hjort et al. (2010), including an excellent and concise review of BNP models beyond the Dirichlet process in Lijoi and Prünster (2010), Hjort (2003), Müller and Rodríguez (2013), Müller and Quintana (2004), Walker et al. (1999), and Walker (2013). Gelman et al. (2014, Part V) includes a discussion of nonparametric Bayesian data analysis. A mathematically rigorous discussion, with an emphasis on asymptotic properties can be found in the forthcoming book by Ghoshal and van der Vaart (2015).

In this text we will not prove any new results and therefore never need to refer to measure theoretic niceties. We refer interested readers to Phadia (2013), who discusses all the same models that also feature in this text. See also Ghosh and Ramamoorthi (2003), Ghoshal (2010), and Ghoshal and van der Vaart (2015) for a mathematically more rigorous discussion. Briefly summarized, assume an underlying probability space $(\Omega, \mathcal{A}, \mu)$ and let S be a complete and separable metric space equipped with the Borel σ-algebra $\mathcal{B}$. Denote by $M(S)$ the space of probability measures on S endowed with the topology of weak convergence which makes it a complete and separable space. Most BNP priors that we introduce in the following discussion are distributions over $M(S)$ or, in other terms, laws of random probability measures i.e. random elements defined on Ω and taking values in $M(S)$.

References

Cox DR (1972) Regression models and life-tables (with discussion). J R Stat Soc Ser B 34:187–220
Gelman A, Carlin JB, Stern HS, Dunson DB, Vehtari A, Rubin DB (2014) Bayesian data analysis. CRC Press, Boca Raton
Ghosh JK, Ramamoorthi RV (2003) Bayesian nonparametrics. Springer, New York
Ghoshal S (2010) The Dirichlet process, related priors and posterior asymptotics. In: Hjort NL, Holmes C, Müller P, Walker SG (eds) Bayesian nonparametrics. Cambridge University Press, Cambridge, pp 22–34
Ghoshal S, van der Vaart A (2015) Fundamentals of nonparametric Bayesian inference. Cambridge University Press, Cambridge
Hjort NL (2003) Topics in nonparametric Bayesian statistics. In: Green P, Hjort N, Richardson S (eds) Highly structured stochastic systems. Oxford University Press, Oxford, pp 455–487
Hjort NL, Holmes C, Müller P, Walker SG (eds) (2010) Bayesian nonparametrics. Cambridge University Press, Cambridge
Klein JP, Moeschberger ML (2003) Survival analysis: techniques for censored and truncated data. Springer, New York
Lijoi A, Prünster I (2010) Models beyond the Dirichlet process. In: Hjort NL, Holmes C, Müller P, Walker SG (eds) Bayesian nonparametrics. Cambridge University Press, Cambridge, pp 80–136
Müller P, Quintana FA (2004) Nonparametric Bayesian data analysis. Stat Sci 19(1):95–110
Müller P, Rodríguez A (2013) Nonparametric Bayesian inference. IMS-CBMS Lecture notes. IMS, Beachwood
Phadia EG (2013) Prior processes and their applications. Springer, New York
Tsiatis AA (2006) Semiparametric theory and missing data. Springer, New York
Walker S (2013) Bayesian nonparametrics. In: Damien P, Dellaportas P, Polson NG, Stephens DA (eds) Bayesian theory and applications. Oxford University Press, Oxford, pp 249–270
Walker SG, Damien P, Laud PW, Smith AFM (1999) Bayesian nonparametric inference for random distributions and related functions (with discussion). J R Stat Soc B 61:485–527

Chapter 2
Density Estimation: DP Models

Abstract We discuss the use of nonparametric Bayesian models in density estimation, arguably one of the most basic statistical inference problems. In this chapter we introduce the Dirichlet process prior and variations of it that are the by far most commonly used nonparametric Bayesian models used in this context. Variations include the Dirichlet process mixture and the finite Dirichlet process. One critical reason for the extensive use of these models is the availability of computation efficient methods for posterior simulation. We discuss several such methods.

Density estimation is concerned with inference about an unknown distribution G on the basis of an observed i.i.d. sample,

$$y_i \mid G \stackrel{iid}{\sim} G, \ i = 1, \ldots, n. \tag{2.1}$$

If we wish to proceed with Bayesian inference, we need to complete the model with a prior probability model π for the unknown parameter G. Assuming a prior model on G requires the specification of a probability model for an infinite-dimensional parameter, that is, a BNP prior.

2.1 Dirichlet Process

2.1.1 Definition

One of the most popular BNP models is the Dirichlet process (DP) prior. The DP model was introduced by Ferguson (1973) as a prior on the space of probability measures.

Definition 1 (Dirichlet Process—DP) Let $M > 0$ and G_0 be a probability measure defined on S. A DP with parameters $(M, \overline{G_0})$ is a random probability measure G defined on S which assigns probability $G(B)$ to every (measurable) set B such that for each (measurable) finite partition $\{B_1, \ldots, B_k\}$ of S, the joint distribution of the vector $(G(B_1), \ldots, G(B_k))$ is the Dirichlet distribution with parameters

$$(MG_0(B_1), \ldots, MG_0(B_k)).$$

Using Kolmogorov's consistency theorem (Kolmogorov 1933), Ferguson (1973) showed that such a process exists. The process is usually denoted as DP (MG_0), or DP(M, G_0). The parameter M is called the precision or total mass parameter, G_0 is the centering measure, and the product $\alpha \equiv MG_0$ is referred to as the base measure of the DP.

An important property of the DP is the discrete nature of G. As a discrete random probability measure we can always write G as a weighted sum of point masses, $G(\cdot) = \sum_{h=1}^{\infty} w_h \delta_{m_h}(\cdot)$, where $w_1, w_2, \ldots$ are probability weights and $\delta_x(\cdot)$ denotes the Dirac measure at x. Another important property of the DP is its large weak support, which means that under mild conditions, any distribution with the same support as G_0 can be well approximated weakly by a DP random probability measure. Formally, let Q be any probability measure with $Q \ll G_0$, that is, Q does not assign positive probability to any event that has probability 0 under G_0. The large support property means that for any finite number of measurable sets $B_1, \ldots, B_m$, and $\epsilon > 0$,

$$\pi\{|G(B_i) - Q(B_i)| < \epsilon, \text{ for } i = 1, \ldots, m\} > 0.$$

That is, the random probability measure G can come arbitrarily close in a weak sense to Q on the sets B_i. In this statement the probability $\pi\{\ldots\}$ refers to the probability model π of G.

The DP arises naturally as an infinite-dimensional analogue of the finite-dimensional Dirichlet prior, as suggested by the defining property. The definition implies several other useful properties of a DP random measure G. Some are easily seen by considering the partition of the sample space given by $\{B, B^c\}$ consisting of an event B and its complement B^c. In particular, G has the same support as G_0, i.e., $\pi(G(B) > 0) = 1$ if and only if $G_0(B) > 0$. Mean and variance of the random probability $G(B)$ for any B are $E[G(B)] = G_0(B)$ and $\text{Var}[G(B)] = G_0(B)[1 - G_0(B)]/(1 + M)$. The latter can be seen from the fact that $(G(B), G(B^c)) \sim \text{Dir}\{MG_0(B), M[1 - G_0(B)]\}$. These results show the effect of the precision parameter in a DP. If M is large, G is highly concentrated about G_0. This explains why M is also known as the precision parameter of a DP prior. Figure 2.1 demonstrates the effects of increasing the precision parameter. As $M \longrightarrow \infty$ the process is essentially G_0.

Stick Breaking Construction An often useful constructive definition of a DP random probability measure is given by Sethuraman (1994) and is based on the discrete nature of the process $G(\cdot) = \sum_{h=1}^{\infty} w_h \delta_{m_h}(\cdot)$. In this construction, the locations m_h are i.i.d. draws from the centering measure G_0, and each weight w_h is defined as a fraction of $\{1 - \sum_{\ell < h} w_\ell\}$, that is, a fraction of what is left after the preceding $h - 1$ point masses. Formally, let $w_h = v_h \prod_{\ell < h}(1 - v_\ell)$ with

2.1 Dirichlet Process

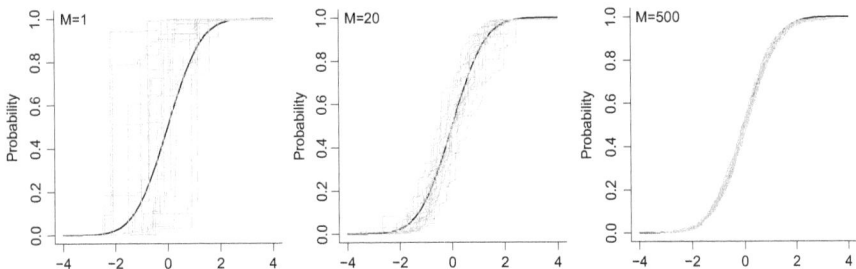

Fig. 2.1 Plots of 15 samples from a DP(MG_0), with $G_0 = N(0, 1)$ a standard normal distribution, for $M = 1, 20$ and 500. In all cases, $G_0 = E(G)$ is overlaid on a plot of the realizations of G

$v_h \stackrel{iid}{\sim} \text{Be}(1, M)$, and $m_h \stackrel{iid}{\sim} G_0$, where $\{v_h\}$ and $\{m_h\}$ are independent. Then

$$G(\cdot) = \sum_{h=1}^{\infty} w_h \delta_{m_h}(\cdot), \tag{2.2}$$

defines a DP(MG_0) random probability measure. The definition of w_h can be pictured as successively breaking fractions v_h of a stick of initially unit length. This representation of a DP random measure is therefore known as "stick-breaking". A consequence of this representation is that if $G \sim \text{DP}(MG_0)$, $m \sim G_0$ and $W \sim \text{Be}(1, M)$, and all of them are independent, then $W\delta_m(\cdot) + (1 - W)G(\cdot)$ follows again a DP(MG_0) distribution.

Finally, the DP has an important conditioning property, which follows immediately from the definition. If A is a (measurable) set with $G_0(A) > 0$ (which implies that $G(A) > 0$ a.s.), then the random measure $G\mid_A$, the restriction of G to A defined by $G\mid_A (B) = G(B \mid A) = G(A \cap B)/G(A)$, is also a DP with parameters M and $G_0\mid_A$, and is independent of $G(A)$. The argument can be extended to more than one set. Thus the DP locally splits into numerous independent DP's.

2.1.2 Posterior and Marginal Distributions

Posterior Updating The DP is conjugate with respect to i.i.d. sampling. That is, under the sampling model (2.1) with a DP on G, the posterior distribution for G is again a DP. The base measure of the posterior DP adds a point mass to the prior base measure at each observed data point y_i. In other words, the posterior DP centering measure is a weighted average of G_0 and the empirical distribution $\hat{f}_n(\cdot) = \frac{1}{n}\sum_{i=1}^{n} \delta_{y_i}(\cdot)$, and the posterior total mass parameter is incremented to $M+n$. In summary,

Result 1 (Ferguson 1973) *Let* $y_1, \ldots, y_n \mid G \overset{iid}{\sim} G$ *and* $G \sim \text{DP}(MG_0)$. *Then,*

$$G \mid y_1, \ldots, y_n \sim DP\left(MG_0 + \sum_{i=1}^{n} \delta_{y_i}\right). \tag{2.3}$$

Example 3 (T-Cell Receptors) Guindani et al. (2014) consider data on counts of distinct T-cell receptors. The diversity of T-cell receptor types is an important characteristic of the immune system. A common summary of the diversity is the clonal-size distribution. The clonal-size distribution is the table of frequencies $\hat{G}_y$ of counts $y = 1, 2, \ldots, n$. For example, $\hat{G}_2 = 11$ means that there were 11 distinct T-cell receptors that were observed twice, etc.

Table 2.1 shows the observed frequencies for one of the cell types considered in Guindani et al. (2014). Consider a model $y_i \sim G$, with prior $G \sim \text{DP}(MG_0)$ on the clonal size distribution. We use $G_0 = \text{Poi}^+(2)$, a Poisson distribution with mean 2, constrained to positive counts, and $M = 1$. Figure 2.2a shows the base measure G_0 together with the posterior mean $E(G \mid y)$. Figure 2.2b shows ten posterior draws $G \sim p(G \mid y)$.

Software note: See the on-line software page for this chapter for R code to implement sampling from (2.3) for Example 3.

Table 2.1 Example 3. Frequencies $\hat{G}_y$ of counts $y_i = 1, 2, \ldots$

Counts y_i	1	2	3	4	≥ 5
Frequencies	37	11	5	2	0

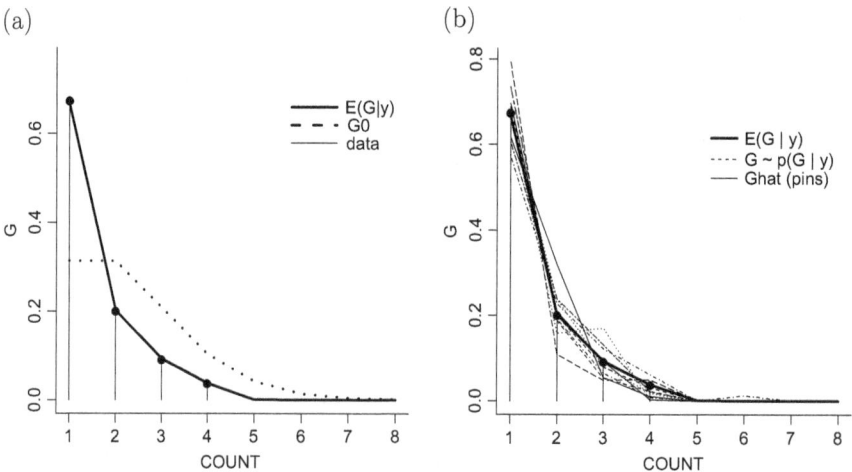

Fig. 2.2 Example 3. Prior mean G_0 (*dotted line*) and posterior mean $E(G \mid x)$ (*solid line*) of the clonal size distribution G (panel **a**), and posterior draws $G \sim p(G \mid y)$ (panel **b**). Only the probabilities at the integer values $y = 1, 2, \ldots$ are meaningful. The points are connected only for a better display

Marginal Distribution A key property of the DP prior is its a.s. discreteness. Consider a random sample, $y_i \mid G \sim G$, i.i.d., $i = 1, \ldots, n$. The discreteness of G implies a positive probability of ties among the y_i. This is at the heart of the Polya urn representation of Blackwell and MacQueen (1973) for the marginal distribution $p(y_1, \ldots, y_n) = \int \prod_{i=1}^n G(y_i) \, d\pi(G)$. The Polya urn specifies the marginal distribution as a product of a sequence of increasing conditionals $p(y_1, \ldots, y_n) = p(y_1) \prod_{i=2}^n p(y_i \mid y_1, \ldots, y_{i-1})$ with

$$p(y_i \mid y_1 \ldots, y_{i-1}) = \frac{1}{M+i-1} \sum_{h=1}^{i-1} \delta_{y_h}(y_i) + \frac{M}{M+i-1} G_0(y_i), \quad (2.4)$$

for $i = 2, 3, \ldots$, and $y_1 \sim G_0$. Since the y_i are i.i.d. given G the marginal joint distribution of $(y_1, \ldots, y_n)$ is exchangeable, i.e., the probabilities remain unchanged under any permutation of the indices. In particular, the complete conditional $p(y_i \mid y_h, h \neq i)$ has the same form as (2.4) for y_n. This will be important later for defining posterior simulation. Another important special case is the (posterior) predictive for a future observation y_{n+1} given data $y_1, \ldots, y_n$. It takes the form of (2.4) for $i = n + 1$.

Later we will rewrite (2.4) more compactly by combining all terms with identical y_i, writing (2.4) in terms of the unique values $y_j^\star$, $j = 1, \ldots, k$, for $k \leq n$ distinct unique values. As $n \to \infty$, the expected number of distinct y's grows as $M \log(n)$ (Korwar and Hollander 1973), which is asymptotically much smaller than n. In the following discussion we will frequently make use of the clustering that is implied by these ties.

2.2 Dirichlet Process Mixture

2.2.1 The DPM Model

The DP generates distributions that are discrete with probability one, making it awkward for continuous density estimation. This limitation can be fixed by convolving its trajectories with some continuous kernel, or more generally, by using a DP random measure as the mixing measure in a mixture over some simple parametric forms. Such an approach was introduced by Ferguson (1983), Lo (1984), Escobar (1988, 1994), and Escobar and West (1995). Let Θ be a typically finite-dimensional parameter space. For each $\theta \in \Theta$, let f_θ be a continuous p.d.f. In many applications a normal kernel $f_\theta(y) = N(y \mid \mu, \sigma)$ is used, with $\theta = (\mu, \sigma)$. Given a probability distribution G defined on Θ, a mixture of f_θ with respect to G has the p.d.f.

$$f_G(y) = \int f_\theta(y) dG(\theta). \quad (2.5)$$

Such mixtures can form a very rich family. For example, a mixture with respect to location and scale $\theta = (\mu, \sigma)$ using $f_\theta(y) = \sigma^{-1} k((y-\mu)/\sigma)$, for some fixed density k, approximates any density in the L_1 sense if σ is allowed to approach 0 (Lo 1984). Thus, a prior on densities may be induced by putting a DP prior on the mixing distribution G. Such models are known as DP mixtures (DPM) models.

The mixture model (2.5), together with a DP prior on the mixing measure G can equivalently be written as a hierarchical model. Assume $y_i \mid G \overset{iid}{\sim} F_G$ as in (2.5). An equivalent hierarchical model is

$$y_i \mid \theta_i \overset{ind}{\sim} f_{\theta_i}$$
$$\theta_i \mid G \overset{iid}{\sim} G \qquad (2.6)$$

and $G \sim \mathsf{DP}(MG_0)$. The hierarchical model introduces new latent variables θ_i specific to each experimental unit. It is easily seen that (2.6) is equivalent to (2.5). Just integrate with respect to θ_i to marginalize the hierarchical model (2.6) with respect to θ_i. The result is exactly the DPM (2.5). Under this hierarchical model, the posterior distribution on G is a mixture of DP's, i.e., $p(G \mid y_1, \ldots, y_n)$ is a mixture of DP models, mixing with respect to the latent θ_i.

Result 2 (Antoniak 1974) *If $y_i \mid \theta_i \overset{ind}{\sim} f_{\theta_i}$, $i = 1, \ldots, n$, $\theta_i \overset{iid}{\sim} G$ and $G \sim \mathsf{DP}(\alpha)$, then*

$$G \mid y \sim \int \mathsf{DP}\left(\alpha + \sum_{i=1}^n \delta_{\theta_i}\right) dp(\theta \mid y), \qquad (2.7)$$

where $\theta = (\theta_1, \ldots, \theta_n)$ and $y = (y_1, \ldots, y_n)$.

Recall that we write $\alpha = MG_0$ for the (un-normalized) base measure. In words, conditional on θ the posterior model is (2.3). Marginalizing with respect to θ, the posterior given y becomes a mixture over (2.3) with respect to the posterior distribution on θ. Because of this result, DPM models are sometimes called mixture of DP models. We find this terminology misleading, since models are not usually named for the properties of their posterior distribution, and therefore avoid it here.

Property (2.7) can be exploited to impute G or certain summaries of G under the posterior distribution by averaging summaries of $\mathsf{DP}(\alpha + \sum \delta_{\theta_i})$ with respect to a posterior sample on θ. Computation further simplifies by noting that for large n we can approximate $G \sim \mathsf{DP}(\alpha + \sum \delta_{\theta_i})$ by $G \propto \alpha + \sum \delta_{\theta_i}$.

The choice of an appropriate kernel depends on the underlying sample space. If the underlying density function is defined on the entire real line, a location-scale kernel is appropriate. On the unit interval, beta distributions form a flexible two-parameter family. On the positive half line, mixtures of gamma, Weibull or log-normal distributions may be used. The use of a uniform kernel leads to random histograms. Petrone and Veronese (2002) motivated a canonical way of viewing the

2.2 Dirichlet Process Mixture

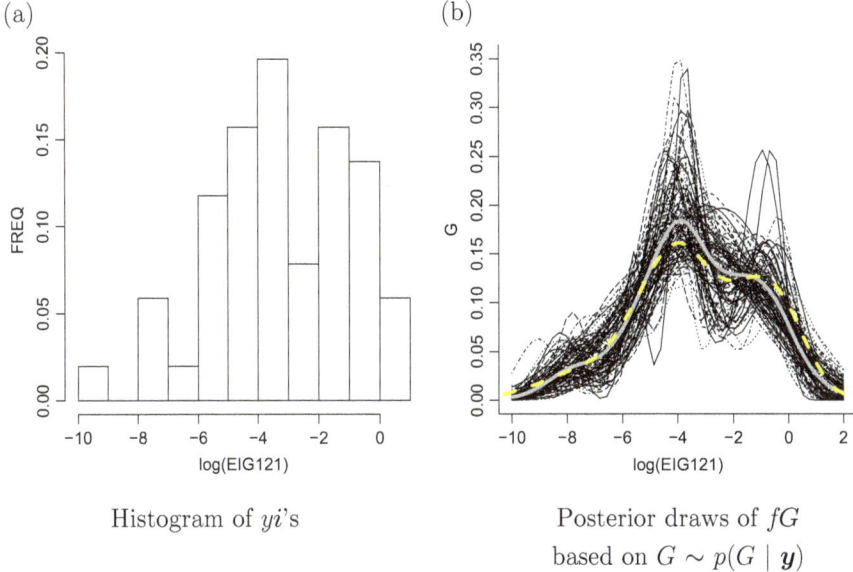

Histogram of y_i's

Posterior draws of f_G
based on $G \sim p(G \mid y)$

Fig. 2.3 Example 4. Data (panel **a**) and posterior inference for G (panel **b**). Panel (**b**) shows 96 posterior draws of the mixture model f_G based on $G \sim p(G \mid y)$ (*thin black curves*) and the posterior mean $E(f_G \mid y)$ (*thick grey curve*). For comparison the figure also shows a kernel density estimate (*dashed thick yellow line*)

choice of a kernel through the notion of a Feller sampling scheme, and called the resulting prior a Feller prior.

Example 4 (Gene Expression Data) Figure 2.3a shows measurements y_i corresponding to EIG121 gene expression for $n = 51$ uterine cancer patients. We assume $y_i \sim f_G$ with a DPM prior as in (2.6). Figure 2.3b shows posterior inference on f_G. Inference is based on 500 iterations of a Gibbs sampler, using an approximation with a finite DP prior. See Sect. 2.4.6.

Software note: Simple R code to implement inference in the DPM model (2.6) for Examples 4 and 3 (continued below) is available in the on-line software appendix for this chapter.

In Example 4 we used the DPM model to estimate a continuous distribution. The convolution with the kernel $f_{\theta_i}(\cdot)$ in (2.6) serves to smooth out the discrete point masses of G to define a continuous distribution. In some examples, the DPM might also be used for extrapolation in inference for a discrete random probability measure. Recall Example 3. We used a DP prior for inference on $G(y)$, $y = 1, 2, \ldots$. This inference ignored an important feature of the experiment. By the nature of the experiment zero counts are censored. That is, $y_i = 0$ is censored. In other words, some rare T-cell receptors that are present in the probe might not be seen, simply because of sampling variation. Let $\hat{G}(y)$ denote the empirical distribution. If we extrapolate $\hat{G}(y)$ in Fig. 2.2 to $y = 0$, we would expect a large number of rare T-cell receptors. However, inference under a DP prior on G does not implement such extrapolation. Consider a straightforward extension of the earlier analysis by using $G \sim \text{DP}(MG_0)$ with $G_0 = \text{Poi}(2)$, now without the constraint to $y \geq 1$. The posterior distribution for the extrapolation is $p(G(0) \mid x) = \text{Be}(MG_0(0), M(1 - G_0(0)) + n)$. This is a direct consequence of Definition 1 and Result 1 with $B_1 = \{0\}$ and $B_2 = \{1, 2, \ldots\}$. There is no notion of extrapolation. Inference on $G(0)$ hinges only on the number of observations n, but does not attempt to extrapolate the trend in $\hat{G}$ as $y \to 0$. In Guindani et al. (2014) we use a DPM to allow for such extrapolation. We use (2.5) with a Poisson kernels $f_{\theta_i}(\cdot)$ centered at the latent θ_i. Figure 2.4 shows inference under this DPM prior.

Example 3 (T-Cell Receptors, ctd.) We now replace the DP prior on G by a DPM model with Poisson kernels, $y_i \sim \text{Poi}(\theta_i)$ and $\theta_i \sim G$ with $G \sim \text{DP}(M G_0)$. Importantly, we drop the constraint $y_i \geq 1$. Instead we assume that T-cell receptor counts are generated as $y_i \sim f_G$, $i = 1, \ldots, k$ for $k \geq n$, with $y_i = 0$ for $i = n+1, \ldots, k$. Without loss of generality we assume that the observed non-zero counts are the first n counts. The last $k - n$ counts are censored. The total number of T-cell receptors k becomes another model parameter. Figure 2.4a shows inference on the estimated distribution $f_G(y) = \int \text{Poi}(y \mid \theta) \, dG(\theta)$ together with posterior draws $f_G \sim p(f_G \mid y)$. The right panel of the same figure shows the implied posterior distribution $p(k \mid y)$.

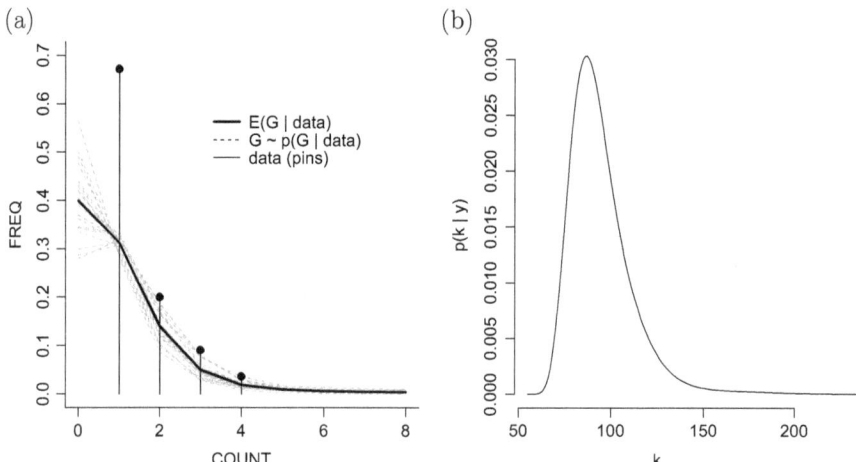

Fig. 2.4 Example 3. Prior mean G_0 (*dotted line*) and posterior mean $E(f_G \mid y)$ (*solid line*) of the clonal size distribution G (panel **a**), and posterior draws $f_G \sim p(f_G \mid y)$. Only the probabilities at the integer values $y = 1, 2, \ldots$ are meaningful. The points are connected only for a better display. Panel (**b**) shows the implied posterior $p(k \mid y)$ for the total number of distinct T-cell receptors

2.2.2 Mixture of DPM

A minor but practically important generalization of the DPM model (2.6) arises when the base measure of the DP prior includes unknown hyper-parameters η and the model is extended with a hyper-prior for η. Similarly, the model could include a hyper-prior on an unknown total mass parameter M. For reference, we state the complete model

$$y_i \mid \theta_i \sim f_{\theta_i}$$
$$\theta_i \mid G \stackrel{iid}{\sim} G$$
$$G \mid \eta, M \sim \mathsf{DP}(M, G_\eta)$$
$$(\eta, M) \sim \pi. \tag{2.8}$$

For example, $G_\eta = \mathsf{N}(m, s)$ with $\eta = (m, s)$ and a normal/inverse gamma prior on (m, s). The posterior characterization (2.7) remains valid, now conditional on η and M. The additional layer in the hierarchical model does not introduce any significant complication in posterior simulation. Implementation of posterior inference for M becomes particularly easy with a gamma prior on M, $M \sim \mathsf{Ga}(a, b)$. We will discuss details later.

2.3 Clustering Under the DPM

An important implication of (2.6) is the fact that the DPM model induces a probability model on clusters, in the following sense. The discrete nature of the DP implies a positive probability for ties among the latent θ_i. Let $\theta_j^\star$, $j = 1, \ldots, k$, denote the $k \leq n$ unique values, let $S_j = \{i : \theta_i = \theta_j^\star\}$, and let $n_j = |S_j|$ denote the number of θ_i tied with $\theta_j^\star$. When n is not understood from the context we include an additional index k_n, n_{nj} etc. The multiset $\rho_n = \{S_1, \ldots, S_k\}$ forms a partition of the set of experimental units $\{1, \ldots, n\}$. Since θ_i are random, the sets S_j are random. In other words, the DPM (2.6) implies a model on a random partition ρ_n of the experimental units. The model $p(\rho_n)$ is also known as the Polya urn. The probability model on ρ_n might seem like an incidental by-product of the construction, but actually many applications of the DPM model focus on this partition ρ_n. The posterior model $p(\rho_n \mid y)$ reports posterior inference on clustering of the data. We will discuss this in more detail later, in Chap. 8.

In the following discussion of posterior simulation for DPM models it is convenient to represent the clustering by an equivalent set of cluster membership indicators, $s_i = j$ if $i \in S_j$, usually with the convention that clusters are labeled by order of appearance, i.e., $s_1 = 1$ by definition, $s_{i_2} = 2$ for the lowest $i_2 > 1$ with $\theta_{i_2} \neq \theta_1$, $s_{i_3} = 3$ for the smallest $i_3 > i_2$ with $\theta_{i_3} \notin \{\theta_1, \theta_{i_2}\}$, etc. Eq. (2.4) implies

$p(s_i \mid s_1, \ldots, s_{i-1})$. Let k_i denote the number of unique θ_ℓ among $\{\theta_1, \ldots, \theta_i\}$ and let $n_{i,j}$ denote the multiplicity of the j-th of these unique values. Note that by definition $\sum_{j=1}^{k_i} n_{ij} = i$. Then

$$p(s_i = j \mid s_1, \ldots, s_{i-1}) = \begin{cases} \frac{n_{i-1,j}}{M+i-1} & \text{for } j = 1, \ldots, k_{i-1} \\ \frac{M}{M+i-1} & j = k_{i-1} + 1. \end{cases} \quad (2.9)$$

Let $s_{-i} = (s_1, \ldots, s_{i-1}, s_{i+2}, \ldots, s_n)$. By exchangeability of the θ_i the conditional (prior) probability $p(s_i = j \mid s_{-i})$ takes the same form as (2.9) for $i = n$. Also, we can now read off the prior $p(\rho_n)$ as

$$p(s) = \prod_{i=2}^{n} p(s_i \mid s_1, \ldots, s_{i-1}) = \frac{M^{k-1} \prod_{j=1}^{k}(n_j - 1)!}{(M+1) \cdots (M+n-1)}. \quad (2.10)$$

Recall that $s_1 = 1$ by definition. For later reference, we state the implied conditional distribution for θ_i that follows from (2.9). Let $\theta_{i,j}^\star$ denote the j-th unique value among $\{\theta_1, \ldots, \theta_i\}$. Noting that $s_i = j$ implies $\theta_i = \theta_{i-1,j}^\star$ and $s_i = k_{i-1} + 1$ implies that $\theta_i \sim G_0$, we have

$$p(\theta_i \mid \theta_1, \ldots, \theta_{i-1}) \propto \sum_{j=1}^{k_{i-1}} n_{i-1,j} \delta_{\theta_{i-1,j}^\star}(\theta_i) + M G_0(\theta_i). \quad (2.11)$$

Finally, note that the DPM (2.6) model is exchangeable in $\theta_1, \ldots, \theta_n$. That is, the model remains invariant under arbitrary changes of the indexing of θ_i. Therefore (2.11) must remain valid also for $p(\theta_i \mid \theta_1, \ldots, \theta_{i-1}, \theta_{i+1}, \ldots, \theta_n)$,

$$p(\theta_i \mid \boldsymbol{\theta}_{-i}) \propto \sum_{j=1}^{k^-} n_j^- \delta_{\theta_j^{\star-}}(\theta_i) + M G_0(\theta_i). \quad (2.12)$$

Here $\boldsymbol{\theta}_{-i}$ denotes $\boldsymbol{\theta}$ without the i-th element θ_i, k^- is the number of unique values in $\boldsymbol{\theta}_{-i}$ and $\theta_j^{\star-}$ is the j-th unique element.

2.4 Posterior Simulation for DPM Models

A critical advantage of using BNP methods compared to a parametric Bayesian analysis is the ability to incorporate uncertainty at the level of distribution functions. However, this flexibility comes at a computational cost. Much of the rapid development of BNP models in the last decades has been a direct result of advances in simulation-based computational methods, particularly Markov Chain Monte Carlo methods (MCMC).

2.4 Posterior Simulation for DPM Models

MCMC algorithms (see Escobar 1988, 1994; Dey et al. 1998; Neal 2000; Griffin and Walker 2011), sequential imputation (Liu 1996; MacEachern et al. 1999), and predictive recursions (Newton et al. 1998; Newton and Zhang 1999) have been used for fitting models with DP priors. In this section we focus the attention on MCMC methods. MCMC methods allow the construction of general purpose algorithms, and have been successfully used for posterior sampling under DP priors in many diverse applications and modeling contexts.

2.4.1 Conjugate DPM Models

Escobar (1988) proposed the first posterior Gibbs sampler for the DPM model (2.6), based on transition probabilities that update θ_i by draws from the complete conditional posterior $p(\theta_i \mid \boldsymbol{\theta}_{-i}, \boldsymbol{y})$. However, this Gibbs sampler can be argued to suffer from a slowly mixing Markov chain.

Most currently used posterior MCMC methods for DPM models are based on a variation proposed by Bush and MacEachern (1996). They use two types of transition probabilities. One updates s_i by draws from the complete conditional posterior probability $p(s_i \mid \boldsymbol{s}_{-i}, \boldsymbol{y})$, after marginalizing with respect to $\boldsymbol{\theta}$. The other type of transition probability generates $\theta_j^\star$ from $p(\theta_j^\star \mid \boldsymbol{s}, \boldsymbol{y})$. We first discuss the latter. This will help us to establish notation that we will need for the other transition probability.

Sampling from $p(\theta_j^\star \mid \boldsymbol{s}, \boldsymbol{y})$: We update $\theta_j^\star$ conditional on the imputed partition $\boldsymbol{s}$ using

$$p(\theta_j^\star \mid \boldsymbol{s}, \boldsymbol{y}) \propto G_0(\theta_j^\star) \prod_{i \in S_j} f_{\theta_j^\star}(y_i). \tag{2.13}$$

Recall that $S_j = \{i : s_i = j\}$ is the j-th cluster under the DPM model. We used that *a priori* $p(\theta_j^\star) = G_0(\theta_j^\star)$. This follows from the stick-breaking definition of the DP random measure. The posterior $p(\theta_j^\star \mid \boldsymbol{s}, \boldsymbol{y})$ is simply the posterior on $\theta_j^\star$ in a parametric model with prior $G_0(\theta)$ and sampling model $f_\theta(y_i)$ for data y_i, $i \in S_j$.

Let $\boldsymbol{y}^\star_j = (y_i\ i \in S_j)$ denote y_i arranged by cluster. We write $p(\theta_j^\star \mid \boldsymbol{s}, \boldsymbol{y})$ also as $p(\theta_j^\star \mid \boldsymbol{y}^\star_j)$. In this notation the conditioning on $\boldsymbol{s}$ is implicit in the selection of the elements in $\boldsymbol{y}^\star_j$.

Sampling from $p(s_i \mid \boldsymbol{s}_{-i}, \boldsymbol{y})$: The probabilities $p(s_i \mid \boldsymbol{s}_{-i}, \boldsymbol{y})$ are derived as follows. First consider $p(\theta_i \mid \boldsymbol{\theta}_{-i}, \boldsymbol{y})$. The prior $p(\theta_i \mid \boldsymbol{\theta}_{-i})$ is (2.12). Recall that $\theta_j^{\star-}$ denote the k^- unique values among $\boldsymbol{\theta}_{-i}$ and similarly for n_j^-. Also, let $\boldsymbol{y}^{\star-}_j = \boldsymbol{y}^\star_j \setminus \{y_i\}$, Multiply with the sampling distribution to get the posterior distribution

$$p(\theta_i \mid \boldsymbol{\theta}_{-i}, \mathbf{y}) \propto \sum_{j=1}^{k^-} n_j^- f_{\theta_j^{*-}}(y_i) \delta_{\theta_j^{*-}}(\theta_i) + M f_{\theta_i}(y_i) G_0(\theta_i). \tag{2.14}$$

Some care is needed, as $f_{\theta_i}(y_i) G_0(\theta_i)$ in the second term is not normalized. Let $H_0(\theta_i) \propto f_{\theta_i}(y_i) G_0(\theta_i)$ with normalization constant $h_0(y_i) \equiv \int f_\theta(y_i) G_0(d\theta)$, i.e.,

$$f_{\theta_i}(x_i) G_0(\theta_i) = h_0(y_i) \, H_0(\theta_i).$$

Note that h_0 is a function of y_i. Recognizing that $\theta_i = \theta_j^{*-}$ implies $s_i = j$ we can write the same conditional as a joint distribution for (θ_i, s_i)

$$p(\theta_i, s_i \mid \boldsymbol{\theta}_{-i}, \mathbf{y}) \propto \sum_{j=1}^{k^-} n_j^- f_{\theta_j^{*-}}(y_i) \delta_j(s_i) \delta_{\theta_j^{*-}}(\theta_i) + M h_0(y_i) \, \delta_{k^-+1}(s_i) H_0(\theta_i).$$

Finally, we marginalize with respect to $\boldsymbol{\theta}$, that is, with respect to θ_i and $\boldsymbol{\theta}_{-i}$. In the last term the marginalization leaves $\int h_0(y_i) H_0(\theta_i) \, d\theta = h_0(y_i)$. In the first k^- terms the marginalization leaves $\int f_{\theta_j^*}(y_i) \, dp(\theta_j^{*-} \mid \mathbf{y}^{*-}_{\ j}) = p(y_i \mid \mathbf{y}^{*-}_{\ j})$. Here $p(\theta_j^{*-} \mid \mathbf{y}^{*-}_{\ j})$ is defined similar to (2.13), just now excluding y_i in the conditioning subset. Note that θ_j^{*-} need not be the same as θ_j^*. When i is a singleton cluster, then removing the i-th unit from the partition might change the indices of other clusters. We get

$$p(\theta_j^{*-} \mid \mathbf{y}^{*-}_{\ j}) \propto G_0(\theta_j^{*-}) \prod_{\ell \in S_j \setminus \{i\}} f_{\theta_j^{*-}}(y_\ell). \tag{2.15}$$

Then

$$p(s_i = j \mid \mathbf{s}_{-i}, \mathbf{y}) \propto \begin{cases} n_j^- \, p(y_i \mid s_i = j, \mathbf{y}^{*-}_{\ j}) & \text{for } j = 1, \ldots, k^- \\ M \, h_0(y_i) & j = k^- + 1. \end{cases} \tag{2.16}$$

The posterior Gibbs sampler is summarized in the following algorithm. It is only practicable for DPM models with conjugate $G_0(\theta)$ and $f_\theta(\cdot)$. Without conjugacy the evaluation of h_0 would typically be analytically intractable. We therefore refer to the algorithm as "MCMC for conjugate DPM".

Algorithm 1: *MCMC for Conjugate DPM.*

1. *Clustering:* For $i = 1, \ldots, n$, draw $s_i \sim p(s_i \mid \mathbf{s}_{-i}, \mathbf{y})$ using (2.16).
2. *Cluster parameters:* For $j = 1, \ldots, k$, generate $\theta_j^* \sim p(\theta_j^* \mid \mathbf{s}, \mathbf{y})$ using (2.13).

One of the limitations of this algorithm is the slow mixing of the implied Markov chain. For example, to split a current cluster, the algorithm has to first create a new singleton cluster and then slowly grow it by adding one member at a time. Jain

2.4 Posterior Simulation for DPM Models

and Neal (2004) proposed a merge-split sampler for conjugate DPM models. Being a merge-split algorithm (see e.g., Phillips and Smith 1996; Richardson and Green 1997), their method updates groups of indices in one update and thus is able to "step over valleys of low probability" and move between high-probability modes. Their algorithm involves a modified Gibbs sampler (restricted Gibbs scans) and, instead of proposing naive random splits of components which are unlikely to be supported by the model, proposes splits that are more probable by sweetening a naive split. The algorithm reallocates the indices involved in the split among two split components through as series of t, Gibbs-style updates. Jain and Neal (2004), recommend a small number of intermediate restricted Gibbs scans, $t = 4$ to 6.

Dahl (2005) proposed an alternative merge-split sampler for conjugate DPM models borrowing ideas from sequential importance sampling. The sampler, referred to as SAMS, proposes splits by sequentially allocating observations to one of two split components using allocation probabilities that are conditional on previously allocated data. The algorithm does not require further sweetening and is, hence, computationally efficient. In addition, no tuning parameter needs to be chosen. While the conditional allocation of observations is similar to sequential importance sampling, the output from the sampler has the correct stationary distribution due to the use of the Metropolis-Hastings ratio. See Dahl (2005) for details on its computation.

2.4.2 Updating Hyper-Parameters

Posterior inference under (2.8) requires some minor generalization of Algorithm 1. Conditional on η and M, the conditional posterior distributions (2.16) and (2.13) remain unchanged, leaving steps 1 and 2 of Algorithm 1 valid. But we add two more steps to update the hyper-parameters. The stick-breaking definition of the DP prior implies that $\theta_j^\star \mid \eta, k \stackrel{\text{iid}}{\sim} G_\eta, j = 1, \ldots, k$, *a priori*, leading to

$$p(\eta \mid \boldsymbol{\theta}^\star) \propto p(\eta) \prod_{j=1}^{k} G_\eta(\theta_j^\star),$$

where p is the prior distribution for η, and η is conditionally independent of s and y, given $\boldsymbol{\theta}^\star$. If p and G_η are a conjugate pair, we can add a Gibbs sampling step to update η by a draw from the complete conditional posterior. In general, a Metropolis-Hastings type transition probability might be needed.

Updating the total mass parameter M becomes easy under a gamma prior, $M \sim \mathsf{Ga}(a, b)$. From (2.10) we find the likelihood for M as

$$p(k \mid M) \propto M^k \Gamma(M) \Gamma(M+n) = M^k \frac{\Gamma(M+n)}{M \Gamma(n)} \int_0^1 \eta^M (1-\eta)^{n-1} \, d\eta,$$

as a function of M. Here, the proportionality constant includes all factors that do not involve M. The last equality exploits the normalizing constant of a $\text{Be}(M+1, n)$ distribution. Escobar and West (1995) use this equality to devise a clever auxiliary variable sampler. We first introduce a latent variable ϕ, such that

$$p(\phi \mid M, k, \ldots) = \text{Be}(M+1, n).$$

Combined with $M \sim \text{Ga}(a, b)$, we get

$$p(M \mid \phi, k) = \pi\, \text{Ga}\{a+k, b - \log(\phi)\} + (1-\pi)\, \text{Ga}\{a+k-1, b - \log(\phi)\},$$

with $\pi/(1-\pi) = (a+k-1)/\{n(b-\log(\phi))\}$.

We include both additional steps to generalize Algorithm 1.

Algorithm 2: *MCMC for Conjugate DPM with hyper-parameters.*

1. *Clustering:* For $i = 1, \ldots, n$, draw $s_i \sim p(s_i \mid \mathbf{s}_{-i}, \mathbf{y})$ using (2.16).
2. *Cluster parameters:* For $j = 1, \ldots, k$, generate $\theta_j^\star \sim p(\theta_j^\star \mid \mathbf{s}, \mathbf{y}, \eta)$.
3. *Hyper-parameters η:* Update hyper-parameters by an appropriate transition probability for η, based on the conditional posterior distribution $p(\eta \mid \boldsymbol{\theta}^\star) \propto p_\eta(\eta) \prod_{j=1}^{k} G_\eta(\theta_j^\star)$.
4. *Total mass parameter:* First generate $\phi \sim \text{Be}(M+1, n)$, evaluate $\pi/(1-\pi) = (a+k-1)/\{n(b-\log(\phi))\}$, and then generate

$$M \mid \phi, k \sim \begin{cases} \text{Ga}\{a+k, b-\log(\phi)\} & \text{with probability } \pi \\ \text{Ga}\{a+k-1, b-\log(\phi)\} & \text{with probability } 1-\pi. \end{cases}$$

2.4.3 Non-Conjugate DPM Models

Algorithm 1 is only practicable when G_0, or G_η, is a conjugate prior for $f_\theta(\cdot)$. For general, possibly non-conjugate choices, the required evaluation of h_0 is usually not analytically tractable. Also sampling from the posterior distribution $p(\theta_j^\star \mid \mathbf{s}, \mathbf{y})$ in (2.13) may be challenging.

West et al. (1994) suggested using either numerical quadrature or a Monte Carlo approximation to evaluate the required integral. If $\int f_\theta(y_j) G_0(d\theta)$ is approximated by an average over m values for θ drawn from G_0, it is also possible to approximate a draw from $p(\theta_j^\star \mid \mathbf{s}, \mathbf{y})$, if required, by drawing from among these m points with probabilities proportional to their likelihood. Unfortunately, this approach is potentially quite inaccurate.

MacEachern and Müller (1998) propose the "no-gaps" algorithm that does allow auxiliary values for θ drawn from G_0 to be used to define a valid Markov chain sampler. Denoting by k the number of distinct elements in $\boldsymbol{\theta}$, they proposed a model

2.4 Posterior Simulation for DPM Models

augmentation of $(\theta_1^\star, \ldots, \theta_k^\star)$ to

$$\{\underbrace{\theta_1^*, \ldots, \theta_k^*}_{\theta_F^*}, \underbrace{\theta_{k+1}^*, \ldots, \theta_n^*}_{\theta_E^*}\},$$

with $\theta_j^\star \sim G_0, j = k+1, \ldots, n$. The augmentation includes the constraint that there will be no gaps in the values of the s_j, i.e., $n_j > 0$ for $j = 1, \ldots, k$, and $n_j = 0$ for $j = k+1, \ldots, n$. Therefore the name, "no gaps", of the algorithm. The additional θ_E^* can be interpreted as potential but not yet used cluster locations, the empty clusters, and θ_F^* can be interpreted as full clusters. In this augmented model the Gibbs sampler simplifies substantially. The evaluation of integrals is replaced by simple likelihood evaluations. Consider updating s_i in Step 1 of Algorithm 1. Assume $s_i = j$ in the currently imputed partition. We need to distinguish two cases.

- If $n_j > 1$, then

$$p(s_i = j \mid s_{-i}, \theta^{\star-}, y) \propto \begin{cases} n_j^- f_{\theta_j^*}(y_i) & j = 1, \ldots, k^- \\ \frac{M}{k^- + 1} f_{\theta_{k^-+1}^*}(y_i) & j = k^- + 1 \end{cases} \quad (2.17)$$

- if $n_j = 1$, i.e., when $s_i = j$ is currently imputed to form a singleton cluster by itself then with probability $(k-1)/k$ leave s_i unchanged. Otherwise remove s_i from the j-th cluster, relabel the θ_j^* to comply with the no-gaps rule, and then update s_i using the same probabilities (2.17).

The probabilities (2.17) follow from a careful analysis of the augmented no-gaps model. See MacEachern and Müller (1998) for details. The no-gaps posterior Gibbs sampler is summarized in the following algorithm.

Algorithm 3: *No-Gaps sampler for nonconjugate DPM.*

1. Clustering: For $i = 1, \ldots, n$, draw $s_i \sim p(s_i \mid s_{-i}, \theta^\star, y)$ using (2.17).
2. Cluster parameters: For $j = 1, \ldots, n$, generate $\theta_j^* \sim p(\theta_j^* \mid s, y)$. For $j > k$, use $p(\theta_j^* \mid s, y) = G_0$.

In step 1, note that θ_j^* remains unchanged when θ_j^* moves from full to empty clusters. Consider a situation where $s_i = j_1$ and $n_{j_1} = 1$, that is, i is the only member in a singleton cluster. Assume now, in step 1 we re-allocate i to another, existing cluster. Closing down the singleton cluster j_1 involves (i) relabeling the remaining clusters into $j = 1, \ldots, k-1$; (ii) the old $\theta_{j_1}^*$ becomes θ_k^*; and finally, (iii) update $k \equiv k-1$. In particular, the currently imputed value $\theta_{j_1}^*$ remains as new 0_{k+1}^*. In step 2, in an actual implementation one need not actually record $\theta_j^*, j = k+1, \ldots, n$. They can be imputed as needed, when the values are required (except for recycled values, like $\theta_{j_1}^*$ above).

The key feature of Algorithm 3 is that it does not require evaluation of the integral h_0 that featured in the MCMC algorithm for conjugate DPM models. The algorithm can be implemented for any model as long as we can generate from G_0 and compute $f_\theta(y_j)$. There is no need for G_0 to be the conjugate prior for F_θ.

As noted by Neal (2000), however, there is a puzzling inefficiency in the algorithm's mechanism for setting $s_j = k^- + 1$, i.e., for assigning an observation to a newly created mixture component. The probability of such a change is reduced from what one might expect by a factor of $k^- + 1$, with a corresponding reduction in the probability of the opposite change. Neal (2000) described a similar algorithm without this inefficiency and proposed three Metropolis-Hastings algorithms with partial Gibbs sampling to update the configurations. We describe it in the following section.

MacEachern and Müller have also developed an algorithm based on a "complete" scheme for mapping $\boldsymbol{\theta}^*$ to $\boldsymbol{\theta}_i$. It requires maintaining n values for $\boldsymbol{\theta}^*$, which may be inefficient for large n. Finally, Dahl (2005) also proposed a version of the SAMS sampler for non-conjugate DPM.

2.4.4 Neal's Algorithm 8

Neal (2000) proposes a Gibbs sampler with auxiliary variables (Algorithm 8 in the paper) that is similar to Algorithm 3, but without the reduced probability for creating new clusters in the algorithm. We commented on this inefficiency before.

Algorithm 8 is based on a clever model augmentation. The DP prior in (2.6) implies in particular a marginal prior $p(\boldsymbol{\theta})$ on the latent θ_i, which after marginalizing w.r.t. G is shown in (2.11). Alternatively we can write $p(\boldsymbol{\theta}) = p(s, \boldsymbol{\theta}^\star) = p(s) p(\boldsymbol{\theta}^\star \mid s)$ instead. Note that model (2.6) really defines a sequence of probability models $p_n(\cdot)$, indexed by the sample size n. Let $\boldsymbol{\theta}_n = (\theta_1, \ldots, \theta_n)$ and let k_n denote the number of unique elements in $\boldsymbol{\theta}_n$. The sequence p_n is coherent in the sense that the marginal on $(\boldsymbol{\theta}_n)$ under $p_{n+1}(\cdot)$ is identical to $p_n(\boldsymbol{\theta}_n)$, or, in short,

$$p_{n+1}(\boldsymbol{\theta}_n) = \int p_{n+1}(\boldsymbol{\theta}_{n+1}) \, d\theta_{n+1} = p_n(\boldsymbol{\theta}_n),$$

with the predictive for the $(n+1)$-st θ_{n+1} given by (2.4) with $i = n+1$.

Neal (2000) augments the sequence of models $p_n(\boldsymbol{\theta})$ to a sequence of augmented models $q_n(\boldsymbol{\theta}_n, \theta^\star_{k_n+1}, \ldots, \theta^\star_{k_n+m})$, with $\theta^\star_{k_n+j} \sim G_0$, $j = 1, \ldots, m$. The model is augmented with m additional latent variables $z_n = (\theta^\star_{k_n+1}, \ldots, \theta^\star_{k_n+m})$ that were not defined in p_n. The clever trick is to link z_n with θ_{n+1} under p_{n+1}. Recall that $n_{n,j} = \sum_{i=1}^{n} I(\theta_i = \theta^\star_j)$ denotes the size of the j-th cluster among $\theta_1, \ldots, \theta_n$ and define

$$q_{n+1}(\theta_{n+1} \mid \boldsymbol{\theta}_n, \theta^\star_{k_n+1}, \ldots, \theta^\star_{k_n+m}) \propto \sum_{j=1}^{k_n} n_{n,j} \delta_{\theta^\star_j}(\theta_{n+1}) + \frac{M}{m} \sum_{j=1}^{m} \delta_{\theta^\star_{k_n+j}}(\theta_{n+1}).$$

(2.18)

2.4 Posterior Simulation for DPM Models

This expression replaces the prior (2.11) in (2.16). In other words, we use one of the $\theta^\star_{k_n+j}$ as θ_{n+1} if $s_{n+1} > k_n$ opens a new cluster. Since $\theta^\star_{k_n+j}$ was generated from G_0, this leaves the implied prior $q_n(\boldsymbol{\theta}_n)$, after marginalizing w.r.t. z_n, unchanged as $q_n(\boldsymbol{\theta}_n) = p_n(\boldsymbol{\theta}_n)$. Thus, when implementing MCMC under the augmented model $q_n(\cdot)$, we could in the end simply drop the augmented parameters and get a sample from the posterior under $p_n(\cdot)$.

The critical difference between (2.11) and (2.18) is that the latter does not require the integration w.r.t. G_0 in (2.16). Instead we get

$$p(s_i = j \mid \mathbf{s}_{-i}, \boldsymbol{\theta}^\star, \mathbf{M}, \mathbf{y}) \propto \begin{cases} \frac{M}{m} f_{\theta^\star_j}(y_i) & j = k^- + 1, \ldots, k^- + m \\ n_j f_{\theta^\star_j}(y_i) & j = 1, \ldots, k^-. \end{cases} \quad (2.19)$$

And there is no special case for $n_j = 1$. The conditional (2.19) replaces (2.16). Note that when $m = 1$, Algorithm 8 of Neal (2000) closely resembles the "no gaps" algorithm of MacEachern and Müller (1998). The main difference is the justification. The main practical difference is that the probability of changing s_j from a component shared with other observations to a new singleton component is approximately $k^- + 1$ times greater with Algorithm 8 and the same is true for the reverse change. When M is small this seems to be a clear benefit, since the probabilities for other changes are affected only slightly. Using a simulated dataset, Neal (2000) also showed that the auxiliary Gibbs sampler (with a properly chosen tuning parameter) has the best computational efficiency of one-at-a-time non-conjugate samplers for DPM models.

Software note: R code to implement transition probabilities under Algorithm 8 is given in the on-line software appendix for this chapter.

2.4.5 Slice Sampler

Walker (2007), Griffin and Walker (2011) and Kalli et al. (2011) developed a slice sampler for the DPM model. The method also applies for other nonparametric Bayes priors. But we focus on the DPM model here. In contrast to the earlier discussed methods, they do not marginalize out the random probability measure G. Recall the stick breaking representation

$$G(\cdot) = \sum_{h=1}^{\infty} w_h \delta_{m_h}(\cdot),$$

with $w_h = v_h \prod_{\ell < h}(1 - v_\ell)$, $v_h \stackrel{iid}{\sim} \text{Be}(1, M)$ and $m_h \stackrel{iid}{\sim} G_0$. Let $\boldsymbol{w}$ and $\boldsymbol{m}$ denote the sequences of w_h and m_h, respectively. We can use this representation to explicitly state the DPM model $f_G(y_i) = \int f_\theta(y_i)\,dG(\theta)$ as

$$p(y_i \mid \boldsymbol{w}, \boldsymbol{m}) = \sum_{h=1}^{\infty} w_h f_{m_h}(y_i). \quad (2.20)$$

Here $p(y_i \mid \boldsymbol{w}, \boldsymbol{m})$ is just a complicated way of writing $f_G(y_i)$. At this moment $p(y_i \mid \boldsymbol{w}, \boldsymbol{m})$ is still an infinite sum, making it difficult to use for computing and posterior simulation. The first trick is to introduce latent variables u_i to reduce (2.20) to a finite sum

$$p(y_i, u_i \mid \boldsymbol{m}, \boldsymbol{w}) = \sum_{h=1}^{\infty} I(u_i < w_h) f_{m_h}(y_i). \quad (2.21)$$

Integration with respect to u_i recovers (2.20), as intended. We verify that indeed only finitely many terms are included in (2.21). Let $C_w(u) = \{h : u < w_h\}$ denote the set of h that index the sum. In constructing $C_w(u_i)$ we only need to consider all indices $\ell < h^\star$, where $h^\star = \min\{h : u_i > 1 - \sum_{\ell=1}^{h} w_\ell\}$. This is the case since $w_h \leq 1 - \sum_{\ell=1}^{h^\star} w_\ell < u_i$ for all $h > h^\star$ (the first inequality simply follows from $\sum w_h = 1$). In particular, the sum is over finitely many terms.

Next we add a latent selection indicator r_i with $p(r_i = h \mid u_i, \boldsymbol{w}) \propto I(u_i < w_h)$, that is, a uniform over $C_w(u_i)$,

$$p(y_i, u_i, r_i \mid \boldsymbol{m}, \boldsymbol{w}) = I(u_i < w_{r_i}) f_{m_{r_i}}(y_i). \quad (2.22)$$

Again, verify by integrating out, i.e., summing over r_i, to find (2.21), and upon integrating u_i finally (2.20), as needed. This is all! The augmented model allows a straightforward Gibbs sampling implementation for posterior simulation.

Under the model augmentation with $\boldsymbol{u}$ and $\boldsymbol{r}$ we get the joint model

$$p(\boldsymbol{y}, \boldsymbol{u}, \boldsymbol{r} \mid \boldsymbol{w}, \boldsymbol{m}) = \prod_{i=1}^{n} I(u_i < w_{r_i}) f_{m_{r_i}}(y_i).$$

We can define a Gibbs sampler with transition probabilities that update w_h, m_h, u_i and r_i by draws from the complete conditional posterior distributions. Recall $w_h = v_h \prod_{\ell < h}(1 - v_\ell)$ and $v_h \sim \mathsf{Be}(1, M)$. Let $A_h = \{i : r_i = h\}$ and $B_h = \{i : r_i > h\}$. Then

$$p(v_h \mid \ldots) = \mathsf{Be}(1 + |A_h|, M + |B_h|) \prod_i I(u_i < w_{r_i}).$$

The product of indicators simply amounts to a lower and upper bound for v_h. Similarly

$$p(m_h \mid \ldots, y) \propto G_0(m_h) \prod_{i \in A_h} f_{m_h}(y_i),$$

etc. We only need to update m_h with non-empty index set A_h. Others can be generated later, only as and when needed. The complete conditional posterior for u_i is a uniform, $p(u_i \mid r_i, w) \sim \mathsf{Unif}(0, w_{r_i})$. Finally, $p(r_i = h \mid u) = \mathsf{Unif}(C_w(u_i))$.

2.4.6 Finite DP

Ishwaran and Zarepour (2000) and Ishwaran and James (2001, 2002) proposed to approximate DPM models by truncating the stick-breaking representation of the DP. The fractions v_h are truncated after H terms by setting $v_H = 1$, leaving

$$G(\cdot) = \sum_{h=1}^{H} w_h \delta_{m_h}(\cdot), \qquad (2.23)$$

with $w_h = v_h \prod_{\ell < h}(1 - v_\ell)$ with $v_h \sim \mathsf{Be}(1, M)$, $h = 1, \ldots, H-1$ and $v_H = 1$. The prior on the point masses remains unchanged, i.e., $m_h \stackrel{iid}{\sim} G_0$, $h = 1, \ldots, H$. We write $G \sim \mathsf{DP}_H(MG_0)$ and DPM_H for a DPM model (2.6) when a DP_H replaces a DP prior,

$$f_G(y) = \sum_{h=1}^{H} w_h f_{m_h}(y). \qquad (2.24)$$

The truncated DP is particularly attractive for posterior computation. Ishwaran and James (2001) show a bound on the approximation error that arises when using inference under a truncated DP to approximate inference under the corresponding DP prior. The main use of the approximation with the DP_H is in posterior simulation for DPM models. Assume $y_i \stackrel{iid}{\sim} F$, $i = 1, \ldots, n$, independently, with a DPM_H prior on F. First we replace the mixture (2.24) of the DPM_H by the following equivalent hierarchical model with latent indicators r_i, $i = 1, \ldots, n$,

$$y_i \mid r_i = h \sim f_{m_h} \quad \text{and} \quad p(r_i = h) = w_h.$$

The latent indicators r_i are different from the cluster membership indicators that we used in (2.9). If k is the number of unique values among the x_i, then $s_i \in \{1, \ldots, k\}$ links the data with the unique values, whereas $r_i \in \{1, \ldots, H\}$ with $H \geq k$ links the data with the point masses in G. Let $r = (r_1, \ldots, r_n)$, $v = (v_1, \ldots, v_{H-1})$ and

$\boldsymbol{m} = (m_1, \ldots, m_H)$. We can then define posterior MCMC simulation with a Gibbs sampler for $p(\boldsymbol{r}, \boldsymbol{w}, \boldsymbol{\theta} \mid \boldsymbol{x})$.

Algorithm 4: *MCMC for* DPM_H.

1. *Clustering:* For $i = 1, \ldots, n$, draw r_i with $p(r_i = h \mid \boldsymbol{v}, \boldsymbol{m}, y_i) \propto w_h f_{m_h}(y_i)$, $h = 1, \ldots, H$.
2. *Weights:* Let $A_h = \sum_i I(r_i = h)$ and $B_h = \sum_i I(r_i > h)$. For $h = 1, \ldots, H-1$, generate $v_h \sim \text{Be}(A_h + 1, B_h + M)$.
3. *Locations:* Let $S_h = \{i : r_i = h\}$ denote the set of observations with $r_i = h$. For $h = 1, \ldots, H$, generate $m_h \sim p(m_h \mid \boldsymbol{y}, \boldsymbol{r}) \propto g_0(m_h) \prod_{i \in S_h} f_{m_h}(y_i)$.

Note that S_h may be empty. If $g_0(m)$ and $f_m(\cdot)$ are chosen as a pair of conjugate prior and likelihood, then updating m_h is straightforward by a draw from the complete conditional posterior $p(m_h \mid \boldsymbol{y}, \boldsymbol{r})$. In the case of non-conjugate g_0 and f_m, we replace the draw from the complete conditional posterior distribution by a Metropolis-Hastings transition probability.

2.5 Generalizations of the Dirichlet Processes

While the DP is arguably one of the most widely used BNP model, its reliance on only two parameters may sometimes be restrictive. One drawback of the DP prior is that it always produces discrete random probability measure. Another undesirable property is that the correlation between the random probabilities of two sets is always negative. In some situations, random probabilities of sets that are close enough are expected to be positively related if some smoothness is assumed. Flexible priors may be constructed by generalizing the way the prior probabilities are assigned.

2.5.1 Tail-Free Processes

The notion of a tail-free (TF) process was introduced by Freedman (1963) and Fabius (1964), and predates that of the DP. Assume that Ω is a complete and separable sample space, e.g. $\Omega = \mathbb{R}$. Let $E = \{0, 1\}$, $E^m = E \times \ldots \times E$, $E^0 = \emptyset$, and $E^* = \bigcup_{m=0}^{\infty} E^m$. We will write $\epsilon \in E^m$ as a binary integer $\epsilon = \varepsilon_1 \cdots \varepsilon_m$. A TF process is defined by allocations of random probabilities to sets in a nested sequence of partitions of the sample space, using $\epsilon \in E^*$ to index partitioning subsets B_ϵ as follows. Let $\pi_0 = \{\Omega\}$, $\pi_1 = \{B_0, B_1\}$, $\pi_2 = \{B_{00}, B_{01}, B_{10}, B_{11}\}$, $\ldots$, be a sequence of nested partition of Ω such that $B_\epsilon = B_{\epsilon 0} \cup B_{\epsilon 1}$ and $B_{\epsilon 0} \cap B_{\epsilon 1} = \emptyset$ for every $\epsilon = \varepsilon_1 \cdots \varepsilon_m \in E^*$. In other words, the π_n are partitions of Ω, with π_{n+1} being a refinement of π_n by splitting each of the partitioning subsets $B_\epsilon \in \pi_n$ into $B_\epsilon = B_{\epsilon 0} \cup B_{\epsilon 1}$.

2.5 Generalizations of the Dirichlet Processes

Assume $\Omega = \mathbb{R}$ and that $B_{\epsilon 0}$ lies below $B_{\epsilon 1}$ and that B_ϵ is a left open right closed interval except for $\epsilon = 1 \cdots 1$, i.e., all ones. Further assume that $\bigcup_{m=0}^{\infty} \pi_m$ is a generator for the Borel σ-field on Ω. Note that this is ensured if the collection of right end points of B_ϵ is dense in Ω. A probability G may then be described by specifying all the conditional probabilities $\{Y_\varepsilon = G(B_{\epsilon 0} \mid B_\epsilon) : \varepsilon \in E^*\}$. A prior for G may thus be defined by specifying the joint distributions of all Y_ε's. The specification may be written in a tree form. The probability distributions at the different levels in the hierarchy can be interpreted as prior specification at different levels of detail. A prior for G is said to be tail-free with respect to the sequence of partitions $\{\pi_m\}_0^\infty$ if the collections $\{Y_\emptyset\}$, $\{Y_0, Y_1\}$, $\{Y_{00}, Y_{01}, Y_{10}, Y_{11}\}$, ..., are mutually independent. Note that variables within the same hierarchy need not be independent; only the variables at different levels are required to be so.

The family of TF processes includes the DP as an important special case. The DP is TF with respect to any sequence of partitions. Indeed, the DP is the only prior that has this distinct property. See Ferguson (1974) and references therein. TF priors satisfy some interesting zero-one laws, namely, the random measure generated by a tail-free process is absolutely continuous with respect to a given finite measure with probability zero or one. This follows from the fact that the criterion of absolute continuity may be expressed as a tail event with respect to a collection of independent random variables and Kolmogorov's zero-one law may be applied (see, Ghosh and Ramamoorthi 2003, for details). Dubins and Freedman (1967), Kraft (1964), and Metivier (1971) gave sufficient conditions for the almost sure continuity and absolute continuity of a tail-free process.

2.5.2 Species Sampling Models (SSM)

The infinite series representation (2.2) gives rise to several generalizations of the DP prior, by changing the distribution of the weights, the support points, or the number of terms. Natural candidates are truncations of the infinite series representation. In this setup, the prior $\sum_{h=1}^{\infty} w_h \delta_{m_h}$, is replaced by $\sum_{h=1}^{N} w_h \delta_{m_h}$ for some appropriately chosen value of N. A popular example is the finite DP (2.23). Another example of this procedure is the ϵ-DP proposed by Muliere and Tardella (1998), where N is chosen such that the total variation distance between the DP and the truncation is bounded by a given $\epsilon > 0$. Another variation is the Dirichlet-multinomial process introduced by Muliere and Secchi (1995). Here the random probability measure is, for some finite N,

$$G(\cdot) = \sum_{h=1}^{N} w_h \delta_{m_h}(\cdot),$$

with

$$(w_1, \ldots, w_N) \mid M, N \sim \text{Dir}(M/N, \ldots, M/N) \text{ and } m_h \mid G_0 \overset{iid}{\sim} G_0, \qquad (2.25)$$

$h = 1, \ldots, N$. Interestingly, as a limit as $N \to \infty$ we can again recover a $\text{DP}(M, G_0)$ prior (Green and Richardson 2001).

More generally, Pitman (1996) described a class of models

$$G(\cdot) = \sum_{h=1}^{\infty} w_h \delta_{m_h}(\cdot) + \left(1 - \sum_{h=1}^{\infty} w_h\right) G_0(\cdot),$$

where, for a continuous distribution G_0, we have $m_1, m_2, \ldots \overset{iid}{\sim} G_0$, assumed independent of the non-negative random variables w_h. The weights w_h are constrained by $\sum_{h=1}^{\infty} w_h \leq 1$ a.s. The model is known as Species Sampling Model (SSM), with the interpretation of w_h as the relative frequency of the i-*th* species in a list of species in a certain population, and m_h as the tag assigned to that species. If $\sum_{h=1}^{\infty} w_h = 1$ the SSM is called *proper* and the corresponding prior random probability measure is discrete. The stick-breaking priors studied by Ishwaran and James (2001) are a special case of SSM, adopting the form $\sum_{h=1}^{N} w_h \delta_{m_h}$, where $1 \leq N \leq \infty$. The weights are defined as $w_h = \prod_{j<h}(1 - v_j) v_h$ with $v_h \sim \text{Be}(a_h, b_h)$, independently, for given sequences $(a_1, a_2, \ldots)$ and $(b_1, b_2, \ldots)$. The finite DP (2.23) is a special case.

Stick-breaking priors are quite general, including not only the Dirichlet-multinomial process and the DP as special cases, but also a two-parameter DP extension, known as the Poisson-Dirichlet process (Pitman and Yor 1997), and the two-parameter beta process (Ishwaran and Zarepour 2000). Additional examples and MCMC implementation details for stick-breaking random probability measures can be found in Ishwaran and James (2001). Further discussion on SSMs appears in Pitman (1996) and Ishwaran and James (2003).

2.5.3 Generalized Dirichlet Processes

The k-dimensional Dirichlet distribution may be viewed as the conditional distribution of $\boldsymbol{p} = (p_1, \ldots, p_k)$ given that $\sum_{j=1}^{k} p_j = 1$, where $p_j = \exp\{-Y_j\}$ and Y_j's are independent exponential variables. In general, if $(Y_1, \ldots, Y_k)$ have a joint density h, the conditional joint density of $(p_1, \ldots, p_{k-1})$ is proportional to

$$h(-\log p_1, \ldots, -\log p_k) p_1^{-1} \cdots p_k^{-1},$$

where $p_k = 1 - \sum_{j=1}^{k-1} p_j$. Hjort (1996) considered

$$h(Y_1, \ldots, Y_k) \propto \prod_{j=1}^{k} \exp\{-\alpha_j Y_j\} g_0(Y_1, \ldots, Y_k),$$

and hence the resulting (conditional) density of $(p_1, \ldots, p_{k-1})$ is proportional to $p_1^{\alpha_1 - 1} \cdots p_1^{\alpha_k - 1} g_0(-\log p_1, \ldots, -\log p_k)$. We may put $g(\boldsymbol{p}) = \exp\{-\lambda \Delta(\boldsymbol{p})\}$, where $\Delta(\boldsymbol{p})$ is a penalty term for roughness. The penalty term helps to maintain positive correlation and hence smoothness. The tuning parameter λ controls the extent to which penalty is imposed for roughness. Under i.i.d. sampling the resulting posterior distribution is conjugate with a posterior mode equivalent to a penalized maximum likelihood estimator.

References

Antoniak CE (1974) Mixtures of Dirichlet processes with applications to Bayesian nonparametric problems. Ann Stat 2:1152–1174
Blackwell D, MacQueen JB (1973) Ferguson distributions via Pólya urn schemes. Ann Stat 1:353–355
Bush CA, MacEachern SN (1996) A semiparametric Bayesian model for randomised block designs. Biometrika 83:275–285
Dahl DB (2005) Sequentially-allocated merge-split sampler for conjugate and nonconjugate Dirichlet process mixture models. Techical Report, Texas AM University
Dey D, Müller P, Sinha D (1998) Practical nonparametric and semiparametric Bayesian statistics. Springer, New York
Dubins LE, Freedman DA (1967) Random distribution functions. In: Proceedings of the fifth Berkeley symposium on mathematics, statistics and probability, vol 2, pp 183–214
Escobar MD (1988) Estimating the means of several normal populations by nonparametric estimation of the distributions of the means. Unpublished doctoral thesis, Deparment of Statistics, Yale University
Escobar MD (1994) Estimating normal means with a Dirichlet process prior. J Am Stat Assoc 89:268–277
Escobar MD, West M (1995) Bayesian density estimation and inference using mixtures. J Am Stat Assoc 90:577–588
Fabius J (1964) Asymptotic behavior of Bayes' estimates. Ann Math Stat 35:846–856
Ferguson TS (1973) A Bayesian analysis of some nonparametric problems. Ann Stat 1:209–230
Ferguson TS (1974) Prior distribution on the spaces of probability measures. Ann Stat 2:615–629
Ferguson TS (1983) Bayesian density estimation by mixtures of normal distributions. In: Siegmund D, Rustage J, Rizvi GG (eds) Recent advances in statistics. Papers in honor of Herman Chernoff on his sixtieth birthday, Bibliohound, pp 287–302
Freedman D (1963) On the asymptotic distribution of Bayes' estimates in the discrete case. Ann Math Stat 34:1386–1403
Ghosh JK, Ramamoorthi RV (2003) Bayesian nonparametrics. Springer, New York
Green PJ, Richardson S (2001) Modelling heterogeneity with and without the Dirichlet process. Scand J Stat 28(2):355–375
Griffin JE, Walker SG (2011) Posterior simulation of normalized random measure mixtures. J Comput Graph Stat 20(1):241–259. doi:10.1198/jcgs.2010.08176

Guindani M, Sepúlveda N, Paulino CD, Müller P (2014) A Bayesian semi-parametric approach for the differential analysis of sequence counts data. Appl Stat 63:385–404

Hjort NL (1996) Bayesian approaches to non- and semiparametric density estimation. In: Bernadro JM, Berger JO, Dawid AP, M SAF (eds) Bayesian statistics, vol 5. Oxford University Press, Oxford, pp 223–253

Ishwaran H, James LF (2001) Gibbs sampling methods for stick-breaking priors. J Am Stat Assoc 96:161–173

Ishwaran H, James LF (2002) Approximate Dirichlet process computing in finite normal mixtures: smoothing and prior information. J Comput Graph Stat 11:508–532

Ishwaran H, James LF (2003) Generalized weighted Chinese restaurant processes for species sampling mixture models. Stat Sin 13:1211–1235

Ishwaran H, Zarepour M (2000) Markov chain Monte Carlo in approximate Dirichlet and beta two-parameter process hierarchical models. Biometrika 87:371–390

Jain S, Neal RM (2004) A split-merge Markov chain Monte Carlo procedure for the Dirichlet Process mixture model. J Comput Graph Stat 13:158–182

Kalli M, Griffin J, Walker S (2011) Slice sampling mixture models. Stat Comput 21:93–105. doi:10.1007/s11222-009-9150-y. http://dx.doi.org/10.1007/s11222-009-9150-y

Kolmogorov AN (1933) Foundations of the theory of probability, 2nd edn. Nathan Morrison, New York

Korwar RM, Hollander M (1973) Contributions to the theory of Dirichlet processes. Ann Probab 1:705–711

Kraft CM (1964) A class of distribution function processes which have derivatives. J Appl Probab 1:385–388

Liu JS (1996) Nonparametric hierarchical Bayes via sequential imputations. Ann Stat 24:911–930

Lo AY (1984) On a class of Bayesian nonparametric estimates I: density estimates. Ann Stat 12:351–357

MacEachern SN, Müller P (1998) Estimating mixture of Dirichlet process models. J Comput Graph Stat 7(2):223–338

MacEachern SN, Clyde M, Liu JS (1999) Sequential importance sampling for nonparametric Bayes models: the next generation. Can J Stat 27:251–267

Metivier M (1971) Sur la construction de mesures aleatoires presque surement absolument continues par rapport a une mesure donnee. Zeitschrift fur Wahrschinlichkeitstheorie und Verwandte Gebiete 20:332–334

Muliere P, Secchi P (1995) A note on a proper Bayesian Bootstrap. Techical Report, Università degli Studi di Pavia, Dipartimento di Economia Politica e Metodi Quantitativ

Muliere P, Tardella L (1998) Approximating distributions of random functionals of Ferguson-Dirichlet priors. Can J Stat 26:283–297

Neal RM (2000) Markov chain sampling methods for Dirichlet process mixture models. J Comput Graph Stat 9:249–265

Newton MA, Zhang Y (1999) A recursive algorithm for nonparametric analysis with missing data. Biometrika 86:15–26

Newton MA, Quintana FA, Zhang Y (1998) Nonparametric Bayes methods using predictive updating. In: Dey D, Müller P, Sinha D (eds) Practical nonparametric and semiparametric Bayesian statistics. Springer, New York, pp 45–62

Petrone S, Veronese P (2002) Nonparametric mixture priors based on an exponential random scheme. Stat Methods Appl 11:1–20

Phillips DB, Smith AFM (1996) Bayesian model comparisons via jump diffusions. In: Gilks WR, Ricahrdson S, Spiegelhalter DJ (eds) Markov chain Monte Carlo in practice. Chapman and Hall, New York

Pitman J (1996) Some developments of the Blackwell-MacQueen urn scheme. In: Ferguson TS, Shapeley LS, MacQueen JB (eds) Statistics, probability and game theory. Papers in honor of David Blackwell. IMS lecture notes - monograph series. IMS, Hayward, pp 245–268

Pitman J, Yor M (1997) The two-parameter Poisson-Dirichlet distribution derived from a stable subordinator. Ann Probab 25:855–900

References

Richardson S, Green PJ (1997) On Bayesian analysis of mixtures with an unknown number of components. J R Stat Soc B 59:731–792

Sethuraman J (1994) A constructive definition of Dirichlet prior. Stat Sin 2:639–650

Walker SG (2007) Sampling the Dirichlet mixture model with slices. Commnun Stat Simul Comput **36**:45–54

West M, Müller P, Escobar MD (1994) Hierarchical priors and mixture models, with application in regression and density estimation. In: Freeman PR, Smith AFM (eds) Aspects of uncertainty. Wiley, New York, pp 363–368

Chapter 3
Density Estimation: Models Beyond the DP

Abstract The ubiquitous use of Dirichlet process models should not discourage researchers from considering interesting features of alternative models. In particular, the Polya tree model turns out to be an attractive choice for some applications. In this chapter we discuss the use of the Polya tree prior and its variations for density estimation. We define the model, introduce computation efficient methods for posterior inference and identify relative advantages and limitations compared with Dirichlet process models.

3.1 Polya Trees

3.1.1 Definition

Recall the discrete nature of a DP random probability measures G, that is, when $G \mid M, G_0 \sim \text{DP}(MG_0)$. For many applications, especially for univariate and low dimensional sample space (of G), an elegant alternative that avoids this limitation is the Polya tree (PT) prior. The PT includes DP models as a special case. But in contrast to the DP, an appropriate choice of the PT parameters allows the user to generate continuous distributions with probability one. The construction of PT priors was originally considered by Ferguson (1974) and Blackwell and MacQueen (1973), and later studied by Mauldin et al. (1992), and Lavine (1992, 1994). The prior can be seen as the De Finneti measure in a generalized Polya urn scheme (Mauldin et al. 1992). The connection with Polya urn schemes justifies the name of PT (see, Monticino 2001, for an illustrative explanation) and allows for direct proofs of many of their properties.

The PT essentially defines a random histogram. Consider the bins of a histogram defined by a partition of the sample space into nonempty, subsets $\{B_\ell, \ell = 0, \ldots, 2^m - 1\}$ (the size of the partition is written as 2^m in anticipation of the upcoming discussion). We could now define random probabilities $G(B_\ell)$ for each bin. Next consider refining the histogram by splitting each bin into two, $B_\ell = B_{\ell 0} \cup B_{\ell 1}$, and define random probabilities for the refined histogram by defining $Y_{\ell 0} = G(B_{\ell 0} \mid B_\ell)$ and $Y_{\ell 1} = 1 - Y_{\ell 0} = G(B_{\ell 1} \mid B_\ell)$. The recursive refinement of bins defines a sequence of nested partitions. This construction is exactly the idea of the PT prior. We create the nested partitions starting from the entire sample space, i.e., $\Omega = B_0 \cup B_1$. Thus the subindices of the partitioning subsets are sequences $\varepsilon = \varepsilon_1 \cdots \varepsilon_m$ of binary indicators $\varepsilon_j \in \{0, 1\}$ and $G(B_{\varepsilon_1 \cdots \varepsilon_m}) = \prod_{j=1}^{m} Y_{\varepsilon_1 \cdots \varepsilon_j}$. The PT prior is the random probability measure G that arises when the $Y_{\varepsilon 0}$'s are independent beta random variables.

Recall from Sect. 2.5.1 the definition of a sequence of nested partitions $\Pi = \{\pi_m; \ m = 0, 1, 2, \ldots\}$. For example, if $\Omega = [0, 1]$ is the unit interval, then we could use $\pi_0 = [0, 1]$, $\pi_1 = \{[0, \frac{1}{2}), [\frac{1}{2}, 1]\}$, $\pi_2 = \{[0, \frac{1}{4}), [\frac{1}{4}, \frac{1}{2}), [\frac{1}{2}, \frac{3}{4}), [\frac{3}{4}, 1]\}$, etc. In general, we use sequences of binary indicators, $\epsilon = \varepsilon_1 \cdots \varepsilon_m$ with $\varepsilon \in \{0, 1\}$ to index the partitioning subsets in the level m partition π_m. That is, $\pi_1 = \{B_{\varepsilon_1}\}$, $\pi_2 = \{B_{\varepsilon_1 \varepsilon_2}\}$, etc. The condition $B_\epsilon = B_{\epsilon 0} \cup B_{\epsilon 1}$ makes π_{m+1} nested within π_m. Since we start with 2 subsets in π_1, we have 2^m subsets in π_m. That is, the index set of the $B_\epsilon \in \pi_m$ is $\epsilon \in \{0, 1\}^m$. Let $E^* = \bigcup_{m=0}^{\infty} \{0, 1\}^m$, with $\{0, 1\}^0 \equiv \emptyset$. Then E^* is the index set of all partitioning subsets in Π.

Definition 2 Let $\Pi = \{\pi_m\}$ be a sequence of nested binary partitions as before and $\mathcal{A} = \{\alpha_\varepsilon : \varepsilon \in E^*\}$ be a collection of nonnegative numbers. A random probability measure G on Ω is said to be a Polya tree with parameters $(\Pi, \mathcal{A})$ if for every $m = 1, 2, \ldots$, and every $\varepsilon = \varepsilon_1 \cdots \varepsilon_m \in E^m$,

$$G(B_{\varepsilon_1 \cdots \varepsilon_m}) = \prod_{j=1}^{m} Y_{\varepsilon_1 \ldots \varepsilon_j}, \qquad (3.1)$$

where the conditional probabilities $Y_{\varepsilon_1 \cdots \varepsilon_{j-1} 0}$ are mutually independent beta random variables

$$Y_{\varepsilon_1 \cdots \varepsilon_{j-1} 0} \sim \text{Be}\left(\alpha_{\varepsilon_1 \cdots \varepsilon_{j-1} 0}, \alpha_{\varepsilon_1 \cdots \varepsilon_{j-1} 1}\right), \qquad (3.2)$$

and $Y_{\varepsilon 1 \cdots \varepsilon_{j-1} 1} = 1 - Y_{\varepsilon_1 \cdots \varepsilon_{j-1} 0}$. We write $G \sim \text{PT}(\Pi, \mathcal{A})$.

From the definition, it follows that a PT process is a special case of a TF process, where besides independence across rows, the random conditional probabilities are also independent within rows and have beta distributions. Degenerate beta distributions are permitted, for instance, by considering $\alpha_{\varepsilon 0} = 0$.

The class of PTs contains the DP, which is characterized by the condition $\alpha_{\varepsilon 0} + \alpha_{\varepsilon 1} = \alpha_\varepsilon$, for every $\varepsilon \in E^*$ (Ferguson 1974). The advantage of a DP over a more general PT is that the DP is the only TF process in which the choice of $\{\pi_m\}$ does not affect inference. An attractive property of the PT model is that conditions can be set on the elements of $\mathcal{A} = \{\alpha_\varepsilon : \varepsilon \in E^*\}$ such that G is absolutely continuous with probability one (see, Ferguson 1974). Dubins and Freedman (1967) showed that when $\alpha_\varepsilon = 1$ continuous singular distributions are generated. Kraft (1964) and Metivier (1971) showed that $\alpha_{\varepsilon_1 \cdots \varepsilon_m} = m^2$ is a sufficient condition to guarantee that the PT assigns probability one to the set of continuous distributions. More general sufficient conditions are given in Theorem 1.121 and Lemma 1.124 on pages 66–68 of Schervish (1995). Any choice $\alpha_{\varepsilon_1 \cdots \varepsilon_m} = c\rho(m)$ with $\rho(m)$ such that $\sum_{m=1}^{\infty} \rho(m)^{-1} < \infty$ guarantees G to be absolutely continuous *a priori*.

3.1.2 Prior Centering

From the TF property and the beta distribution of the Y_ε's it is possible to find expressions for the moments of $G(B_\varepsilon)$. For example, the mean and the variance are given by the following expressions. For every $\varepsilon \in E^*$ let $\mu_{\varepsilon 0} = E(Y_{\varepsilon 0})$, $\mu_{\varepsilon 1} = 1 - E(Y_{\varepsilon 0})$, $s_{\varepsilon 0} = E(Y_{\varepsilon 0}^2)$ and $s_{\varepsilon 1} = E([1-Y_{\varepsilon 0}]^2)$ denote the first and second moments of a $\text{Be}(\alpha_{\varepsilon 0}, \alpha_{\varepsilon 1})$ distribution. Then

$$\text{E}\{G(B_{\varepsilon_1 \cdots \varepsilon_m})\} = \prod_{j=1}^{m} \mu_{\varepsilon_1 \cdots \varepsilon_j}, \quad \text{Var}\{G(B_{\varepsilon_1 \cdots \varepsilon_m})\} = \prod_{j=1}^{m} s_{\varepsilon_1 \cdots \varepsilon_j} - \prod_{j=1}^{m} \mu_{\varepsilon_1 \cdots \varepsilon_j}^2. \quad (3.3)$$

In practice, it is difficult to elicit the family $\mathcal{A}$ and the partitions Π for a PT model. Here, the moment conditions from above help. The moment conditions imply some default choices that allow centering of $G \mid \Pi, \mathcal{A} \sim \text{PT}(\Pi, \mathcal{A})$ at some desired prior mean $E(G) = G_0$ for a PT random probability measure defined on the entire real line or a subset of it.

Prior Centering by Π: $\text{PT}(G_0, \mathcal{A})$ Lavine (1992) proposed the following choice to center the PT around a given centering probability measure G_0. In short, fix Π as the dyadic quantiles of G_0 and use $\alpha_{\varepsilon 0} = \alpha_{\varepsilon 1}$, for every $\varepsilon \in E^*$.

For a formal description of the construction, let G_0^{-1} denote the inverse cumulative density function (c.d.f.) of G_0, and define the partitioning subsets $B_{\varepsilon_1 \cdots \varepsilon_m} \in \pi_m$ as the intervals defined by the quantiles $G_0^{-1}(k/2^m)$, $k = 0, 1, \ldots 2^m$. Let $N(\varepsilon)$ denote the integer with base-2 representation $\varepsilon = \varepsilon_1 \cdots \varepsilon_m \in E^m$, that is, interpret ε as the digits of a base-2 integer N. Then, for every for $\varepsilon = \varepsilon_1 \cdots \varepsilon_m \in E^m$, set

$$B_{\varepsilon_1 \cdots \varepsilon_m} = \left[G_0^{-1}\left(\frac{N(\varepsilon)}{2^m}\right), G_0^{-1}\left(\frac{N(\varepsilon)+1}{2^m}\right) \right).$$

Also, take $\alpha_{\varepsilon 0} = \alpha_{\varepsilon 1}$ for all $\varepsilon \in E^*$. Then

$$E[G(B_{\varepsilon_1 \cdots \varepsilon_m})] = \prod_{j=1}^{m} E(Y_{\varepsilon_1 \cdots \varepsilon_j}) = \frac{1}{2^m} = G_0(B_{\varepsilon_1 \cdots \varepsilon_m}).$$

Thus G_0 has a similar role as the centering distribution in a DP. We write $G \sim \text{PT}(G_0, \mathcal{A})$. Later, when we include hyper-parameters η in $G_{0,\eta}$ we will write Π^η to indicate the sequence of random partitions that we constructed in this centering.

Prior Centering by $\mathcal{A}$: $\text{PT}(\Pi, G_0)$ Alternatively, one can fix Π and select $\mathcal{A}$ to achieve the desired prior expectation, $E\{G(B_{\varepsilon_1 \cdots \varepsilon_m})\} = G_0(B_{\varepsilon_1 \cdots \varepsilon_m})$. For every $\varepsilon \in E^*$, consider the split of B_ε into $B_\varepsilon = B_{\varepsilon 0} \cup B_{\varepsilon 1}$. The desired prior centering is achieved with

$$\alpha_{\varepsilon j} \propto G_0(B_{\varepsilon j}), \quad j = 0, 1$$

Again it follows that $E\{G(B_{\varepsilon_1\cdots\varepsilon_m})\} = G_0(B_{\varepsilon_1\cdots\varepsilon_m})$ for every $\varepsilon_1\cdots\varepsilon_m \in E^m$. We write $G \mid \Pi, G_0 \sim \mathsf{PT}(\Pi, G_0)$.

Canonical Choices for $\alpha_{\varepsilon_1\cdots\varepsilon_m}$ in $\mathsf{PT}(G_0, \mathcal{A})$ Consider now the first construction, $G \sim \mathsf{PT}(G_0, \mathcal{A})$ to center a PT prior. Once the PT is centered around a probability measure, G_0, the family $\mathcal{A} = \{\alpha_\varepsilon : \varepsilon \in E^*\}$ determines how much G can deviate from G_0, much like the role of the total mass parameter M in a DP. Likewise, $\mathcal{A}$ determines how quickly prior shrinkage towards G_0 is washed out by the likelihood. In contrast to the DP prior, the PT has infinitely many parameters, specified in $\mathcal{A}$, which may be used to describe the prior belief. To mitigate the need of extensive prior elicitation, a default method is usually adopted, where one chooses α_ε depending only on the length of the binary string ε. Lavine (1992) proposes $\alpha_{\varepsilon_1\cdots\varepsilon_m} = m^2$ as a canonical choice. Walker and Mallick (1997) and Paddock (1999) used $\alpha_{\varepsilon_1\cdots\varepsilon_m} = cm^2$, with $c > 0$. Berger and Guglielmi (2001) considered this family and others of the form $\alpha_{\varepsilon_1\cdots\varepsilon_m} = c\rho(m)$. Specifically, the choice $\rho(m) = 8^m$ satisfies a consistency theorem of Barron et al. (1999).

By considering different values of c, Hanson and Johnson (2002) found that the family $\alpha_{\varepsilon_1\cdots\varepsilon_m} = cm^2$ was sufficiently rich to capture interesting features of the distributions under consideration. For future reference, we denote this family as $\mathcal{A}_c$. That is

$$\mathcal{A}_c = \{\alpha_\varepsilon = cm^2, \ \varepsilon = \varepsilon_1\cdots\varepsilon_m \in E^\star\}.$$

Hanson and Johnson (2002) proved two results that indicate broadly the effect that c has on inference. Consider a PT random measure on $\mathbb{R}$, using $G \sim \mathsf{PT}(G_0, \mathcal{A}_c)$, that is, a PT prior that is centered at $E(G) = G_0$ by using dyadic quantiles of G_0 to define the nested sequence of partitions. Assume $y_1, \ldots, y_n \mid G \overset{iid}{\sim} G$, and let $\boldsymbol{y} = (y_1, \ldots, y_n)$. Hanson and Johnson (2002) showed that

$$G((-\infty, t]) \mid \boldsymbol{y} \xrightarrow{c \to \infty} G_0((-\infty, t]),$$

and

$$G((-\infty, t]) \mid \boldsymbol{y} \xrightarrow{c \to 0} \sum_{j=1}^n p_j I(y_j < t)$$

in distribution, where $(p_1, \ldots, p_n) \sim \mathrm{Dirichlet}(1, \ldots, 1)$. The same results are obtained for the DP as the precision parameter M tends to ∞ and 0, respectively. Figure 3.1 demonstrates the effects of increasing the precision parameter. As is the case for the DP prior, when $c \longrightarrow \infty$ the PT process defines a random probability measure that is essentially degenerate at G_0.

3.1 Polya Trees

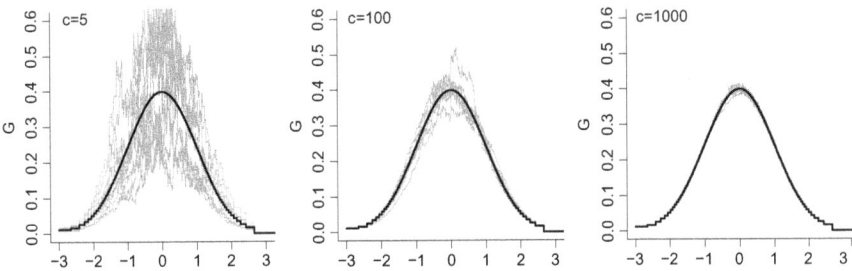

Fig. 3.1 Plots of $n = 10$ density g_i samples from $G_i \sim \mathsf{PT}(G^o, \mathcal{A}^c)$, $i = 1, \ldots, n$, centered on a standard normal distribution G^o, for $c = 5, 100$ and 1000. In all cases, $E(g_i)$ is overlaid over a plot of the realizations of g_i

3.1.3 Posterior Updating and Marginal Model

Mauldin et al. (1992) and Lavine (1992, 1994) catalogue properties of the PT, including a conjugacy result. In words, the PT is a conjugate prior on a random probability measure G under i.i.d. sampling, $y_1, \ldots, y_n \mid G \overset{iid}{\sim} G$. The posterior $p(G \mid y_1, \ldots, y_n)$ is again a PT, with updated beta parameters. The parameter α_ε is incremented by 1 for each $y_i \in B_\varepsilon$. Let $n_\varepsilon = \sum_{i=1}^n I(y_i \in B_\varepsilon)$ denote the number of observations in a partitioning subset B_ε.

Result 3 *Suppose that* $y_1, \ldots, y_n \mid G \overset{iid}{\sim} G$, *and* $G \sim \mathsf{PT}(\Pi, \mathcal{A})$. *Then*

$$G \mid y \sim \mathsf{PT}(\Pi, \mathcal{A}^\star) \tag{3.4}$$

where the updated beta parameters $\alpha_\varepsilon^\star \in \mathcal{A}^\star$ *are* $\alpha_\varepsilon^\star = \alpha_\varepsilon + n_\varepsilon$.

Lavine (1992) provided an expression for the marginal model $p(y_1, \ldots, y_n)$, when $y_1, \ldots, y_n \mid G \overset{iid}{\sim} G$ and a PT prior is assumed for G, that is, $p(y_1, \ldots, y_n) = \int \prod_{i=1}^n G(y_i) \, dp(G)$, with a PT prior on G. Assume a centered PT, with $G \mid G_0, \mathcal{A} \sim \mathsf{PT}(G_0, \mathcal{A})$ or with $G \mid \Pi, G_0 \sim \mathsf{PT}(\Pi, G_0)$. Let g_0 denote the p.d.f. of G_0. We need some notation to locate an observation y in partitioning subsets at various levels of the nested partition. For every $m = 1, 2, \ldots$, let $\epsilon_m(y_i) = \varepsilon_1 \cdots \varepsilon_m \in E^m$ denote the index of the level m subset that contains y_i, i.e., $y_i \in B_{\varepsilon_1 \cdots \varepsilon_m}$. Also, let $m^*(y_i)$ denote the lowest level m such that y_i is the only data point in $B_{\epsilon_m(y_i)}$, among $y_1, \ldots, y_i$. Finally, let

$$n_\varepsilon^{(j)} = \sum_{i=1}^{j-1} I(y_i \in B_\varepsilon) \quad \text{and} \quad \alpha_\varepsilon^{\star(j)} = \alpha_\varepsilon + n_\varepsilon^{(j)}$$

denote the number of observations $y_1, \ldots, y_{j-1}$ that lie in B_ε and the beta parameters updated with these counts, respectively.

Result 4 *The marginal distribution of a random sample* $(y_1, \ldots, y_n)$ *is given by*

$$p(y_1, \ldots, y_n) = \left\{\prod_{i=1}^n g_0(y_i)\right\} \prod_{j=2}^n \prod_{m=1}^{m^*(y_j)} \frac{\alpha^{\star(j)}_{\epsilon_m(y_j)}}{\alpha^{\star(j)}_{\epsilon_m(y_j)}} \cdot \frac{\alpha_{\epsilon_{m-1}(y_j)0} + \alpha_{\epsilon_{m-1}(y_j)1}}{\alpha^{\star(j)}_{\epsilon_{m-1}(y_j)0} + \alpha^{\star(j)}_{\epsilon_{m-1}(y_j)1}}. \tag{3.5}$$

We refer to Berger and Guglielmi (2001) and Hanson and Johnson (2002) for more discussion. In particular, Berger and Guglielmi (2001) use the marginal model to evaluate Bayes factors. The proof of (3.5) is straightforward. The innermost product over the factors involving $\alpha^\star$, that is, $\prod_m \alpha^{\star(j)}_{\epsilon_m(y_j)}/\{\alpha^{\star(j)}_{\epsilon_{m-1}(y_j)0} + \alpha^{\star(j)}_{\epsilon_{m-1}(y_j)1}\}$, is the posterior predictive probability $p(y_j \in B_\epsilon \mid y_1, \ldots, y_{j-1})$ for $\varepsilon = \epsilon_m(y_j)$. It follows from (3.4) applied for $p(G \mid y_1, \ldots, y_{j-1})$, and (3.3), substituting $E(Y_\varepsilon) = \alpha_{\varepsilon 0}/(\alpha_{\varepsilon 0} + \alpha_{\varepsilon 1})$. Conditional on $y_j \in B_\epsilon$, the conditional prior predictive distribution is G_0 restricted to B_ϵ, i.e., has density $g_0(y_j) \frac{1}{G_0(B_\epsilon)}$. By construction, $G_0(B_\epsilon) = E[G(B_\epsilon)]$, the prior mean, which in turn can be written as a similar product of factors, $\prod_{m=1}^{m^*(y_j)} \alpha_{\epsilon_m(y_j)}/\{\alpha_{\epsilon_{m-1}(y_j)0} + \alpha_{\epsilon_{m-1}(y_j)1}\}$, now involving the prior parameters α_ε.

The argument remains valid under either prior centering, $\mathsf{PT}(G_0, \mathcal{A})$ as well as $\mathsf{PT}(\Pi, G_0)$. In the earlier case, with $\alpha_{\varepsilon_1 \cdots \varepsilon_m} = cm^2$ and $G_0(B_{\varepsilon_1 \cdots \varepsilon_m}) = 1/2^m$ by definition of B_ε as the quantile sets under G_0, the expression can be further simplified to

$$p(y_1, \ldots, y_n) = \left\{\prod_{i=1}^n g_0(y_i)\right\} 2^m \prod_{j=2}^n \prod_{m=1}^{m^*(y_j)} \frac{cm^2 + n^{(j)}_{\epsilon_m(y_j)}}{2cm^2 + n^{(j)}_{\epsilon_{m-1}(y_j)}}. \tag{3.6}$$

Expressions (3.6) and (3.5) remain valid also when the base measure G_0 is indexed with unknown hyper-parameters, that is, when the base measure is $G_{0,\eta}$. See the upcoming discussion in Sect. 3.2.1.

Example 4 (Gene Expression, ctd.) We implement density estimation for the gene expression data given before, in Example 4. We assume $y_i \mid G \overset{\text{iid}}{\sim} G$, $i = 1, \ldots, n$, with

$$G \sim \mathsf{PT}(G_0, \mathcal{A})$$

with $\alpha_{\varepsilon_1 \cdots \varepsilon_m} = cm^2$ and $G_0 = \mathsf{N}(\mu, \sigma^2)$. For the moment we fix $(\mu, \sigma) = (-3, 4)$ and $c = 3$. Figure 3.2b summarizes the inference (we will describe panel (a) later).

Software note: R code for Fig. 3.2b is shown in the software appendix for this chapter. The code implements Algorithm 5, shown below.

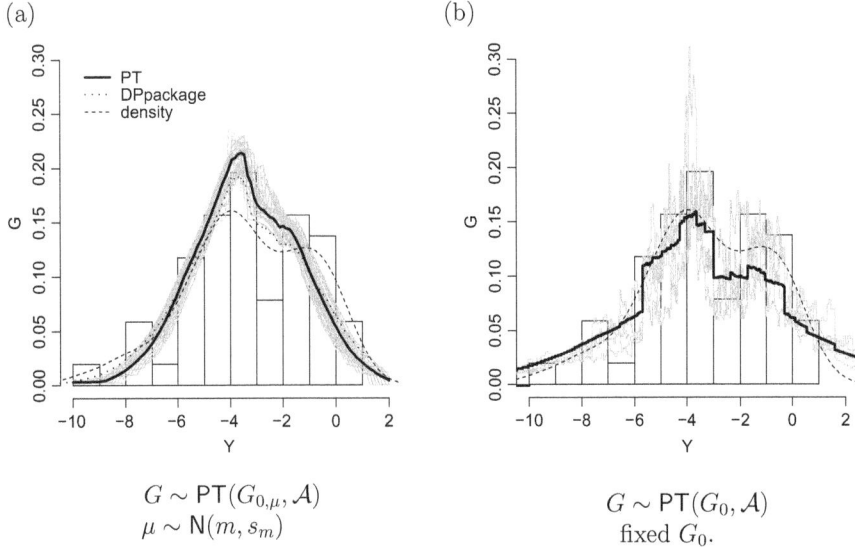

Fig. 3.2 Example 4. Posterior inference for G under PT prior, $G \sim \text{PT}(G_0, \mathcal{A})$, with $G_0 = \text{N}(\mu, \sigma^2)$. In panel (**a**) we use a hyper-prior on μ. In panel (**b**) G_0 is fixed. For comparison, panel (**a**) also shows a kernel density estimate (*dashed, thin line*) and an estimate with an additional hyper-prior $p(c)$ on the precision parameter in $\alpha_{\varepsilon_1 \cdots \varepsilon_m} = cm^2$ (marked "DPpackage"). In both panels, posterior draws are also overlaid as *greyed out lines*. See the discussion in Sect. 3.3

3.2 Variations of the Polya Tree Processes

3.2.1 Mixture of Polya Trees

Although the prior mean distribution function may have a smooth Lebesgue density, the randomly sampled densities from a simple PT are very rough, being nowhere differentiable (see, Fig. 3.1). Barron et al. (1999) noted that the posterior predictive densities of future observations computed under a PT prior have noticeable jumps at the boundaries of partitioning subsets and that a choice of centering distribution G_0 that is particularly unlike the sample distribution of the data will make convergence of the posterior very slow. Note also that a practical implementation requires some meaningful elicitation of the centering distribution. Often a class of target measures can be identified, like the normal family, but it is hard to choose a single member of the family.

To overcome these difficulties it is natural to consider a centering measure which contains unspecified parameters, $G_{0,\eta}$, and a further prior on these hyper-parameters, π. The resulting hierarchical prior is a mixture of Polya trees (MPT). The additional parameter leads to inference that averages out jumps to yield smooth densities (Hanson and Johnson 2002). Note, however, that the TF property is lost.

Of particular interest is the situation where η is a scale parameter and G is forced to have median zero. Such models are of interest for residual distributions.

Hanson and Johnson (2002, Theorem 1) show that a MPT model with a prior on a scale parameter η in the base measure $G_{0,\eta}$ implies a continuous predictive distribution (except at 0). The result is under i.i.d. sampling, $y_1, \ldots, y_n \mid G \overset{iid}{\sim} G$, with a PT prior $G \mid \eta \sim \mathsf{PT}(G_{0,\eta}, \mathcal{A})$ using $\alpha_{\varepsilon_1 \cdots \varepsilon_m} = cm^2$, and a hyper-prior $\pi(\eta)$. The PT is constrained to 0 median (to be suitable as residual distribution in a regression model) and $g_{0,\eta}$ is assumed to be continuous in $\mathbb{R}$. There are two more technical conditions to the result. We need the existence of a bound $L(\eta)$ such that $g_{0,\eta}(y) < L(\eta)$ for every $y \in \mathbb{R}$ and $\int [L(\eta)]^j \pi(\eta) d\eta < \infty$ for $j = n, n+1$. Under these conditions the predictive distribution $p(y_{n+1} \mid y_1, \ldots, y_n)$ is continuous everywhere except at 0. By using similar arguments as in Hanson and Johnson (2002) it is possible to prove that when η is a location parameter the posterior expected density is continuous everywhere.

Another possible way of creating a MPT model is to keep the partition fixed and vary the α_ε parameters. As the partitions do not vary, the resulting density is discontinuous everywhere, just like a usual PT. This kind of MPT was considered by Berger and Guglielmi (2001) for testing a parametric family against the nonparametric alternative using a Bayes factor.

Example 4 (Gene Expression, ctd.) We now relax the setup of the PT prior for the gene expression data. We continue to use $y_1, \ldots, y_n \mid G \overset{iid}{\sim} G$, with

$$G \mid \eta \sim \mathsf{PT}(G_{0,\eta}, \mathcal{A}),$$

where $G_{0,\eta} = \mathsf{N}(\mu, \sigma^2)$. But now we implement an MPT, mixing with respect to $\eta = (\mu, \sigma^2)$. We assume

$$\mu \sim \mathsf{N}(m, s_m^2),$$

with $m = -3$, $s_m = 2$ and σ fixed at $\sigma = 4$. In this implementation we still fix c. However, including a Metropolis-Hastings step to update c would be straightforward. See the R code in the online appendix for this chapter.

Figure 3.2a summarizes the inference. The solid line, marked "PT" shows the density estimate under the MPT model. For comparison the figure also shows the density estimate with respect to mixing on both μ and σ, as well as over c. Inference is implemented using the R package *DPpackage*. The density estimate is marked as "DPpackage" in the plot. Also for comparison, the figure shows a kernel density estimate, marked as "density".

Software note: Inference for density estimation with PT and MPT priors is implemented in DPpackage, in the function PTdensity(·). For an example, see the R code for this example in the on-line software appendix for this chapter.

3.2.2 Partially Specified Polya Trees

Computation with PT priors might be hindered by the need to update the infinite number of parameters which describe the tree. The finite Polya tree (FPT), which is also known as "partially specified Polya tree" (Lavine 1994), is an alternative to address this concern. The finite PT is constructed to be identical to the PT up to a finite pre-specified level J. However, the PT parameters in the set $\{\alpha_\varepsilon : \varepsilon \in E^*\}$ are updated only up to this level J in the FPT.

Lavine (1994) discusses two scenarios for which it might be reasonable to update only to a pre-specified level J. The first scenario is when the parameters in $\{\alpha_\varepsilon : \varepsilon \in E^*\}$ are constructed to increase rapidly enough as the level of the tree increases. The posterior updating of the distributions of Y_ε beyond level J does not affect the prior strongly. The second scenario in which FPT are appealing arises from concerns related to prior elicitation. It might be possible to elicit prior information about parameters near the top of the PT and information about aspects of the distribution such as shape and modality, but it could be unreasonable to expect to elicit meaningful prior distributions for each and every parameter of the PT prior.

Lavine (1994) detailed how such a level can be chosen by placing bounds on the posterior predictive distribution at a point. Hanson and Johnson (2002) suggested the rule of thumb $J \approx \log_2(n)$ and Hanson (2006) suggested $J \approx \log_2(n/N)$, where N is a "typical" number of observations falling into each set at level J when there is reasonable comfort in the centering family.

We write $G \sim \mathsf{FPT}(G_{0,\eta}, \mathcal{A}_c, J)$ for a FPT that truncates a $\mathsf{PT}(G_{0,\eta}, \mathcal{A}_c)$ at level J. Recall that in our earlier notation $\mathcal{A}_c$ is defined by setting $\alpha_{\varepsilon_1 \cdots \varepsilon_m} = cm^2$.

3.3 Posterior Simulation for Polya Tree Models

3.3.1 FTP and i.i.d. Sampling

Recall that the PT prior is conjugate under i.i.d. sampling (Result 3). Consider $y_1, \ldots, y_n \mid G \overset{\text{iid}}{\sim} G$, with a finite PT prior $G \sim \mathsf{FPT}(G_0, \mathcal{A}_c, J)$. That is, the PT prior is centered around a distribution G_0 by fixing the partitioning subsets as dyadic quantile sets under G_0 and we only consider the first J levels of nested partitions. Recall the earlier discussion, in Sect. 3.1.2. Recall that $\mathcal{A}_c$ refers to using $\alpha_{\varepsilon_1 \cdots \varepsilon_m} = cm^2$. In summary, the model is given by

$$y_1, \ldots, y_n \mid G \overset{\text{iid}}{\sim} G, \qquad G \sim \mathsf{FPT}(G_0, \mathcal{A}_c, J).$$

For the moment we fix c as well as the centering measure G_0.

We state an explicit algorithm for posterior inference under this model. The algorithm implements the prior centering of the $\mathsf{FPT}(G_0, \mathcal{A}_c, J)$ prior and carries out the posterior updating of Result 3. Assume $\Omega = \mathbb{R}$, and let $B_{\varepsilon_1\cdots\varepsilon_m} = [L_{\varepsilon_1\cdots\varepsilon_m}, R_{\varepsilon_1\cdots\varepsilon_m})$, with $B_{0\cdots 0} = (-\infty, R_{0\cdots 0})$. Let $N(\epsilon)$ denote the integer with dyadic representation ϵ, and let $q(z) = G_0^{-1}(z)$ denote the inverse c.d.f. of the desired centering measure G_0. Below we will use indexing of vectors with binary integers $\epsilon = \varepsilon_1\cdots\varepsilon_m$. In an implementation, for example, in R, it is convenient to map ϵ to decimal integer indices $j = 1,\ldots,2^m$.

Algorithm 5: *Posterior simulation under a finite PT prior.*

1. *Construct Π:* For $m = 1,\ldots,J$ and for all $\epsilon \in E^m$,
   let $R_\epsilon = q\left(2^{-m}(N(\epsilon) + 1)\right)$ *(right subset boundaries)*
2. *Evaluate $\mathcal{A}^\star$:* For $m = 1,\ldots,J$,

   1. for all $\epsilon \in E^m$, let $\alpha_\epsilon = \alpha_\epsilon^\star = cm^2$ *(initializing $\alpha_\epsilon^\star$)*
   2. for $i = 1,\ldots,n$

      - $\epsilon_m(y_i) = \min\{\epsilon \in E^m : R_\epsilon \geq y_i\}$ *(index of the level m subset containing y_i)*
      - $\alpha_{\epsilon_m(y_i)}^\star \mathrel{+}= 1$ *(building up $\alpha_\epsilon^\star = \alpha_\epsilon + n_\epsilon$ for all subsets)*

3. *Posterior simulation:*

   1. For $m = 0,\ldots,J-1$ and for all $\epsilon \in E^m$ let

   $$Y_{\epsilon 0} \sim \mathrm{Be}(\alpha_{\epsilon 0}^\star, \alpha_{\epsilon 1}^\star) \quad \text{and} \quad Y_{\epsilon 1} = 1 - Y_{\epsilon 0}.$$

   2. $G(B_{\varepsilon_1\cdots\varepsilon_J}) = \prod_{m=1}^J Y_{\varepsilon_1\cdots\varepsilon_m}$.

   For large J, use $G(B_{\varepsilon_1\cdots\varepsilon_J})$ to plot G at printer resolution.

For example, Step 1 could be implemented in R by setting up a list (R[[1]],...,R[[J]]) with R[[m]] = q(2^(-m)*(1:2^m)), using, e.g., q(z)=qnorm(z,m=m,sd=s) for $G_0 = N(m,s)$ (substitute some large number, say 99, for $q(1.0)$).

Algorithm 6: *Posterior expectation under a finite PT prior.* Start with steps 1 and 2 in Algorithm 5 to evaluate $\alpha_\epsilon^\star$. Then evaluate

$$E\{G(B_{\varepsilon_1\cdots\varepsilon_J}) \mid y\} = \prod_{m=1}^J E(Y_{\varepsilon_1\cdots\varepsilon_m} \mid y) = \prod_{m=1}^J \frac{\alpha_{\varepsilon_1\cdots\varepsilon_m}^\star}{\alpha_{\varepsilon_1\cdots\varepsilon_{m-1}0}^\star + \alpha_{\varepsilon_1\cdots\varepsilon_{m-1}1}^\star}.$$

For large J, $E\{G(B_{\varepsilon_1\cdots\varepsilon_J}) \mid y\}$ plots $E(G \mid y)$ at printer resolution.

Algorithm 6 can be adapted for a PT, without restriction to a finite level J of nested partitions, by replacing the loop over $m = 1,\ldots,J$ by an iteration until $n_\varepsilon = 0$.

3.3.2 PT and MPT Prior Under i.i.d. Sampling

Consider again $y_1,\ldots,y_n \mid G \overset{\mathrm{iid}}{\sim} G$, now with a PT prior $G \mid \eta \sim \mathrm{PT}(G_{0,\eta}, \mathcal{A}_c)$. That is, the PT prior is centered around a distribution $G_{0,\eta}$ with unknown hyper-

3.3 Posterior Simulation for Polya Tree Models

parameters. As before, the partitioning subsets as dyadic quantile sets under $G_{0,\eta}$. In summary, the model is given by

$$y_1, \ldots, y_n \mid G \overset{iid}{\sim} G,$$
$$G \mid c, \eta \sim \mathsf{PT}(G_{0,\eta}, \mathcal{A}_c) = \mathsf{PT}(\Pi^\eta, \mathcal{A}_c), \qquad (3.7)$$

completed with a hyper-prior, π, for c and η,

$$(c, \eta) \sim \pi.$$

Here we used Π^η to indicate the nested partitions that are used in the centered $\mathsf{PT}(G_{0,\eta}, \mathcal{A}_c)$ model. The notation highlights the dependence of the sequence of nested partitions on the hyper-parameters η.

MCMC for the Marginal Posterior $p(\eta, c \mid y)$ It is possible to marginalize (3.7) with respect to G and base the inference on the predictive distribution $p(y_1, \ldots, y_n \mid c, \eta)$. Recall Eq. (3.5). Note that $\alpha_\varepsilon^{\star(j)}$ in Eq. (3.5) is now a function of c and the partition sequence Π^η is a function of the hyper-parameters η. The marginalization removes the need for sampling the infinite-dimensional process G. The problem is that the infinite-dimensional G can of course only be represented approximately, with some finite approximation (such as the FPT). However, after marginalization, sampling from the infinite-dimensional process G is no longer required, and inference is exact up to MCMC error. In summary, substituting (3.5) for the marginal, the joint posterior distribution is

$$p(\eta, c \mid y) \propto p(y_1, \ldots, y_n \mid c, \eta) \pi(c, \eta) =$$

$$\left\{ \prod_{i=1}^n g_{0,\eta}(y_i) \right\} \prod_{j=2}^n \prod_{m=1}^{m^*(y_j)} \frac{\alpha_{\varepsilon_m(y_j)}^{\star(j)}}{\alpha_{\varepsilon_m(y_j)}^{\star(j)}} \cdot \frac{\alpha_{\varepsilon_{m-1}(x_j)0}^{\star(j)} + \alpha_{\varepsilon_{m-1}(y_j)1}^{\star(j)}}{\alpha_{\varepsilon_{m-1}(x_j)0}^{\star(j)} + \alpha_{\varepsilon_{m-1}(y_j)1}^{\star(j)}} \pi(c, \eta), \qquad (3.8)$$

and could be further simplified for a $\mathsf{PT}(G_0, \mathcal{A}_c)$ by substituting (3.6),

$$p(\eta, c \mid y) \propto \left\{ \prod_{i=1}^n g_{0,\eta}(y_i) \right\} \prod_{j=2}^n \prod_{m=1}^{m^*(y_j)} \frac{2cm^2 + 2n_{\varepsilon_m(y_j)}^{(j)}}{2cm^2 + n_{\varepsilon_{m-1}(y_j)}^{(j)}} \pi(c, \eta).$$

Hanson and Johnson (2002) use (3.8) to implement inference in a median regression model with a PT prior for the residual errors. They implement a Metropolis-Hastings algorithm to obtain posterior inference based on the simplified expression.

We state an explicit step-by-step algorithm to evaluate (3.8) for a FPT. Write
$p(y_1, \ldots, y_n \mid c, \eta) = \{\prod_{i=1}^n g_{0,\eta}(y_i)\} \psi(\mathbf{y})$ with

$$\psi(\mathbf{y}) = \prod_{j=2}^n \prod_{m=1}^{m^*(y_j)} \frac{\alpha_{\epsilon_m(y_j)}^{\star(j)}}{\alpha_{\epsilon_{m-1}(y_j)0}^{\star(j)} + \alpha_{\epsilon_{m-1}(y_j)1}^{\star(j)}} \cdot \frac{\alpha_{\epsilon_{m-1}(y_j)0} + \alpha_{\epsilon_{m-1}(y_j)1}}{\alpha_{\epsilon_m(y_j)}}.$$

Keep in mind that the partitioning subsets $B_{\varepsilon_1 \cdots \varepsilon_m}$ are quantile sets of $G_{0,\eta}$, and thus $\alpha_\epsilon^{\star(j)}$ are implicitly functions of η and c. In the algorithm below, we build up the counts $n^{\star(j)}(\epsilon)$ and the posterior parameters $\alpha^\star(\epsilon)$ over $j = 2, \ldots, n$, starting with initial values for $j = 1$.

Algorithm 7: *Marginal distribution $p(\mathbf{y})$ under a FPT prior.* Start with steps 1. and 2. of Algorithm 5 to evaluate $\alpha_\epsilon^\star$ and α_ϵ.
Marginal distribution: We evaluate $\psi(\mathbf{y})$ only.

1. Initialize $L = 0$; for $m = 1, \ldots, J$ and $j = 2, \ldots, n$ and for all $\epsilon \in E^m$ initialize $n_\epsilon^{(j)} = I\{\epsilon = \epsilon_m(y_1)\}$
2. For $j = 2, \ldots, n$

   For $m = 1, \ldots, J$

   - if $n_{\epsilon_{m-1}(y_j)}^{(j)} > 0$ then
     - Let $\epsilon_0 = \epsilon_{m-1}(y_j)0$ and $\epsilon_1 = \epsilon_{m-1}(y_j)1$ (last digit in $\epsilon_m(y_j)$ replaced by 0 and 1)
     - $po = \alpha_{\epsilon_m(y_j)}^{\star(j)}/(\alpha_{\epsilon_0}^{\star(j)} + \alpha_{\epsilon_1}^{\star(j)})$, and $pr = \alpha_{\epsilon_m(y_j)}/(\alpha_{\epsilon_0} + \alpha_{\epsilon_1})$
     - $L \mathrel{+}= \log(po/pr)$
   - $n_{\epsilon_m(y_j)}^{(\ell)} \mathrel{+}= 1$, $\ell = j+1, \ldots, n$ (building up $n^{(\ell)}$)

3. Return $\log \psi(\mathbf{y}) = L$.

FPT and Conditionally Conjugate Models An alternative strategy is to consider an FPT by terminating and updating the partition Π^η up to a finite level J. Under i.i.d. sampling, the posterior distribution on the random probability measure is described in Result 3.

The FPT becomes attractive when the random probability measure is part of a larger model. Lavine (1994) described the use of the FPT to model the residual errors in a regression problem. Inference can then make use of a Gibbs sampler algorithm for the PT probabilities. That is, conditional on the parameters of the regression mean function, posterior inference reduces to the conjugate problem of inference for density estimation under i.i.d. sampling (of the residuals). The posterior for the conditional probabilities in the FPT reduces to independent beta distributions. And, vice versa, conditional on the FPT, posterior inference for the parameters of the regression mean function reduces to a standard parametric inference problem. Also, Eq. (3.8) remains valid, with m^* capped at J.

3.3.3 Posterior Inference for Non-Conjugate Models

Hanson (2006) developed posterior MCMC algorithms when the conjugacy property of the PT is lost, that is, when we use sampling models different from i.i.d. sampling, using a FPT with nested partitions up to level J. The finite truncation of the nested partition sequence makes it possible to consider explicit expressions for the p.d.f., c.d.f., quantile functions of the random probability measure, or hazard rates. This, in turn, facilitates the development of MCMC transition probabilities, even when conjugacy is lost. Details depend on the model. In the following discussion we only assume that evaluation of the likelihood is possible if the p.d.f., the c.d.f., the hazard function, or quantile functions of the random probability measure G were known, and pointwise evaluation were feasible.

To formally state the proposed transition probabilities, we introduce notation for the random probabilities of the partitioning subsets at the finest level of the FTP. Let

$$\mathcal{Y}^J = \{Y_{\varepsilon_1 \cdots \varepsilon_m}, \ m = 1, \ldots, J \text{ and } \varepsilon_j \in \{0, 1\}\}$$

denote the set of random conditional probabilities up to level J in an FPT. Set $p_{\varepsilon_1 \cdots \varepsilon_m} \equiv G(B_{\varepsilon_1 \cdots \varepsilon_m}) = \prod_{m=1}^{J} Y_{\varepsilon_1 \cdots \varepsilon_m}$. In an FPT

$$\boldsymbol{p} = \{p_{\varepsilon_1 \cdots \varepsilon_J} : \ \varepsilon_j \in \{0, 1\}, \ j = 1, \ldots, J\}$$

are the 2^J level J probabilities at the finest level of partition.

We can then use $p_{\varepsilon_1 \cdots \varepsilon_J}$ to evaluate the likelihood for the observed data. For example, assume that evaluation of the likelihood function were to require the p.d.f. of the random probability measure G. Recall that $\boldsymbol{\epsilon}_J(y) = \varepsilon_1 \cdots \varepsilon_J$ denotes the index of the level J partitioning the subset $B_{\varepsilon_1 \cdots \varepsilon_J}$ that contains y. Let $g_{0,\eta}(y)$ denote the p.d.f. of the centering distribution $G_{0,\eta}$ evaluated at y. The p.d.f. g of $G \mid \eta, c \sim \mathsf{FPT}(G_{0,\eta}, c, J)$ can then be written as a function of the conditional probabilities $\mathcal{Y}^J$ as

$$g(y) = p_{\varepsilon_1 \cdots \varepsilon_J} \cdot 2^J g_{0,\eta}(y) \quad \text{with} \quad \varepsilon_1 \cdots \varepsilon_J = \boldsymbol{\epsilon}_J(y).$$

The factor 2^J arises from $1/G_{0,\eta}(B_{\varepsilon_1 \cdots \varepsilon_J})$, remembering that $B_{\varepsilon_1 \cdots \varepsilon_m}$ were defined as dyadic quantiles under $G_{0,\eta}$. Recall that $p_{\varepsilon_1 \cdots \varepsilon_J}$ is defined as a product of random conditional probabilities in $\mathcal{Y}^J$. Hanson (2006) gives similar expressions for the c.d.f. of G and the quantile functions G^{-1}. Both are easily determined based on g. Those expressions can be used to construct the likelihood and latent variable distribution in different settings. Hanson (2006) considers simple Metropolis-Hastings updates of the elements of $\mathcal{Y}_J$, where the candidates $(\tilde{Y}_{\varepsilon_1 \cdots \varepsilon_m 0}, \tilde{Y}_{\varepsilon_1 \cdots \varepsilon_m 1})$ are generated from a beta distribution with parameters $(hY_{\varepsilon_1 \cdots \varepsilon_m 0}, hY_{\varepsilon_1 \cdots \varepsilon_m 1})$, with $h > 0$.

3.4 A Comparison of DP Versus PT Models

Much of the recent BNP literature has concentrated on the development of new models with less emphasis given to the practical advantage of the new proposals. In general, the full support of the models and the extremely weak conditions under which the different models have been shown to imply consistent posterior inference might well trap the unwary into a false sense of security, by suggesting that good estimates of the probability models can be obtained in a wide range of settings. More research seems to be needed in that direction.

Early papers on PT's (Lavine 1992; Walker and Mallick 1997, 1999) show "spiky" and "irregular" density estimates. However, these papers picked a very small precision c (in the definition of $\alpha_{\varepsilon_1\cdots\varepsilon_m} = cm^2$) and used a fixed centering distribution (without a random scale σ) that was often much more spread out than what the data warranted. The MPT prior automatically centers the prior at a reasonable centering distribution and smooths over partition boundaries. We argue that both MPT and DPM are competitor models, with appealing properties regarding support and posterior consistency, and that performance of each should be evaluated in real-life applications with finite sample sizes. We will illustrate this point by means of the analyses of simulated data. Other comparisons can be found in Hanson (2006), Hanson et al. (2008) and Jara et al. (2009).

We compared MPT and DPM estimates using "perfect samples" (data are percentiles of equal probability from the distribution, approximating expected order statistics) from four densities, motivated by Figures 2.1 and 2.3 in Efromovich (1999). Both models were fit under more or less standard prior specifications for samples of size $n = 500$. Specifically, the MPT model was fit in DPpackage (Jara et al. 2011) using the PTdensity function with a baseline measure $G_{0,\eta} = \mathsf{N}(\mu, \sigma^2)$, and the following prior settings: $J = 6$, $c \sim \mathsf{Ga}(10, 1)$, and $\pi(\mu, \sigma) \propto \sigma^{-1}$ (Jeffreys' prior under the normal model). The DPM model was fit using the DPdensity function included in DPpackage (Jara et al. 2011). This function fits the DPM model considered by Escobar and West (1995),

$$y_i|\mu_i, \tau_i \stackrel{iid}{\sim} \mathsf{N}(\mu_i, \tau_i^{-1}), \quad (\mu_i, \tau_i)|G \stackrel{iid}{\sim} G, \quad G|\alpha, G_{0,\eta} \sim DP(\alpha G_{0,\eta}),$$

where the centering distribution, $G_{0,\eta}$ is the conjugate normal/gamma model, i.e., $G_{0,\eta}(\mu, \tau) \equiv \mathsf{N}(\mu \mid m, (k\tau)^{-1}) \times \mathsf{Ga}(\tau \mid a_\tau, b_\tau)$. The model was fit by assuming $a_\tau = 2$ and $b_\tau = 1$ and, $m \sim \mathsf{N}(0, 10^5)$, $k \sim \mathsf{Ga}(0.5, 50)$ and $\alpha \sim \mathsf{Ga}(1, 1)$.

Figure 3.3 shows the true models and the density estimates under the DPM and MPT models, along with a histogram of the data. Although it is difficult to see differences between the estimates under the DPM and MPT models across true models, the density estimates under the MPT are a bit rougher than under DPM, but there are no obvious partitioning effects or unruly spikes where there should not be. More importantly, either method can perform better than the other depending on the data generating mechanism; both can do a good job.

3.4 A Comparison of DP Versus PT Models

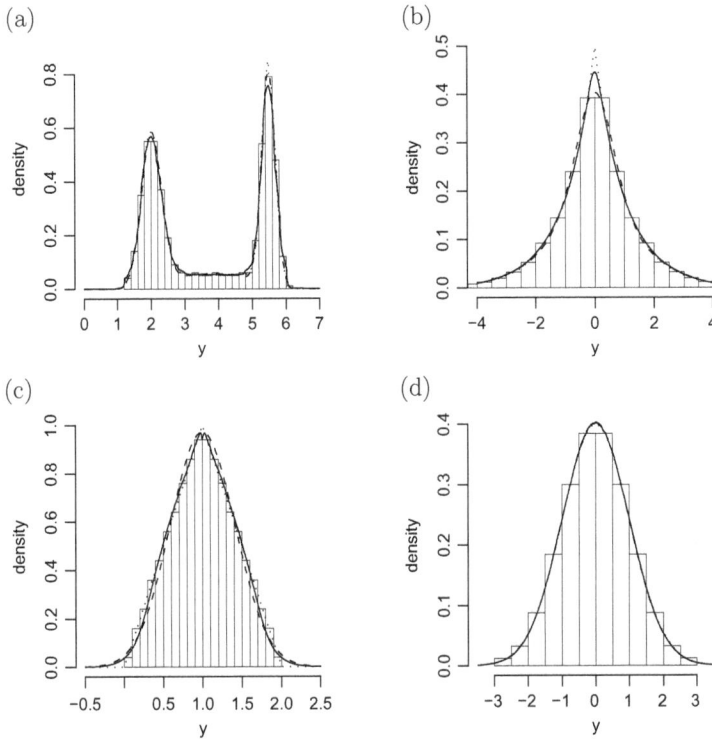

Fig. 3.3 Simulated data: The estimated density functions under the MPT and DPM models are displayed as *solid and dashed lines*, respectively. The data generating model is represented as *dotted lines*. Panels (**a**), (**b**), (**c**) and (**d**) display the density estimates, true model and the histogram of the simulated data under a mixture of normals and uniform, double exponential, triangle and standard normal distribution, respectively

When the true model is a mixture of two normals and a uniform distribution, the L_1 distance between the MPT estimates and the true model was $L_1 = 0.056$, while for the DPM, we find $L_1 = 0.034$. When the true model was a double exponential distribution, the MPT model outperformed the DPM. In this case $L_1 = 0.025$ and $L_1 = 0.060$ for the MPT and DPM model, respectively. A similar behavior was observed when the model under consideration had a triangular shape. In this case, $L_1 = 0.051$ and $L_1 = 0.096$ for the MPT and DPM model, respectively. Finally, when the data generating mechanism was a standard normal distribution, both models performed equally well; $L_1 = 0.009$ for both MPT and DPM. From the plots in Fig. 3.3 and the L_1 distances, the MPT appears to be a serious competitor to the DPM model, doing (two times) better or as well in three out of four cases.

3.5 NRMI

3.5.1 Other Generalizations of the DP Prior

Many alternative priors for random probability measures have been proposed. Many can be characterized as natural generalizations or simplifications of the DP prior. Ishwaran and James (2001) propose generalizations and variations based on the stick-breaking definition (2.2), including the finite DP that was introduced before, in Sect. 2.4.6 for approximating inference under a DP prior. The DP_K was defined by truncating the sequence of fractions v_h in (2.2). Besides truncation, the beta priors for v_h in (2.2) can be replaced by any $v_h \sim \text{Be}(a_h, b_h)$, without complicating posterior simulations. In particular, $v_h \sim \text{Be}(1 - a, b + ha)$ defines the Poisson-Dirichlet process, also referred to as Pitman-Yor process, with parameters a, b (Pitman and Yor 1997).

Alternatively we could focus on other defining properties of the DP to motivate generalizations. For example, the DP can be defined as a normalized gamma process (Ferguson 1973). The gamma process is a particular example of a much wider class of models known as completely random measures (CRM) (Kingman 1993, Chap. 8). Consider any non-intersecting measurable subsets $A_1, \ldots, A_k$ of the desired sample space. The defining property of the CRM μ is that $\mu(A_j)$ be mutually independent. The gamma process is a CRM with $\mu(A_j) \sim \text{Ga}(M\mu_0(A), 1)$, mutually independent, for a probability measure μ_0 and $M > 0$. Normalizing μ by $G(A) = \mu(A)/\mu(S)$ defines a DP prior with base measure proportional to μ_0. Replacing the gamma process by any other CRM defines alternative BNP priors for random probability measures.

Such priors are known as normalized random measures with independent increments (NRMI) and were first described in Regazzini et al. (2003) and include a large number of BNP priors. A recent review of NRMI's appears in Lijoi and Prünster (2010). Besides the DP prior, other examples are the normalized inverse Gaussian (NIG) of Lijoi et al. (2005) and the normalized generalized gamma process (NGGP), discussed in Lijoi et al. (2007). The construction of the NIG in many ways parallels the DP prior. Besides the definition as a CRM, a NIG process G can also be characterized by a normalized inverse Gaussian distribution (Lijoi et al. 2005) for the joint distribution of random probabilities $(G(A_1), \ldots, G(A_k))$, and just as in the DP case, the probabilities for cluster arrangements defined by ties under i.i.d. sampling are available in closed form. For the DP, we will still consider this distribution in more detail in the next section. The NIG, as well as the DP are special cases of the NGGP.

3.5.2 Mixture of NRMI

Two recent papers (Barrios et al. 2013; Favaro and Teh 2013) discuss mixture models with an NRMI prior on the mixing measure, similar to (7.5), but with any other NRMI prior replacing the specific DP prior. Both discuss the specific case of the normalized generalized Gaussian process (NGGP), which is attractive as it includes the DP as well as several other examples as special cases.

They describe practicable implementations of posterior simulation for such mixture model, based on a characterization of posterior inference in NRMIs discussed in James et al. (2009) who characterize $p(G \mid y)$ under i.i.d. sampling $y_1, \ldots, y_n \mid G \overset{iid}{\sim} G$, from a random probability measure G with NRMI prior. Both describe algorithms specifically for the NGGP, conditioning on the same latent variable U that is introduced as part of the description in James et al. (2009). Favaro and Teh (2013) describe what can be characterized as a modified version of the Polya urn. The Polya urn defines the marginal distribution of $(y_1, \ldots, y_n)$ under the DP prior, after marginalizing with respect to G. We discuss the marginal model under the DP in more detail in Sects. 2.3 and 8.2. A similar approach is described in Argiento et al. (2010). In contrast, Barrios et al. (2013) describe an approach that includes sampling of the random probability measure. This is particularly useful when desired inference summaries require imputation of the unknown probability measure. The methods of Barrios et al. (2013) are implemented in the R package BNPdensity, which is available in the CRAN package repository (http://cran.r-project.org/).

References

Argiento R, Guglielmi A, Pievatolo A (2010) Bayesian density estimation and model selection using nonparametric hierarchical mixtures. Comput Stat Data Anal 54(4):816–832

Barrios E, Lijoi A, Nieto-Barajas LE, Prünster, I (2013) Modeling with normalized random measure mixture models. Stat Sci 28:313–334

Barron A, Schervish MJ, Wasserman L (1999) Posterior distributions in nonparametric problems. Ann Stat 27:536–561

Berger J, Guglielmi A (2001) Bayesian testing of a parametric model versus nonparametric alternatives. J Am Stat Assoc 96:174–184

Blackwell D, MacQueen JB (1973) Ferguson distributions via Pólya urn schemes. Ann Stat 1:353–355

Dubins LE, Freedman DA (1967) Random distribution functions. In: Proceedings of the fifth Berkeley symposium on mathematics, statistics and probability, vol 2, pp 183–214

Efromovich S (1999) Nonparametric curve estimation: methods, theory and applications. Springer, New York

Escobar MD, West M (1995) Bayesian density estimation and inference using mixtures. J Am Stat Assoc 90:577–588

Favaro S, Teh YW (2013) MCMC for normalized random measure mixture models. Stat Sci 28:335–359

Ferguson TS (1973) A Bayesian analysis of some nonparametric problems. Ann Stat 1:209–230

Ferguson TS (1974) Prior distribution on the spaces of probability measures. Ann Stat 2:615–629
Hanson T, Johnson WO (2002) Modeling regression error with a mixture of Polya trees. J Am Stat Assoc 97:1020–1033
Hanson T, Kottas A, Branscum A (2008) Modelling stochastic order in the analysis of receiver operating characteristic data: Bayesian nonparametric approaches. J R Stat Soc Ser C 57:207–225
Hanson TE (2006) Inference for mixtures of finite Polya tree models. J Am Stat Assoc 101(476):1548–1565
Ishwaran H, James LF (2001) Gibbs sampling methods for stick-breaking priors. J Am Stat Assoc 96:161–173
James LF, Lijoi A, Prünster I (2009) Posterior analysis for normalized random measures with independent increments. Scand J Stat 36(1):76–97
Jara A, Hanson T, Lesaffre E (2009) Robustifying generalized linear mixed models using a new class of mixture of multivariate Polya trees. J Comput Graph Stat 18:838–860
Jara A, Hanson TE, Quintana FA, Müller P, Rosner GL (2011) DPpackage: Bayesian semi- and nonparametric modeling in R. J Stat Softw 40(5):1–30
Kingman JFC (1993) Poisson processes. Oxford University Press, New York
Kraft CM (1964) A class of distribution function processes which have derivatives. J Appl Prob 1:385–388
Lavine M (1992) Some aspects of Polya tree distributions for statistical modeling. Ann Stat 20:1222–1235
Lavine M (1994) More aspects of Polya tree distributions for statistical modeling. Ann Stat 22:1161–1176
Lijoi A, Prünster I (2010) Models beyond the Dirichlet process. Cambridge University Press, Cambridge, pp 80–136
Lijoi A, Mena RH, Prünster I (2005) Hierarchical mixture modeling with normalized inverse-Gaussian priors. J Am Stat Assoc 100(472):1278–1291
Lijoi A, Mena RH, Prünster I (2007) Controlling the reinforcement in Bayesian non-parametric mixture models. J R Stat Soc Ser B (Stat Methodol) 69(4):715–740
Mauldin RD, Sudderth WD, Williams SC (1992) Polya trees and random distributions. Ann Stat 20:1203–1221
Metivier M (1971) Sur la construction de mesures aleatoires presque surement absolument continues par rapport a une mesure donnee. Zeitschrift fur Wahrscheinlichkeitstheorie und Verwandte Gebiete 20:332–334
Monticino M (2001) How to construct a random probability measure. Int Stat Rev 69:153–167
Paddock SM (1999) Randomized Polya trees: Bayesian nonparametrics for multivariate data analaysis. Unpublished doctoral thesis, Inistitute of Statistics and Decision Sciences, Duke University
Pitman J, Yor M (1997) The two-parameter Poisson-Dirichlet distribution derived from a stable subordinator. Ann Probab 25:855–900
Regazzini E, Lijoi A, Prünster I (2003) Distributional results for means of normalized random measures with independent increments. Ann Stat 31(2):560–585
Schervish MJ (1995) Theory of statistics. Springer, New York
Walker SG, Mallick BK (1997) Hierarchical generalized linear models and frailty models with Bayesian nonparametric mixing. J R Stat Soc Ser B 59:845–860
Walker SG, Mallick BK (1999) A Bayesian semiparametric accelerated failure time model. Biometrics 55(2):477–483

Chapter 4
Regression

Abstract Regression problems naturally call for nonparametric Bayesian methods when one wishes to relax restrictive parametric assumptions on the mean function, the residual distribution or both. We introduce suitable nonparametric Bayesian methods to facilitate such generalizations, including priors for random mean functions, the use of nonparametric density estimation for residual distributions and finally nonparametric Bayesian methods for fully nonparametric regression when both mean function and residual distribution are modeled nonparametrically. The latter includes approaches where the complete shape of the response distribution is allowed to change as a function of the predictors, which is also known as density regression. We introduce the popular dependent Dirichlet process model and several other alternatives.

4.1 Bayesian Nonparametric Regression

Consider the generic regression problem of explaining an outcome y_i as a function of a covariate $x_i \in \mathcal{X}$. For the moment we assume that both, outcome and covariate, are univariate, and state the regression problem as

$$y_i = f(x_i) + \epsilon_i \tag{4.1}$$

$i = 1, \ldots, n$. Here f is an unknown centering function and ϵ_i are residuals, usually assumed to be independent. In many cases, f would indicate the mean response, or alternatively, f could mark a given quantile, such as the median. If the function f and the residual distribution are indexed by a finite dimensional parameter vector θ, then the problem reduces to traditional parametric regression, for example, normal linear regression. Without the restriction to finite dimensional θ we are led to nonparametric extensions of (4.1).

This definition of nonparametric regression as a relaxation of the parametric model makes it natural to distinguish three types of nonparametric regression models: (i) when a nonparametric prior is used to model the residuals distribution, i.e., when $\epsilon_i \mid G \overset{iid}{\sim} G$ and a BNP prior is specified for G; (ii) when a nonparametric prior is assumed on the mean function f; or (iii) when a nonparametric prior is used on the set of conditional distributions, i.e., when $y_i \mid \mathcal{G}, x_i \overset{\text{ind}}{\sim} G_{x_i}$ with a BNP prior on the family $\mathcal{G} = \{G_x, \ x \in \mathcal{X}\}$. We refer to these three approaches as nonparametric residual distributions, nonparametric mean functions, and fully nonparametric regression, respectively. The latter is also known as density regression.

4.2 Nonparametric Residual Distribution

Inference under BNP regression with nonparametric residuals reduces essentially to BNP density estimation. Assume $f(\cdot) = f_\theta(\cdot)$ is a parametric mean function, indexed by a (finite-dimensional) parameter vector θ with prior π, and $\epsilon_i \mid G \overset{\text{iid}}{\sim} G$, with a BNP prior on G. Posterior inference is most conveniently implemented by MCMC simulation with two transition probabilities. Conditional on a currently imputed parameter vector θ, inference on G reduces to density estimation for $\epsilon_i \equiv y_i - f_\theta(x_i)$. We can use posterior simulation for BNP density estimation to define a transition probability that updates G conditional on θ. In a second step, we condition on the currently imputed probability measure G and update θ, using posterior simulation in a regression model with known residual distribution G. Iterating between the two steps defines posterior MCMC simulation.

To avoid lack of interpretability of the mean function f, nonparametric residual distributions need to be restricted, for instance, to have zero-mean or zero-median. This makes the PT prior particularly attractive, as it can easily be specified such that G has zero-median with probability one. Walker and Mallick (1999) propose a PT prior model for a residual distribution in an accelerated failure time model. That is, in a regression of log event times $y_i = \log(t_i)$ on a vector of risk factors x_i. They assume a PT prior for the residual distribution with the median-zero restriction. A minor limitation of the model is the persistence of partition boundaries in predictive inference. Hanson and Johnson (2002) address this problem by using mixture of PT priors, still centered at median 0. Schörgendorfer et al. (2013) extend this model for testing the suitability of logistic regression with dichotomized continuous outcomes. Hanson and Johnson (2004) use a DP prior for the (multiplicative, before the log transform) residual distribution in an accelerated failure time model. See Sect. 6.3 for related discussion. Other constraints on G can also be used. For example, Kottas and Gelfand (2001) use a DP scale mixture of uniforms to represent a unimodal residual distribution in a regression model.

Example 5 (Old Faithful Geyser) Azzalini and Bowman (1990) analyzed a data set concerning eruptions of the Old Faithful geyser in Yellowstone National Park in Wyoming. The data record eruption durations and intervals between subsequent

4.3 Nonparametric Mean Function

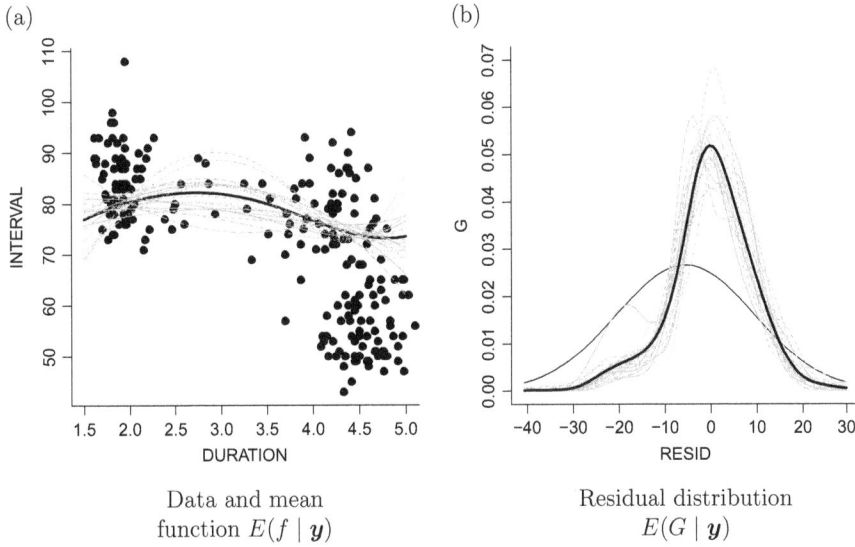

Data and mean function $E(f \mid y)$ Residual distribution $E(G \mid y)$

Fig. 4.1 Example 5. Data and fitted regression curve (panel **a**) and estimated residual distribution (panel **b**). The *thin grey lines* show posterior draws for f (panel **a**) and G (panel **b**)

eruptions, collected continuously from August 1st until August 15th, 1985. Of the original 299 observations we removed 78 observations which were taken at night and only recorded durations as "short", "medium" or "long". We implement inference for a semi-parametric regression (4.1) with a finite DP prior. That is, we assume $\epsilon_i \mid G \overset{iid}{\sim} G$ and $G \sim \mathsf{DP}_H$. Let x_i denote the duration of the preceding eruption, centered to zero-mean and let $z^+ = z$ for $z > 0$ and $z^+ = 0$ for $z \le 0$. We use a linear function of x_i, x_i^2 and $(x_i^3)^+$ as the regression mean function $f(x_i)$ in (4.1). Figure 4.1a plots the data and a fitted nonlinear mean function $E(f \mid y)$. Panel (b) shows the estimated residual distribution $\overline{G}_\epsilon$, together with some posterior draws for G. The posterior mean $\overline{G}_\epsilon$ is shifted to achieve a zero-mean. Let $\mu(G)$ denote the mean of a probability measure G. Then $\overline{G}_\epsilon = E(G \mid y) - \mu\left[E(G \mid y)\right]$. Similarly, the plotted random G are shifted by the same offset. The left skewed nature of G and $\overline{G}_\epsilon$ accommodates the observations in the right lower part of panel (a). For comparison, panel (b) also shows the base measure $G^\star$ of the DP prior.

Software note: R code for Fig. 4.1 is shown in the software appendix to this chapter.

4.3 Nonparametric Mean Function

4.3.1 Basis Expansions

Many approaches do not define the probability model directly on f. Consider a function basis $\mathcal{F} = \{\varphi_k\}$ and let θ denote the set of coefficients with respect to that basis, i.e.,

$$f(\cdot) = \sum_{k=1}^{K} \theta_k \varphi_k(\cdot). \tag{4.2}$$

Defining a probability model on θ implicitly defines a probability model on the unknown mean function. Note that a fully nonparametric prior requires $K = \infty$. In practice, the sum is truncated in some fashion, e.g. the most highly oscillatory φ_k are not included. A good choice of the basis allows us to use an informative prior on the space of basis coefficients. An orthonormal basis can lead to particularly easy posterior inference. Assuming independent normal residuals and equally spaced data implies (approximately) orthogonal columns in the design matrix, and thus a likelihood function that factors across basis coefficients. Together with an independent prior this can be exploited to achieve *a posteriori* independence, making inference particularly simple. This construction is sometimes used, for example, with wavelet bases.

Wavelets

A wavelets basis $\mathcal{F} = \{\phi_{j_0,k}, \psi_{jk}; j \geq j_0, k \in \mathbb{Z}\}$ is a set of orthonormal functions that are defined as shifted and scaled versions of two underlying functions ϕ and ψ, as $\psi_{jk}(x) = 2^{j/2} \psi(2^j x - k)$ and similarly for ϕ_{jk}. Also, $\int \phi_{jk} = 1$ and $\int \psi_{jk} = 0$.

The nature of this function basis is easiest understood by considering a specific example. The Haar wavelet basis defines $\phi_{00}(x) = I(x \in [0, 1])$ as an indicator of the interval $[0, 1]$, and $\psi_{00} = I(x \in [0, 0.5)) - I(x \in [0.5, 1])$, i.e. a step function that switches between 1 and -1 on the left and right half interval. See Fig. 4.2. The set $A_j = \{\phi_{jk}, k \in \mathbb{Z}\}$ approximates a given function f as a step function on a grid of intervals of length 2^{-j}. The functions ψ_{jk} are the orthogonal complement of A_{j+1} and A_j.

Let

$$f(x) = \sum_{k \in \mathbb{Z}} c_{j_0,k} \phi_{j_0,k} + \sum_{j=j_0}^{J} \sum_{k \in \mathbb{Z}} d_{jk} \psi_{jk}(x) \tag{4.3}$$

define the representation of f with respect to the wavelet basis A_J. The practical attraction of wavelet bases is the availability of superfast algorithms to compute the

4.3 Nonparametric Mean Function

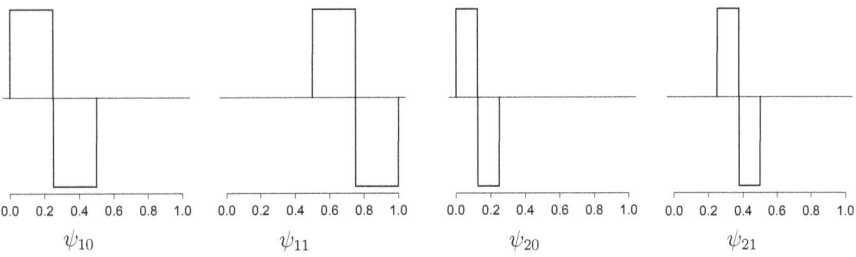

Fig. 4.2 Haar wavelet basis: ψ_{jk} for $j = 1, 2$.

coefficients c_{jk} and d_{jk} given a function, and vice versa. In words, the algorithm proceeds as follows. We start with the function evaluated on a dense equally spaced grid, $f_k = f(k2^{-J})$. Note that ϕ_{Jk} is a narrowly rescaled version of the original ϕ function and integrates to 1. Thus, for sufficiently large J we approximate $2^J c_{Jk} \approx f_k$. In the following argument we drop the scale 2^J, noting that the argument remains valid as long as we also drop the scale when using the reverse algorithm to reconstruct f, starting from c_{0k} and d_{jk}. Starting with c_{Jk} we iteratively proceed for $j = J - 1$ through j_0 to find $\{c_{jk}, d_{jk}; k \in Z\}$. To obtain c_{jk} and d_{jk} from $c_{j+1,k}$, we only need a set of coefficients that define ϕ_{jk} and ψ_{jk} as functions of $c_{j+1,k}$. It can be argued that these coefficients remain the same across j, i.e., we only need to iteratively apply one filter to obtain the coefficients $c_{j_0,k}$ and another filter to obtain $d_{jk}, j_0 \leq j \leq J$ from $c_{Jk} \approx f_k$. The two filters are $h(\cdot)$ and $g(\cdot)$ in the pyramid scheme shown below. It can be shown that $g(\cdot)$ uses the same coefficients as $h(\cdot)$, only with alternating signs. By a symmetric argument we can reconstruct the function f_k from the set of wavelet coefficients by iterative application of the same filters. Also, working with a compactly supported function, we can use a periodic extension of the function to the entire real line. Wavelet coefficients beyond a certain shift k can then be argued to be identical repetitions of other coefficients, and we can thus restrict computations to a finite range of shifts k.

Algorithm 8: *Pyramid Scheme for the Discrete Wavelet Transform.* *Let $(h(\ell), \ell = 1, \ldots, L)$ denote the wavelet filter for the chosen wavelet basis, and let $g(\ell) = (-1)^\ell h(L - 1 - \ell)$ denote the mirror filter. The filter length L varies across different wavelet bases.*

1. *Let $c_{Jk} = f(k\, 2^{-J})$.*
2. *For $j = J - 1, \ldots, j_0$ compute $c_{jk} = \sum_n h(n - 2k) c_{j+1,n}$ and $d_{jk} = \sum_n g(n - 2k) c_{j+1,n}$*
3. *The coefficients $\{c_{j_0,k}, d_{jk}\}$ define the representation of f with respect to the wavelet basis A_{j_0}.*

Reconstruction operates with the inverse filter $c_{jn} = \sum_k h(n - 2k) c_{j-1,k} + \sum_k g(n - 2k) d_{j-1,k}$, starting with $j = j_0 + 1$.

Assuming a prior probability model for the coefficients d_{jk} implicitly puts a prior probability model on a random function f. Typical prior probability models for wavelet coefficients include positive probability mass at zero. Usually this prior probability mass depends on the scale j, $p(d_{jk} = 0) = \pi_j$. Given a non-zero coefficient, an independent prior with level dependent variances is assumed, for example, $d_{jk}|d_{jk} \neq 0 \sim \mathsf{N}(0, \tau_j^2)$. In summary

$$d_{jk} \sim \pi_j \delta_0(\cdot) + (1 - \pi_j)\mathsf{N}(\cdot \mid 0, \tau^2). \tag{4.4}$$

Appropriate choice of π_j and τ_j achieves posterior rules for the wavelet coefficients d_{jk}, which closely mimic the usual wavelet thresholding and shrinkage rules (Chipman et al. 1997; Vidakovic 1998). Clyde and George (2000) discuss the use of empirical Bayes estimates for the hyperparameters in such models.

Posterior inference is greatly simplified by the orthonormality of the wavelet basis. Consider a regression model $y_i = f(x_i) + \epsilon_i$, $i = 1, \ldots, n$, with equally spaced data x_i, for example, $x_i = i/n$. Substitute a wavelet basis representation (4.3), let y, d and ϵ denote the data vector, the vector of all wavelet coefficients and the residual vector, respectively. Also, let B denote the design matrix of the wavelet basis functions evaluated at the x_i. Then we can write the regression in matrix notation as $y = Bd + \epsilon$. The discrete wavelet transform of the data evaluates $\hat{d} = B^{-1}y$, using the computationally highly efficient pyramid scheme algorithm. Assuming independent normal errors, $\epsilon_i \mid \sigma^2 \overset{iid}{\sim} \mathsf{N}(0, \sigma^2)$, orthogonality of the design matrix B implies $\hat{d}_{jk} \sim \mathsf{N}(d_{jk}, \sigma^2)$, independently across (j, k). Assuming *a priori* independent d_{jk} leads to *a posteriori* independence of the wavelet coefficients d_{jk}. In other words, we can consider one univariate inference problem $p(d_{jk}|y)$ at a time. Even if the prior probability model for d is not marginally independent across d_{jk}, it typically assumes independence conditional on hyper-parameters, still leaving a considerable simplification of posterior simulation.

Example 6 (Doppler Function) Donoho and Johnstone (1994) consider a battery of test functions to evaluate performance of wavelet shrinkage methods. One of them is the Doppler function $f(x) = \sqrt{x(1-x)} \sin[(2.1\pi)/(x+0.05)]$, for $0 \leq x \leq 1$. We generated $n = 100$ observations with $y_i = f(x_i) + \epsilon_i$, with noise $\epsilon_i \overset{iid}{\sim} \mathsf{N}(0, 0.05^2)$ and unequally spaced x_i. The simulated data, together with the estimated mean function $\bar{f}(x) = E[f_\theta(x)|y]$ are shown in Fig. 4.3. Figure 4.4 shows the posterior distributions for some of the wavelet coefficients d_{jk}.

The above detailed explanation serves to highlight two critical assumptions. Posterior independence, conditional on hyper-parameters or marginally, only holds for equally spaced data and under *a priori* independence over d_{jk}. In most applications prior independence is a technically convenient assumption, but does not reflect genuine prior knowledge. However, incorporating assumptions about prior dependence is not excessively difficult either. Starting with an assumption about dependence of $f(x_i)$, $i = 1, \ldots, n$, Vannucci and Corradi (1999) show that a straightforward two dimensional wavelet transform can be used to derive the corresponding covariance matrix for the wavelet coefficients d_{jk}.

In the absence of equally spaced data the convenient mapping of the raw data y_i to the empirical wavelet coefficients $\hat{d}_{jk}$ is lost. The same is true for inference problems other than regression where wavelet decomposition is used to model random functions. Typical examples are the unknown density in a density estimation

4.3 Nonparametric Mean Function

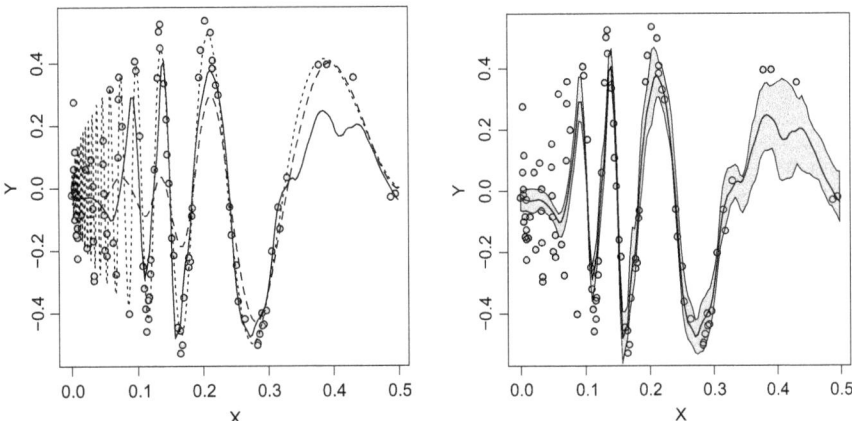

Fig. 4.3 Example 6. The posterior estimated mean function $\bar{f}(x) = E[f_\theta(x)|y]$ (*solid curve*). For comparison, the *dashed line* shows a smoothing spline (cubic B-spline, using the Splus function `smooth.spline()`), and the *thin dotted curve* shows the true mean function $f(x)$ used for the simulation. The *circles* are the data points (x_i, y_i), $i = 1, \ldots, 100$

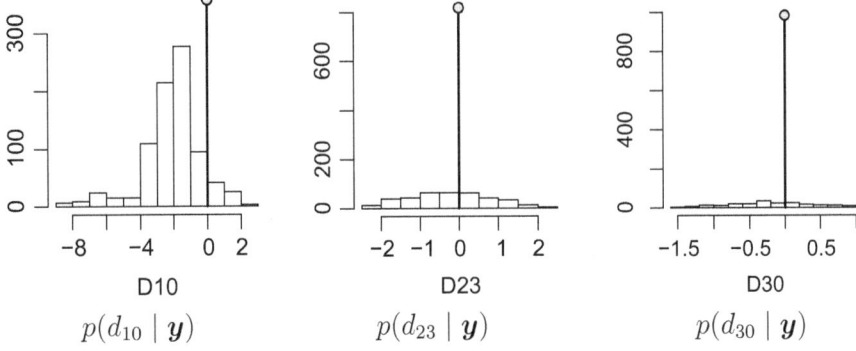

Fig. 4.4 Example 6. Posterior distributions for some wavelet coefficients d_{jk}. Note the point mass at 0

(Müller and Vidakovic 1998), or the spectrum in a spectral density estimation. In either case evaluation of the likelihood $p(y \mid d)$ requires reconstruction of the random function $f(\cdot)$. Although a technical inconvenience, this does not hinder the practical use of a wavelet basis. The superfast wavelet decomposition and reconstruction algorithms still allow computationally efficient likelihood evaluation even with the original raw data.

Example 5 (Old Faithful Geyser, ctd.) Figure 4.1 showed a regression of duration y_t on waiting time x_t, using a non-parametric prior for the residual distribution. Figure 4.5 shows the same regression, but now with a non-parametric mean function, using a wavelet-based prior on f and normal residuals, $\epsilon_i \sim N(0, \sigma^2)$.

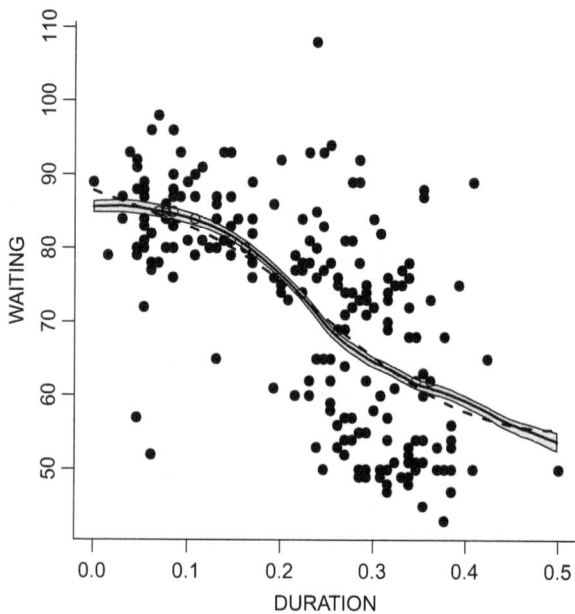

Fig. 4.5 Example 5. Inference on a nonparametric mean function f in (4.1) under a wavelet-based prior for f. The *solid line* shows $E(f \mid y)$. The *grey shaded* bands show pointwise central 50 % credible intervals. For comparison the *dashed line* shows a cubic spline fit

Morris and Carroll (2006) build functional mixed effects models with hierarchical extensions of (4.3) and (4.4) across multiple functions.

Neural Networks

Neural networks can be used to define a BNP prior for an unknown regression function f. In particular, we will focus on feed-forward neural networks (FFNN) that represent f as a mixture of logistic functions. A FFNN model with p input nodes, one hidden layer with M hidden nodes, one output node and activation functions Ψ is a model relating p explanatory variables $x = (x_1, \ldots, x_p)$ and a response variable y of the form

$$\hat{y}(x) = \sum_{j=1}^{M} \beta_j \Psi(x' \gamma_j + \eta_j) \tag{4.5}$$

with $\beta_j \in \mathbb{R}$, $\gamma_j \in \mathbb{R}^p$. The terms η_j are designated biases and may be assimilated to the rest of the γ_j vector if we consider an additional input with constant value one, say $x_0 = 1$. Cybenko (1989) and others show that when Ψ is a sigmoidal function, finite sums of the form (4.5) are dense in $\mathcal{C}(I_p)$, the set of real continuous functions in the p-dimensional unit cube. For their proof, they assume that $M \to \infty$ as the approximation gets better.

The typical setup for FFNNs is the following. Given regression data $D = \{(x_1, y_1), \ldots, (x_N, y_N)\}$ and fixed M, choose $\beta = (\beta_1, \ldots, \beta_M), \gamma = (\gamma_0, \ldots, \gamma_M)$ according to a least squares criterion $\min_{\beta, \gamma} \sum_{i=1}^{N}(y_i - \hat{y}(x_i))^2$, either via *backpropagation* (Rumelhart and McClelland 1986), an implementation of steepest descent, or other optimization methods such as quasi-Newton or simulated annealing. Hence, at least implicitly, we are assuming a normal error model and we are viewing a nonlinear parametric regression problem. A regularization term in the objective function avoids data overfitting. Alternatively, Müller and Ríos-Insua (1998) cast regression with a neural network as a Bayesian inference problem and discuss suitable posterior simulation methods.

Other Basis Expansions

Wavelets or neural networks are not the only basis expansions used for nonparametric regression models. Many alternative basis functions are used, for example the orthogonal Legendre polynomials, sines and cosines (Lenk 1999) and fractional polynomials (Bové and Held 2011); the latter is implemented in the bfp package for R. In such expansions, priors that increasingly shrink coefficients associated with the more oscillatory or "curvy" basis functions are common. Setting coefficients to zero for coefficients beyond a cutoff yields a standard linear model, ably fit through, for example, the INLA or DPpackage packages for R, or simply hand-coded.

Example 5 (Old Faithful Geyser, ctd.) One version of Lenk's (1999) model for the geyser data takes $y_i \sim N(\mu_i, \sigma^2)$ where

$$\mu_i = \mu + \beta_0 x_i + \sum_{j=1}^{J} \beta_j \cos\left\{\frac{\pi(x_i - x_{(1)})}{x_{(n)} - x_{(1)}}\right\}. \tag{4.6}$$

The prior is $p(\mu) = N(0, 1000)$, $\beta_0 \sim N(0, \tau^2)$, and $\beta_j \sim N(0, \tau^2/j)$ for $j = 1, \ldots, J$. Further taking $\sigma^{-2} \sim Ga(a, b)$ and $\tau^{-2} \sim Ga(c, d)$ gives the full conditional $\beta|\tau, \sigma \sim N_{J+2}(M\sigma^{-2}X'y, M)$ where $M = [X'X\sigma^{-2} + D_\tau]^{-1}$, $\sigma^{-2}|\beta, \tau \sim Ga(a + 0.5n, b + 0.5||y - X\beta||^2)$, and $\tau^{-2}|\beta, \sigma \sim Ga(c + 0.5(J + 1), d + 0.5(\beta_0^2 + \sum_{j=1}^{J} j\beta_j^2))$. Here D_τ is a diagonal matrix with the prior precisions of $\mu, \beta_0, \beta_1, \ldots, \beta_J$ on the diagonal. Figure 4.6a shows a fit of the cosine expansion mean function with 95 % CI to the geyser data with $a = b = c = d = 0.001$.

4.3.2 B-Splines

A very flexible and popular basis expansion approach is based on a spline basis, or B-splines (De Boor 2001). A B-spline is a particular piecewise-differentiable polynomial of a given degree d, typically $d = 2$ or $d = 3$ for a quadratic or cubic B-spline. In one dimension the polynomials comprising the B-spline differ

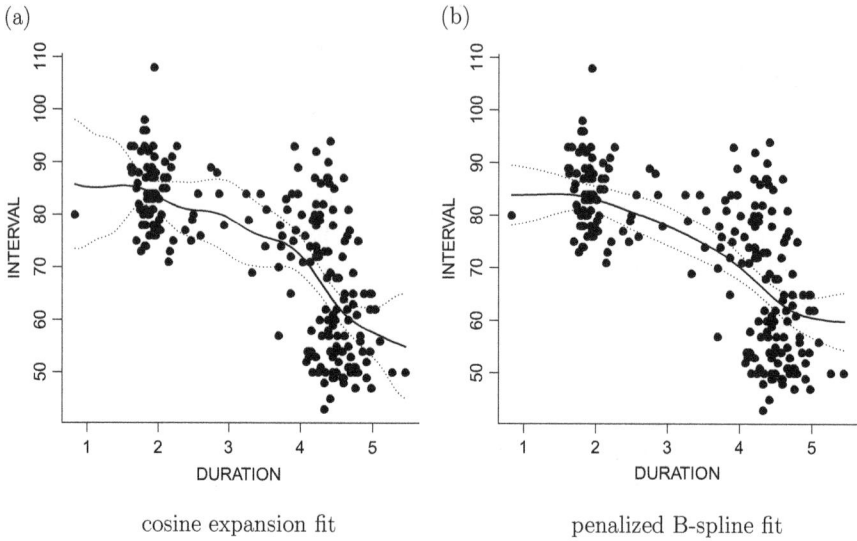

Fig. 4.6 Example 5. Fitted mean function using cosine (panel **a**) and penalized B-spline basis (panel **b**) expansions

between an increasing sequence of points, termed knots. The overall polynomial is continuous ($d \geq 1$) or differentiable ($d \geq 2$) over the range of the knots. Knots can be equispaced yielding a cardinal B-spline or else irregularly-spaced. Computation is especially easy for equispaced knots and so we focus on that here; generalizations can be found in Kneib (2006).

The quadratic B-spline "mother" basis function is defined on $[0, 3]$

$$\varphi(x) = \begin{cases} 0.5x^2 & 0 \leq x \leq 1 \\ 0.75 - (x - 1.5)^2 & 1 \leq x \leq 2 \\ 0.5(3 - x)^2 & 2 \leq x \leq 3 \\ 0 & \text{otherwise} \end{cases}.$$

Say the number of basis functions is J. The B-spline basis functions are shifted, rescaled versions of φ. The j-th basis function is $B_j(x) = \varphi\left(\frac{x - x_{(1)}}{\Delta} + 3 - j\right)$ where $\Delta = \frac{x_{(n)} - x_{(1)}}{J - 2}$. The B-spline model for the mean is $f(x) = \sum_{j=1}^{J} \theta_j B_j(x)$. Note that the B-spline includes polynomials of the same or lower degree as special cases; e.g. a quadratic B-spline includes all constant, linear, and parabolic functions over $[a, b]$.

B-splines are typically used with a rather large number J of basis functions, e.g. 20–40. A global level of smoothness is incorporated into a B-spline model by encouraging neighboring coefficients to be similar; the more regular the coefficients are, the less wiggly $f(\cdot)$ is. Classical spline estimation proceeds by maximizing $\sum(y_i - f(x_i))^2$ subject to the "wiggliness" penalty $\int_a^b |f''(x)|^2 dx \leq c$ for some $c > 0$. This is equivalent to maximizing a penalized log-likelihood. Borrowing from Eilers

4.3 Nonparametric Mean Function

and Marx (1996), Lang and Brezger (2004) recast and developed this idea into a Bayesian framework. Let $D_2 \in \mathbb{R}^{(J-2) \times J}$ and $D_1 \in \mathbb{R}^{(J-1) \times J}$ be defined as

$$D_2 = \begin{bmatrix} 1 & -2 & 1 & 0 & \cdots & 0 \\ 0 & 1 & -2 & 1 & \cdots & 0 \\ \vdots & \vdots & \ddots & \ddots & \ddots & \vdots \\ 0 & 0 & \cdots & 1 & -2 & 1 \end{bmatrix} \text{ and } D_1 = \begin{bmatrix} 1 & -1 & 0 & \cdots & 0 \\ 0 & 1 & -1 & \cdots & 0 \\ \vdots & \vdots & \ddots & \ddots & \vdots \\ 0 & 0 & \cdots & 1 & -1 \end{bmatrix}.$$

For equispaced, quadratic (and cubic) B-splines the penalty can be written as

$$\int_a^b |f''(x)|^2 dx = ||D_2 \theta \Delta||^2.$$

Optimization with the D_2 penalty is equivalent to assuming a second order random-walk prior, that is, the improper prior $D_2\theta \sim N_{J-2}(0, \lambda^{-1} I_{J-2})$. As λ becomes large, $f''(x)$ is forced toward zero and $f(x)$ becomes linear. Alternatively, a first order random walk prior is given by $D_1\theta \sim N_{J-1}(0, \lambda^{-1} I_{J-1})$. When λ is large, adjacent basis functions are forced closer and $f'(x)$ is forced toward zero, yielding a constant $f(x)$.

Example 5 (Old Faithful Geyser, ctd.) Let the i-th row of the design matrix X be

$$[B_1(x_i) \cdots B_J(x_i)].$$

Taking $\sigma^{-2} \sim \text{Ga}(a,b)$, $\lambda \sim \text{Ga}(c,d)$, and using the D_1 penalty gives the full conditional $\theta | \lambda, \sigma \sim N_J(M\sigma^{-2} X'y, M)$ where $M = [X'X\sigma^{-2} + \lambda D_1 D_1']^{-1}$, $\sigma^{-2}|\beta, \tau \sim \text{Ga}(a+0.5n, b+0.5||y-X\theta||^2)$, and $\lambda | \theta, \sigma \sim \text{Ga}(c+0.5(J-1), d+0.5||D_1\theta||^2)$. Figure 4.6b shows a penalized B-spline fit to the Geyser data with $a = b = c = d = 0.001$ using the D_1 penalty.

For multivariate $x_i = (x_{i1}, \ldots, x_{ip})$, the classical linear model $y_i = x_i'\beta + \epsilon_i$ can be generalized to a so-called additive model, $y_i = \sum f_j(x_{ij}) + \epsilon_i$, where $f_1(\cdot), \ldots, f_p(\cdot)$ are functions to be estimated. See Lang and Brezger (2004) and Brezger and Lang (2006). These models are further generalized to outcomes y_i from non-normal distributions that are members of the exponential family (e.g. Poisson, Bernoulli, gamma, etc.) through generalized additive models (Hastie and Tibshirani 1990). Two common examples are Poisson regression with a log-link $y_i \overset{ind}{\sim} \text{Pois}(e^{\eta_i})$ and Bernoulli regression with the logit link $y_i \overset{ind}{\sim} \text{Bern}\{e^{\eta_i}/(1+e^{\eta_i})\}$, where $\eta_i = \sum_{j=1}^{J_i} f_j(x_{ij})$. These models are fit via B-splines in the free-standing program `BayesX` or in the `PSgam` function in `DPpackage`.

Example 7 (Nitrogen Oxide Emissions) Brinkman (1981) considers data on nitrogen oxide emissions from a single-cylinder engine. The data are available, for example, in the R package `lattice` as data set `ethanol`. The concentration of nitrogen oxides (NO and NO2) in micrograms/J was recorded for various settings

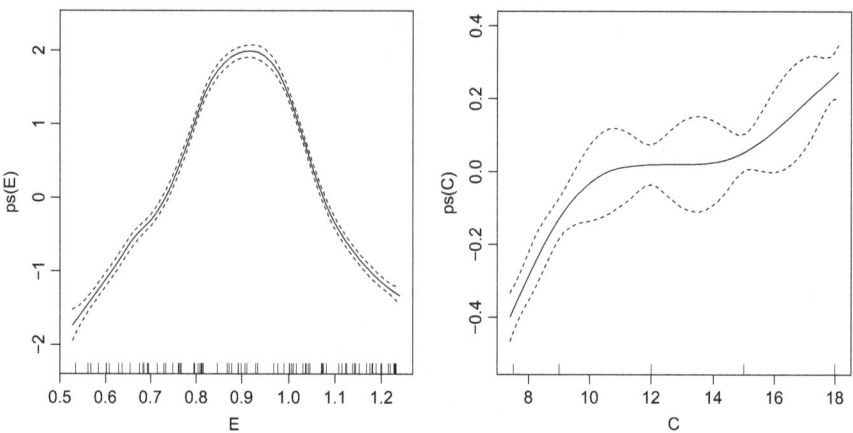

Fig. 4.7 Example 7, generalized additive model with normal errors. *Left panel* is $f_E(\cdot)$ and *right panel* is $f_C(\cdot)$

of the equivalence ratio, which measures the richness of the air/ethanol mixture, and the compression ratio of the engine. Denote these three continuous variables as NOx, E, and C. In all, $n = 88$ engine runs were recorded. The model to be fit is $\text{NOx}_i = f_E(E_i) + f_C(C_i) + \epsilon_i$ where $\epsilon_i \stackrel{iid}{\sim} N(0, \tau^{-1})$. Figure 4.7 shows the estimated functions f_E and f_C.

Software note: Generalized additive models are easily fit using the PSgam function in DPpackage. Alternatively, the R package R2BayesX could be used. Both model the transformations $f_j(\cdot)$ as penalized B-splines. Figure 4.7 shows a fit from the PSgam function in DPpackage under a default, vague prior specification using quadratic B-splines with a second-order random-walk penalty prior.

4.3.3 Gaussian Process Priors

Besides basis representations like (4.2), another commonly used BNP prior for a random mean function $f(\cdot)$ is the Gaussian process (GP) prior. Let $\mu(x)$, $x \in \mathbb{R}^d$ denote a given function and let $r(x_1, x_2)$ for $x_j \in \mathbb{R}^d$ denote a covariance function, i.e., the $(n \times n)$ matrix R with $R_{ij} = r(x_i, x_j)$ is positive definite for any set of distinct $x_i \in \mathbb{R}^d$.

Definition 3 (Gaussian Process) A random function $f(x)$ with $x \in \mathbb{R}^d$ has a GP prior if for any finite set of points $x_i \in \mathbb{R}^d$, $i = 1, \ldots, n$, the function evaluated at those points is a multivariate normal random vector,

$$(f(x_1), \ldots, f(x_n))' \sim N\left((\mu(x_1), \ldots, \mu(x_n))', R\right).$$

Here $R = [r(x_i, x_j)]$ is the $n \times n$ covariance matrix. We write $f \sim \text{GP}(\mu(x), r(x, y))$. The GP can be used as a prior for the unknown mean function in (4.1). Assuming normal residuals, the posterior distribution for $f = (f(x_1), \ldots, f(x_n))$ is multivariate normal again. Similarly, $f(x)$ at new locations x_{n+i} that were not recorded in the data is characterized by multivariate normal distributions again. See O'Hagan (1978) for an early discussion of GP priors, and Kennedy and O'Hagan (2001) for a discussion of Bayesian inference for GP models in the context of modeling output from computer simulations.

Fully Bayesian GP regression can be very computationally demanding, as the inverse of a large-dimensional covariance matrix needs to be computed at each iteration of a Gibbs sampler or a maximization routine. As one solution to this dilemma Gramacy and Lee (2008) posit treed Gaussian processes: the predictor space is partitioned into a number of smaller regions—see Sect. 4.3.4—and independent GP's are fit to each subregion, leading to a nonstationary process over the entire predictor space. The overall inversion of a large matrix is replaced by a number of smaller, computationally feasible inversions. Posterior inference is efficiently handled in the tgp package for R. Other approaches to reducing the dimensionality of the problem include predictive processes (Banerjee et al. 2008) and random projections (Banerjee et al. 2013). Generalized additive models using Gaussian processes are considered by Shively et al. (1999).

Example 5 (Old Faithful Geyser, ctd.) Figure 4.8 shows a default treed Gaussian process fit coupled with 95 % prediction intervals for the geyser data.

Software note: R code to call the tgp package commands is shown in the software appendix to this chapter.

4.3.4 Regression Trees

Chipman et al. (1998) and Denison et al. (1998) developed the Bayesian CART (classification and regression tree) model for non-parametric regression. The idea is compelling. Consider a generic regression problem (4.7) with a multivariate covariate vector $x_i = (x_{ij}, j = 1, \ldots, p)$. For the moment we drop the i index, considering a generic covariate vector x. We partition the covariate space into small enough rectangular regions R described by thresholds on the covariates x_j, such that $E(y \mid x \in R) \approx f_R$ is approximately constant over each rectangular region.

The partition is described by a tree T. The leaves of the tree correspond to the rectangular regions and are labeled with the mean response f_R. The tree T is a recursive structure $T = (j, t, T_0, T_1)$ of splitting rules consisting of a covariate

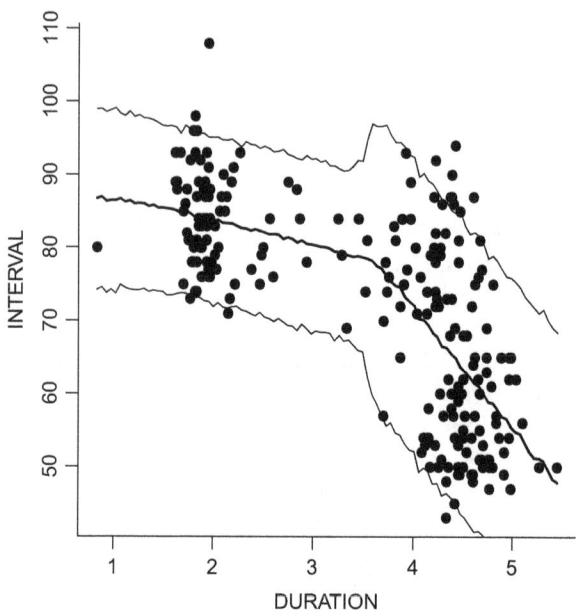

Fig. 4.8 Example 5. Treed Gaussian processes, mean plus 90 % prediction interval for new response

index j and a threshold t that identify a splitting rule $x_j < t$ and two nested trees (T_0, T_1) with the tree T_0 defining the branch $x_j < t$ and T_1 defining the branch $x_j \geq t$. The recursion ends with final leaves that contain a value f_ℓ instead of a tree T_ℓ. Chipman et al. (1998) and Denison et al. (1998) describe prior probability models on T and posterior MCMC simulation. Posterior simulation requires transdimensional MCMC, as the inclusion of new splits and the deletion of existing splits change the dimension of the parameter space. For a more parsimonious model the constant mean response f_R in each leaf can be replaced by any parametric model $p(y \mid x \in R) = f_{\theta_R}(y)$, where θ_R are parameters specific to each leaf.

An extension of CART to a sum of many CART trees, i.e., a forest of regression trees, is defined in the BART (Bayesian additive regression tree) proposed by Chipman et al. (2010). The idea of BART is to use many small trees to approximate the desired mean function. The BART is implemented in an easy to use R package `BayesTree`.

4.4 Fully Nonparametric Regression

A general statement of the generic regression problem (4.1) characterizes regression as

$$y_i \mid x_i \overset{\text{ind}}{\sim} G_{x_i} \qquad (4.7)$$

4.4 Fully Nonparametric Regression

with a family $\mathcal{G} = \{G_x;\ x \in \mathcal{X}\}$ of probability measures indexed by $x \in \mathcal{X}$. The model is completed with a BNP prior on $\mathcal{G}$. Under this setup regression reduces to inference on a family of related random probability measures $\mathcal{G}$. A meaningful prior on $\mathcal{G}$ needs to include dependence of the G_x's, including some notion of continuity across x.

4.4.1 Priors on Families of Random Probability Measures

Perhaps the most popular prior model for a family of random probability measures is the dependent DP (DDP). It was originally introduced by MacEachern (1999), with many variations defined in later papers. The basic idea is simple. Recall the stick breaking construction (2.2) of a DP random probability measure $G_x \sim \text{DP}(M, G_x^*)$. In anticipation of the upcoming generalization we write the stick breaking definition as

$$G_x(\cdot) = \sum_{h=0}^{\infty} w_h \delta_{m_{xh}}(\cdot),$$

with point masses at locations $m_{xh} \overset{iid}{\sim} G_x^*$ and weights $w_h = v_h \prod_{\ell < h}(1 - v_\ell)$ for i.i.d. beta fractions $v_h \overset{iid}{\sim} \text{Be}(1, M)$. By the following construction, the model is easily generalized to a joint prior for $\mathcal{G}$, keeping a DP prior as the marginal for G_x, for every $x \in \mathcal{X}$, but introducing the desired dependence across x. To ensure the marginal DP prior we have to keep the i.i.d. prior on m_{xh} across h. But we are free to introduce dependence of m_{xh} across x (for every h). Let $m_h = (m_{hx}, x \in \mathcal{X})$ denote the family of random variables m_{xh} for fixed h. That is, m_h is a stochastic process indexed by x.

Definition 4 (Dependent DP, DDP) Let $\mathcal{G} = \{G_x;\ x \in \mathcal{X}\}$ denote a family of random probability measures indexed by $x \in \mathcal{X}$. We say that $\mathcal{G}$ is a dependent DP (DDP) if, for every $x \in \mathcal{X}$,

$$G_x(\cdot) = \sum_{h=0}^{\infty} w_h \delta_{m_{xh}}(\cdot), \tag{4.8}$$

with a stick-breaking prior on the weights, $w_h = v_h \prod_{\ell < h}(1 - v_\ell)$ for i.i.d. beta fractions $v_h \overset{iid}{\sim} \text{Be}(1, \alpha)$. The locations $m_h = (m_{hx},\ x \in \mathcal{X})$, $h = 1, 2, \ldots$, are mutually independent realizations of a stochastic process $\{S(x);\ x \in \mathcal{X}\}$ indexed by x. We write $\mathcal{G} \sim \text{DDP}(\alpha, S)$, where S identifies the stochastic process across x.

For example, S could be a Gaussian process with index set $\mathcal{X}$. In this definition we used the same weights w_h across x. Notice the single h subindex on the weights in (4.8). In a more general DDP model the weights are replaced by w_{xh}, with dependence across x. We refer to (4.8) as the varying location DDP, to the alternative model with w_{xh} and m_h as the varying weight DDP, and the general model with w_{xh}, m_{xh} as the varying weight and location DDP.

Posterior Simulation Under a DDP model

The DDP prior is often combined with a sampling model similar to the DPM (2.6), as

$$y_i \mid \theta_i \sim f_{\theta_i}$$
$$\theta_i \mid x_i = x, \mathcal{G} \sim G_x$$
$$\mathcal{G} \sim \text{DDP} \qquad (4.9)$$

Posterior MCMC proceeds similar to inference under the DPM model. Before we discuss details we introduce notation and construct clusters similar to the discussion in Sect. 2.4. First we replace $\theta_i \sim G_x$ by a latent indicator $r_i \in \mathbb{N}$. The indicators r_i select one of the point masses in (4.8), as

$$\theta_i = m_{r_i x_i} \quad \text{and} \quad p(r_i = h) = w_h.$$

Next let $\{r_1^\star, \ldots, r_k^\star\}$ denote the $k \leq n$ unique values r_i, and let $S_j = \{i : r_i = r_j^\star\}$, $j = 1, \ldots, k$. We index clusters by appearance, that is, $r_1^\star = r_1$ etc. We denote with $n_j = |S_j|$ the size of the j-th cluster. Next let $\boldsymbol{m}_j^\star = (m_{hx_i}, h = r_j^\star, i \in S_j)$. That is, $\boldsymbol{m}_j^\star$ is a vector of the n_j sampled observations m_{hx} for $h = r_j^\star$. Also, we introduce cluster membership indicators $s_i \in \{1, \ldots, k\}$ with $s_i = j$ when $i \in S_j$. Note the difference between the indicators r_i and s_i. The earlier refer to unique point masses in the random probability measure (4.8), whereas the latter refer to the finite list of clusters.

Now we are ready to state the transition probabilities for posterior MCMC simulation. The stochastic process in Definition 4 implies a finite dimensional prior $p(\boldsymbol{m}_j^\star)$. For example, when $S(x)$ is a Gaussian process, then $p(\boldsymbol{m}_j^\star)$ is the multivariate normal given in Definition 3. We only discuss the conjugate case. Let $\boldsymbol{y}_j^\star = (y_i, i \in S_j)$ denote the data arranged by clusters and let $\boldsymbol{y}_j^{\star-} = \boldsymbol{y}_j^\star \setminus \{y_i\}$. And analogously for $\boldsymbol{x}_j^\star$ and $\boldsymbol{x}_j^{\star-}$, and n_j and n_j^-. We assume that $p(\boldsymbol{m}_j^\star \mid \boldsymbol{y}_j^\star, \boldsymbol{x}_j^\star)$ and $p(y_i \mid s_i = j, \boldsymbol{y}_j^{\star-}, x_i, \boldsymbol{x}_j^{\star-})$ are available in closed form. By a slight abuse of notation we include the fixed covariates x_i in the conditioning set to highlight the dependence on these covariates.

For example, under a GP prior on m_{hx} with normal sampling, $f_\theta(y_i) = N(\theta, \sigma^2)$ (with fixed σ^2), $p(\boldsymbol{m}_j^\star \mid \boldsymbol{y}_j^\star, \boldsymbol{x}_j^\star)$ is a multivariate normal again and $p(y_i \mid s_i = j, x_i, \boldsymbol{y}_j^{\star-}, \boldsymbol{x}_j^{\star-})$ is the normal posterior predictive distribution for an $(n_j^- + 1)$-st observation at x_i conditional on the n_j^- observations $\boldsymbol{y}_j^{\star-}$ at locations $\boldsymbol{x}_j^{\star-}$. See, for example Sect. 1.3.1. in Müller and Rodríguez (2013).

Posterior MCMC for a DDP model (4.9) proceeds exactly like Algorithm 1, using (2.16) with $p(y_i \mid s_i = j, \mathbf{y}_j^{\star-}, x_i, \mathbf{x}_j^{\star-})$ replacing $p(y_i \mid s_i = j, \mathbf{y}_j^{\star-})$. Similarly $h_0(y)$ is replaced by

$$h_0(y_i \mid x_i) = \int f_{m_{hx_i}}(y) \, dp(m_{hx_i})$$

where $p(m_{hx})$ is the marginal prior on m_{hx} under the assumed stochastic process. In summary

$$p(s_i = j \mid \mathbf{s}_{-i}, \mathbf{y}, \mathbf{x}) \propto \begin{cases} n_j^- \, p(y_i \mid s_i = j, x_i, \mathbf{y}_j^{\star-}, \mathbf{x}_j^{\star-}) & \text{for } j = 1, \ldots, k^- \\ M \, h_0(y_i \mid x_i) & j = k^- + 1. \end{cases} \quad (4.10)$$

Here k^- is the number of clusters after removing i.

Algorithm 9: *MCMC for a Conjugate DDP Mixture Model.*

1. Clustering: For $i = 1, \ldots, n$, draw $s_i \sim p(s_i \mid \mathbf{s}_{-i}, \mathbf{y}, \mathbf{x})$ using (4.10).
2. Cluster parameters: For $j = 1, \ldots, k$, generate $\mathbf{m}_j^\star \sim p(\mathbf{m}_j^\star \mid \mathbf{s}, \mathbf{y}^\star{}_j, \mathbf{x}^\star{}_j)$.

4.4.2 ANOVA DDP and LDDP

The perhaps simplest form of dependent prior on $\{m_{xh}, x \in \mathcal{X}\}$ is a normal linear ANCOVA model. De Iorio et al. (2004) use this construction to define the ANOVA DDP. Assuming, for example, $x = (u, v)$ is a pair of two factors, $u \in \{0, \ldots, n_u\}$ and $v \in \{0, \ldots, n_v\}$, the model could be

$$m_{xh} = \mu_h + a_u + b_v$$

with $\mu_h \sim N(0, \sigma_\mu^2)$, $a_0 = b_0 = 0$ and $a_u \sim N(0, \tau_u^2)$ for $u = 1, \ldots, n_v$, $b_v \sim N(0, \tau_v^2)$ for $v = 1, \ldots, n_v$. In general, letting $\mathbf{d}_x$ denote a design vector for covariates x and collecting all ANOVA effects in a parameter vector $\boldsymbol{\beta}$, the ANOVA DDP model defines dependent $\{m_{xh}, x \in \mathcal{X}\}$ as a linear model $m_{xh} = \boldsymbol{\beta}' \mathbf{d}_x$ with $\boldsymbol{\beta} \sim N(\boldsymbol{\mu}_b, S_b)$.

Definition 5 (ANOVA DDP) Let $x = (x_1, \ldots, x_p)$ denote a vector of categorical covariates $x_j \subset \{0, \ldots, n_j\}$, and let $\mathbf{d}_x$ denote $(q \times 1)$ design vector for x. Let $\mathcal{G} = \{G_x; x \in \mathcal{X}\}$ denote a family of random probability measures

$$G_x(\cdot) = \sum_{h=1}^{\infty} w_h \delta_{m_{xh}}(\cdot), \quad (4.11)$$

indexed by x. An ANOVA DDP prior for $\mathcal{G}$ is induced when $w_h = v_h \prod_{\ell < h}(1 - v_\ell)$, $v_h \stackrel{iid}{\sim} \text{Be}(1, M)$ and

$$m_{hx} = \boldsymbol{\beta}'_h \boldsymbol{d}_x, \quad \text{with} \quad \boldsymbol{\beta}_h \sim p^o(\boldsymbol{\beta}_h).$$

We write $\{G_x;\ x \in \mathcal{X}\} \sim \text{ANOVA DDP}(M, p^o)$. When we want to highlight that the design vector includes a continuous covariate we also write ANCOVA DDP.

Example 8 (Breast Cancer) De Iorio et al. (2009) illustrate inference under the ANOVA DDP model with the analysis of data from a cancer clinical trial described in Rosner (2005). The primary outcome in the study was event free survival. The trial enrolled $n = 761$ women, and recorded several baseline covariates, including treatment dose, estrogen receptor (ER) status and tumor size (TS). Treatment dose is coded as a categorical variable with HI = 1 for high dose and HI = −1 for low dose. Similarly, ER status is coded as ER = 1 for ER positive and ER = −1 for ER negative; and tumor size is coded as a continuous variable, standardized to mean 0 and variance 1. Additionally, the model includes an interaction term for dose/ER status (HI*ER) coded as 1 for high dose and positive ER status, and 0 otherwise. Figure 4.9a shows the data as Kaplan-Meier survival curves separately for patients arranged by ER status and treatment dose. Panel b of the same figure shows the estimated survival functions under the ANOVA DDP regression model.

We will revisit the ANOVA-DDP again later, in Sect. 6.3.2 and in Sect. 7.3.2, in different applications. A variation of the model is included in the R package DPpackage as the LDDP (linear dependent Dirichlet process) model.

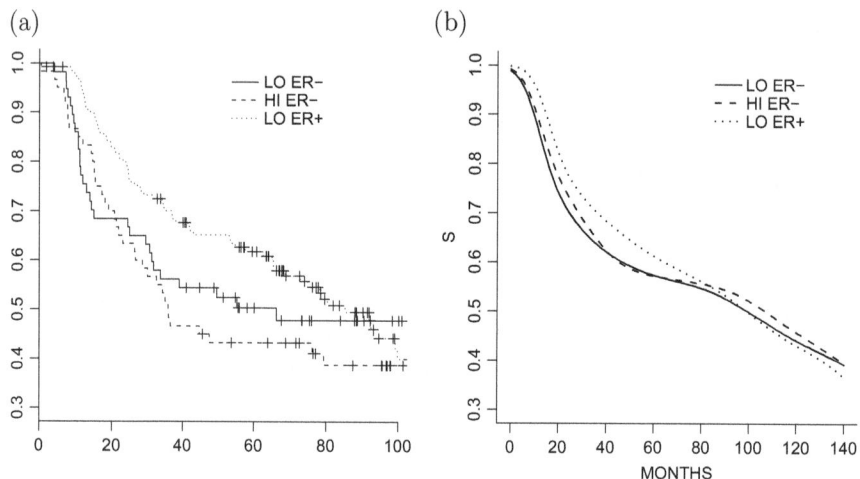

Fig. 4.9 Example 8. Data and posterior estimated G_x under a DDP ANOVA model for overall survival with $\boldsymbol{x}_i = (HI, ER, TS)$. (**a**) Data. (**b**) $E(S_x \mid \boldsymbol{y})$

4.4 Fully Nonparametric Regression

Definition 6 (Linear Dependent Dirichlet Process) Under the setup of Definition 5, define

$$G_x(\cdot) = \sum_{h=1}^{\infty} w_h \mathsf{N}(\cdot \mid \boldsymbol{\beta}'_h \boldsymbol{d}_x, \sigma_h^2). \tag{4.12}$$

with base measure $p^o(\boldsymbol{\beta}_h) = \mathsf{N}(\mu_b, S_b)$, $p^o(\sigma_h^2) = \mathsf{Ga}(\tau_1^2/2, \tau_2^2/2)$ and hyperprior $M \sim \mathsf{Ga}(a, b)$. We write $\{G_x, x \in \mathcal{X}\} \sim \mathsf{LDDP}(p_0)$.

The LDDP model defines a variation of the ANOVA-DDP by adding a convolution with a normal kernel in the definition of G_x and including a hyper-prior on the total mass M.

In the previous example the design vector $\boldsymbol{d}_x$ in $m_{hx} = \boldsymbol{\beta}' \boldsymbol{d}_x$ was

$$\boldsymbol{d}_x = (1, \mathrm{ER}, \mathrm{HI}, \mathrm{TS}, \mathrm{HI} \cdot \mathrm{ER}).$$

Alternatively we could model m_{hx} with, for example, a B-spline basis. In the next example $\boldsymbol{d}_x$ includes B-spline basis functions to allow for flexible modeling of m_{hx} as a function of x.

Example 5 (Old Faithful Geyser, ctd.) We fit a regression of waiting time (y_i, INTERVAL) on the duration of the preceding eruption (x_i, DURATION). We use the LDDP model, modeling m_{hx} as a B-spline expansion (as a function of x). This is achieved by defining the design vector $\boldsymbol{d}_x$ as six B-spline basis functions. We use the implementation in `DPpackage`, with the additional normal kernel in (4.12). Figure 4.10 shows the estimated interval density at the first and third quartiles of DURATION, i.e. $x = 1.97$ and $x = 4.47$ under this ANOVA DDP model.

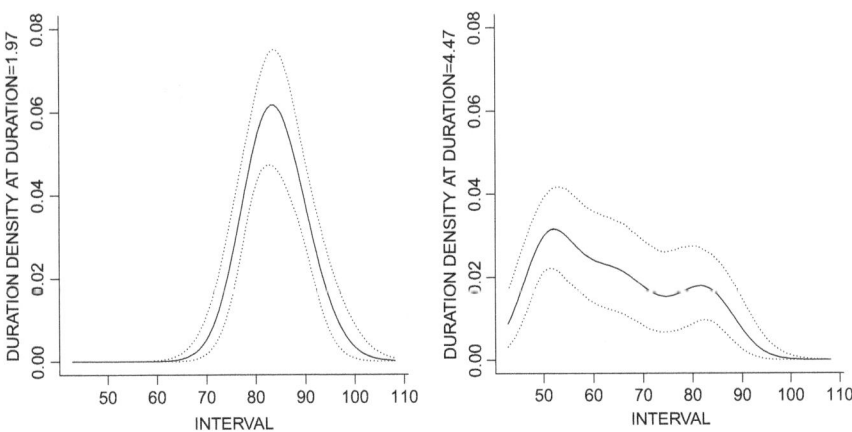

Fig. 4.10 Example 5. Conditional DDP mixture density estimates at the first and third quartile of the predictor

Posterior MCMC for the ANOVA DDP Model

We discuss posterior simulation for the ANOVA DDP model (4.12) with additional normal residuals. The model can be written as

$$G_x(\cdot) = \int \mathsf{N}(\cdot \mid \boldsymbol{\beta}'d_x, \sigma^2)\, dF(\boldsymbol{\beta}, \sigma^2)$$

with

$$F(\cdot) = \sum_h w_h \delta_{\boldsymbol{\beta}_h, \sigma_h^2}(\cdot),$$

and w_h generated by the stick breaking prior and $(\boldsymbol{\beta}_h, \sigma_h^2) \sim p^o$, i.i.d. That is, the ANOVA DDP model can be alternatively written as a DPM of ANOVA models. This representation allows the use of any of the many approaches that have been proposed to implement posterior inference for DPM models. See Sect. 2.4 for a brief review.

4.4.3 Dependent PT Prior

Linear Dependent Tail-Free Process (LDTFP) Similar to the DDP, the PT prior can be extended to a prior on a family $\{G_x,\ x \in \mathcal{X}\}$ of probability measures. One construction is the LDTFP of Jara and Hanson (2011). The LDTFP replaces the beta prior (3.2) by a logistic regression on covariates. We will discuss the LDTFP in more detail later, as a model for survival regression in Sect. 6.3.3. The LDTFP model is implemented for standard regression data in the `LDTFPdensity` function in `DPpackage`.

Example 5 (Old Faithful Geyser, ctd.) Recall Example 5. Figure 4.11 shows the estimated interval density at the duration first and third quartiles, i.e. $x = 1.97$ and $x = 4.47$ based on the LDTFP. The median trend is modeled using a B-spline with six basis functions, as are the conditional probabilities of the tail-free process.

Dependent PT (DPT) A similar construction is the DPT proposed in Trippa et al. (2011). The construction leaves the marginal PT prior for G_x intact. That is, the random splitting probabilities in the binary tree for one random probability measure remain marginally beta distributed. Let $Y_{\varepsilon 0}(x) = G_x(B_{\varepsilon 0} \mid B_\varepsilon)$ denote the random splitting probability for the partitioning subset $B_\varepsilon = B_{\varepsilon 0} \cup B_{\varepsilon 1}$. The desired dependence is introduced by making $Y_\varepsilon(x)$ dependent across $x \in \mathcal{X}$. The partitioning subsets B_ε are the same across x. For the moment drop the index ε. The construction exploits the representation of a beta random variable as a ratio of gamma random variables, writing $Y(x) = C^+(x)/[C^+(x) + C^-(x)]$ where $C^+(x)$ and $C^-(x)$ are two independent gamma random variables. The trick is to define C^+ and C^- in a way that induces the desired dependence across x. This is achieved by introducing

4.4 Fully Nonparametric Regression

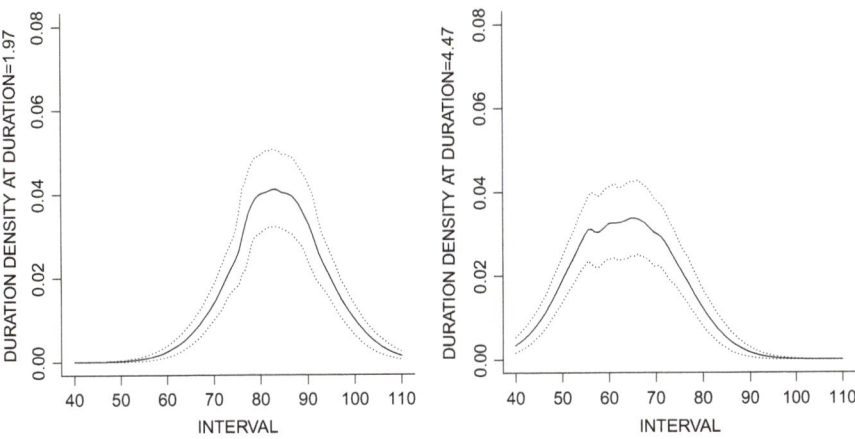

Fig. 4.11 Example 5. Conditional LDTP density estimates at the first and third quartile of the predictor

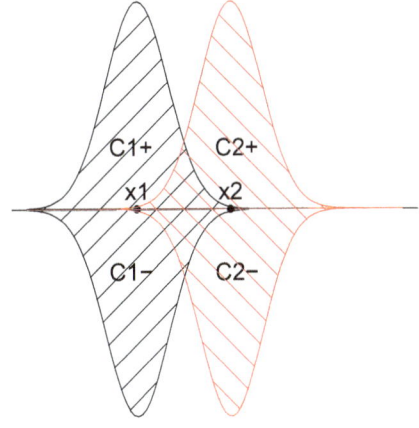

Fig. 4.12 Construction of dependent beta random variables $Y(x_1)$ and $Y(x_2)$. Let $C^+(x_j)$ denote the measure of the kernel S_j^+ under a gamma process, $j = 1, 2$. And similar for $C^-(x_j)$. Then $Y(x_j) = C^+(x_j)/(C^+(x_j) + C^-(x_j))$ defines a beta distributed random variable and induces the desired dependence across x

a gamma process $\mathsf{GaP}(\cdot)$ on $\mathcal{X} \times \mathbb{R}$. Define $C^+(x)$ as the random measure under the gamma process $\mathsf{GaP}(\cdot)$ for an area centered around x, say an area circumscribed by a kernel $S^+(x)$ centered at x. Similarly $C^-(x)$ is defined as the random measure under the gamma process of the area circumscribed by another kernel $S^-(x)$. The definition of S^- and S^+ as non-overlapping sets keeps C^- and C^+ independent, as needed. The construction is illustrated in Fig. 4.12. Note how the two kernels are placed on $\mathcal{X} \times [0, \infty)$ and $\mathcal{X} \times (-\infty, 0]$, respectively, giving rise to independent $C^+(x) = \mathsf{GaP}(S^+(x))$ and $C^-(x) = \mathsf{GaP}(S^-(x))$. Now consider two covariates, x_1

and x_2. As x_2 moves closer to x_1 the kernels centered at x_1 and x_2 have increasingly more overlap, leading to correlated $Y_\epsilon(x_1)$ and $Y_\epsilon(x_2)$, as desired.

4.4.4 Conditional Regression

With a slight abuse of statistical inference the general regression problem of inference on $f(\cdot)$ in (4.7) can be reduced to a density estimation problem. We proceed as if the pairs (x_i, y_i) were independent random samples from a joint distribution $(x_i, y_i) \sim G$, and report inference on G. The implied conditional distributions $\{G_x(y) = G(y \mid x); x \in \mathcal{X}\}$ solve the regression problem. Let $f_G(x) = E_G(y \mid x)$ denote the conditional mean under G as a function of x. The posterior distribution $p(f_G \mid \mathbf{y})$ provides the desired inference on the regression mean curve. We characterized the construction as a slight abuse of statistical inference, because the likelihood function in the augmented model for the pairs (x_i, y_i) includes a sampling model for x_i, even when there might be nothing random about the covariates x_i.

Müller et al. (1996) and Park and Dunson (2010) propose this approach using a DP mixture model for inference on the unknown joint distribution G. Regression curves f_G estimated under this approach take the form of locally weighted linear regression lines, similar to traditional kernel regression in classical nonparametric inference. Considering (x_i, y_i) as an i.i.d. sample—wrongly—introduces an additional factor $\prod G(x_i)$ in the likelihood $\prod G(x_i, y_i) = \prod G(x_i) G(y_i \mid x_i)$ and thus provides only approximate inference.

Consider DP mixture of normal kernels, mixing with respect to location and scale. Write the DPM as a hierarchical model as in (2.6),

$$(x_i, y_i \mid \mu_i, \Sigma_i) \stackrel{\text{ind}}{\sim} \mathsf{N}(\mu_i, \Sigma_j)$$
$$\theta_i \equiv (\mu_i, \Sigma_i) \mid G \sim G \quad \text{and} \quad G \sim \mathsf{DP}(MG_0). \qquad (4.13)$$

Let $\theta_j^\star = (\mu_j^\star, \Sigma_j^\star), j = 1, \ldots, k$, denote the unique values of θ_i, $i = 1, \ldots, n$, with multiplicities n_j. Let $f(y \mid x, \theta_j^\star)$ denote the conditional normal density in y given x under the multivariate normal $\mathsf{N}(\mu_j^\star, \Sigma_j^\star)$ and let $s(x \mid \theta_j^\star)$ denote the marginal normal density in x under $\mathsf{N}(\mu_j^\star, \Sigma_j^\star)$. Similarly, let $f_0(y \mid x)$ and $s_0(x)$ denote the implied conditional and marginal when $\theta^\star$ is generated from $G^\star(\theta^\star)$, i..e., $f_0(y \mid x) = \int f(y \mid x, \theta) \, dG^\star(\theta)$ and $s_0(x) = \int s(x \mid \theta) \, dG^\star(\theta)$.

Now consider (2.11) for a future observation θ_{n+1}, add an additional convolution with $p(y_{n+1} \mid \theta_{n+1})$ and write (x, y) as short for (x_{n+1}, y_{n+1}). We get the predictive distribution

$$p(y \mid x, \theta_1^\star, \ldots, \theta_k^\star) \propto M \, s_0(x) f_0(y \mid x) + \sum_{j=1}^{k} n_j s(x \mid \theta_j^\star) f(y \mid x, \theta_j^\star). \qquad (4.14)$$

4.4 Fully Nonparametric Regression

The predictive $p(y \mid x, \theta_1^\star, \ldots, \theta_k^\star)$ takes the form of a locally weighted mixture of linear regressions, each regression line being indexed by a unique $\theta_j^\star$, and the weights being the normal kernels $n_j s(x \mid \theta_j^\star)$. Plus one term corresponding to the base measure G_0. Inference under (4.14) is implemented in the DPpackage function DPcdensity. Model (4.14), that is, conditional regression under a DPM model for the augmented response vector (x_i, y_i) is also known as WDDP (weight dependent Dirichlet process).

Park and Dunson (2010) point out that such inference can be interpreted as replacing the original Polya urn prior on the random partition by what would be the posterior conditional on x_i, $i = 1, \ldots, n$, only. They refer to the random partition implied by $p(G \mid \mathbf{x})$ as the *predictor dependent product partition model*. That is, the factors M and n_j that would appear in the predictive distribution for y in a model without covariates x_i, are replaced by $M s_0(x)$ and $n_j s(x \mid \theta_j^\star)$.

Example 5 (Old Faithful Geyser, ctd.) Figure 4.13 shows the estimated mean function $f(\cdot)$ as a conditional regression function in a bivariate density estimation for $G(x, y)$. The bivariate density estimation is implemented as a DP mixture of normals (4.13).

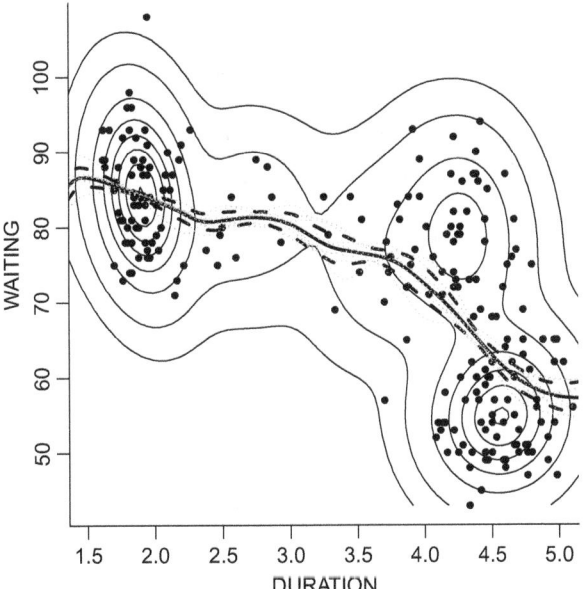

Fig. 4.13 Example 5. Estimated joint density $\overline{G}(x, y)$ (*contour lines*), and conditional mean process $f_G(x) = E[G(y \mid x, \text{data})]$. The *dashed lines* show pointwise posterior standard deviations. *Dotted grey lines* show random draws $f_g \sim p(f_G \mid \mathbf{y})$

References

Azzalini A, Bowman AW (1990) A look at some data on the old faithful geyser. Appl Stat 39:357–365

Banerjee A, Dunson DB, Tokdar ST (2013) Efficient Gaussian process regression for large datasets. Biometrika 100:75–89

Banerjee S, Gelfand AE, Finley AO, Sang H (2008) Gaussian predictive process models for large spatial data sets. J R Stat Soc Ser B 70:825–848

Bové DS, Held L (2011) Bayesian fractional polynomials. Stat Comput 21:309–324

Brezger A, Lang S (2006) Generalized structured additive regression based on Bayesian p-splines. Comput Stat Data Anal 50:967–991

Brinkman N (1981) Ethanol fuel—a single-cylinder engine study of efficiency and exhaust emissions. SAE Trans 90:1410–1424

Chipman HA, Kolaczyk ED, McCulloch RE (1997) Adaptive Bayesian wavelet shrinkage. J Am Stat Assoc 92:1413–1421

Chipman HA, George EI, McCulloch RE (1998) Bayesian CART model search. J Am Stat Assoc 93(443):935–948

Chipman HA, George EI, McCulloch RE (2010) BART: Bayesian additive regression trees. Ann Appl Stat 4:266–298

Clyde M, George E (2000) Flexible empirical Bayes estimation for wavelets. J R Stat Soc Ser B 62:681–698

Cybenko G (1989) Approximation by superposition of a sigmoidal function. Math Cont Sys Sig 2:303–314

De Boor C (2001) A practical guide to splines. Applied mathematical sciences, vol 27. Springer, New York

De Iorio M, Müller P, Rosner GL, MacEachern SN (2004) An ANOVA model for dependent random measures. J Am Stat Assoc 99(465):205–215

De Iorio M, Johnson WO, Müller P, Rosner GL (2009) Bayesian nonparametric non-proportional hazards survival modelling. Biometrics 65:762–771

Denison DGT, Mallick BK, Smith AFM (1998) A Bayesian CART algorithm. Biometrika 85(2):363–377

Donoho DL, Johnstone IM (1994) Minimax risk over l_p-balls for l_q-error. Probab Theory Relat Fields 99:277–304

Eilers PHC, Marx BD (1996) Flexible smoothing with B-splines and penalties. Stat Sci 11(2):89–121

Gramacy RB, Lee HKH (2008) Bayesian treed Gaussian process models with an application to computer modeling. J Am Stat Assoc 103:1119–1130

Hanson T, Johnson WO (2002) Modeling regression error with a mixture of Polya trees. J Am Stat Assoc 97:1020–1033

Hanson T, Johnson WO (2004) A Bayesian semiparametric AFT model for interval-censored data. J Comput Graph Stat 13:341–361

Hastie T, Tibshirani R (1990) Generalized additive models. Chapman and Hall, New York

Jara A, Hanson TE (2011) A class of mixtures of dependent tailfree processes. Biometrika 98:553–566

Kennedy MC, O'Hagan A (2001) Bayesian calibration of computer models. J R Stat Soc Ser B (Stat Methodol) 63(3):425–464.

Kneib T (2006) Mixed model based inference in structured additive regression. Ludwig-Maximilians-Universität München. http://nbn-resolving.de/urn:nbn:de:bvb:19-50112

Kottas A, Gelfand AE (2001) Bayesian semiparametric median regression modeling. J Am Stat Assoc 96:1458–1468

Lang S, Brezger A (2004) Bayesian P-splines. J Comput Graph Stat 13:183–212

Lenk PJ (1999) Bayesian inference for semiparametric regression using a Fourier representation. J R Stat Soc Ser B 61:863–879

References

MacEachern S (1999) Dependent nonparametric processes. In: ASA Proceedings of the section on Bayesian statistical science. American Statistical Association, Alexandria

Morris JS, Carroll RJ (2006) Wavelet-based functional mixed models. J R Stat Soc Ser B Stat Methodol 68(2):179–199

Müller P, Ríos-Insua D (1998) Issues in Bayesian analysis of neural network models. Neural Comput 10:571–592

Müller P, Rodríguez A (2013) Nonparametric Bayesian Inference. IMS-CBMS lecture notes. IMS, Beachwood

Müller P, Vidakovic B (1998) Bayesian inference with wavelets: density estimation. J Comput Graph Stat 7:456–468

Müller P, Erkanli A, West M (1996) Bayesian curve fitting using multivariate normal mixtures. Biometrika 83:67–79

O'Hagan T (1978) Curve fitting and optimal design for prediction. J R Stat Soc Ser B (Methodol) 40(1):1–42.

Park JH, Dunson D (2010) Bayesian generalized product partition models. Stat Sin 20:1203–1226

Rosner GL (2005) Bayesian monitoring of clinical trials with failure-time endpoints. Biometrics 61:239–245

Rumelhart D, McClelland J (1986) Parallel distributed processing. MIT Press, Cambridge

Schörgendorfer A, Branscum A, Hanson T (2013) A Bayesian goodness of fit test and semiparametric generalization of logistic regression with measurement data. Biometrics 69:508–519

Shively TS, Kohn R, Wood S (1999) Variable selection and function estimation in additive nonparametric regression using a data-based prior. J Am Stat Assoc 94:777–794

Trippa L, Müller P, Johnson W (2011) The multivariate beta process and an extension of the Polya tree model. Biometrika 98(1):17–34

Vannucci M, Corradi F (1999) Covariance structure of wavelet coefficients: theory and models in a Bayesian perspective. J R Stat Soc Ser B Methodol 61:971–986

Vidakovic B (1998) Nonlinear wavelet shrinkage with Bayes rules and Bayes factors. J Am Stat Assoc 93:173–179

Walker S, Mallick B (1999) A Bayesian semiparametric accelerated failure time model. Biometrics 55:477–483

Chapter 5
Categorical Data

Abstract We discuss nonparametric Bayesian methods that are suitable for inference with binary, ordinal and general categorical data. Modeling for such data becomes particularly interesting in the presence of covariates, when non- and semi-parametric Bayesian models can generalize the link function in a generalized linear model setup, the regression on covariates or both. An important application arises in inference for diagnostic screening and related inference for ROC (receiver-operator characteristic) curves. We include some discussion of a rapidly growing literature on non-parametric Bayesian inference for ROC curves.

5.1 Categorical Responses Without Covariates

5.1.1 Binomial Responses

We start with an example to illustrate a number of key issues of a BNP approach for binary outcomes.

Example 9 (Baseball Data) Albright (1993) describes a dataset involving the complete sequence of hits and outs for a number of players from both American and National Baseball Leagues over the 1987–1990 seasons. The data are available from: http://www.kelley.iu.edu/albright/Free_downloads.htm. Albright assumes the operational definition of a success to mean a player moving through the bases. We stick to that definition, and therefore, a success consists of either a hit, walk or sacrifice. From this large dataset, we consider now the total number of successes for the subset of $n = 129$ players from both leagues who were at bat at least on 500 occasions during the 1987 season. Denote by y_i, $i = 1, \ldots, n$, the number of successes for the ith player. The simplest possible model for these data would assume just a single success probability, common to all players, that is, $y_1, \ldots, y_n \mid \theta \stackrel{\text{iid}}{\sim} \text{Bin}(\ell_i, \theta)$, $\theta \sim \text{Be}(a, b)$, where ℓ_i is the total number of at-bats for player i and (a, b) are fixed hyperparameters, e.g., $a = b = 1$. The posterior distribution $p(\theta \mid y)$ is a $\text{Be}(28178, 49494)$ distribution. Of course, this would be ridiculously precise inference that fails to accommodate any notion of variation of success probabilities across players. The posterior $p(\theta \mid y)$ is essentially a point mass at the posterior mean $28178/77672 = 0.36$.

In Example 9, a hierarchical model with subject-specific success rates, θ_i, provides for more variability across players

$$y_i \mid \theta_i \stackrel{\text{ind}}{\sim} \text{Bin}(\ell_i, \theta_i), \quad \theta_i \mid a, b \stackrel{\text{iid}}{\sim} \text{Be}(a, b), \quad (a, b) \sim \pi, \tag{5.1}$$

where $i = 1, \ldots, n$, $a, b > 1$, and π is a suitable prior distribution for (a, b). We choose $\pi(a, b) = \pi(a)\pi(b)$, where a and b are i.i.d. with $\text{Ga}(0.001, 0.001)$ distributions. The hierarchical model allows for the success probabilities to vary across players, and the hyper-parameters a, b allow for learning about the level of borrowing strength across players, that is, how diverse the rates can be across players. However, the $\text{Be}(a, b)$ prior still represents a strong prior assumption, as it implies that the distribution of player strengths is unimodal. It fails to allow for population heterogeneity that could lead to a multimodal distribution of θ_i across the population of players. A generalization that removes such restrictions is a typical application of BNP priors. One possible nonparametric alternative appears in Liu (1996), who considers a hierarchical model,

$$y_i \mid \theta_i \stackrel{\text{ind}}{\sim} \text{Bin}(\ell_i, \theta_i), \quad \theta_i \mid F \stackrel{\text{iid}}{\sim} F, \quad F \sim \text{DP}(MF_0), \tag{5.2}$$

where $i = 1, \ldots, n$ and F_0 is the $\text{Be}(a, b)$ distribution. The same prior assumption for (a, b) as in the parametric case may be used. Model (5.2) replaces the beta prior of the parametric hierarchical model by a random probability measure F. From a data analysis perspective, the important feature of the model is the representation of arbitrary distributions of success rates across the population. Figure 5.1 contrasts the estimated distributions in Example 9 under the parametric hierarchical model versus the multimodal estimate $E(F \mid y)$ under the BNP model. There is a second important feature to the model that is often exploited in data analysis. Recall the discrete nature of the DP random probability measure F and the implied clustering in DP mixture models that we discussed in Sect. 2.3. The DP mixture model $y_i \mid F \stackrel{\text{ind}}{\sim} \int \text{Bin}(\ell_i, \theta_i) F(d\theta_i)$ and $F \sim \text{DP}(MF_0)$ implies a partition of players into clusters of equal values $\theta_i = \theta_j^\star$ for $k \leq n$ unique values $\{\theta_1^\star, \ldots, \theta_k^\star\}$. Recall the cluster membership indicators $s_i = j$ that were introduced in Sect. 2.3. Let $s_i = j$ if $\theta_i = \theta_j^\star$, that is $\theta_{s_i} = \theta_j^\star$ with $\theta_j^\star \stackrel{\text{iid}}{\sim} \text{Be}(a, b)$. The implied grouping is then defined by the prior distribution on the indicators $s_1, \ldots, s_n$, which follows the Polya urn scheme (Sect. 2.3). The fact that F_0 is conjugate to the binomial likelihood makes it possible to easily implement any of the posterior simulation schemes discussed in Sect. 2.4, or the sequential importance sampling algorithm used in Liu (1996).

Example 9 (ctd.) We implemented inference under the DP mixture model (5.2). Figure 5.1 compares the results of fitting both, the hierarchical parametric model (5.1) and the nonparametric model (5.2) to the at-bat performance of a group of players during the 1987 season. The top panels show a histogram of the (empirical) proportion of successes at the end of the season, with smoothed versions of the corresponding posterior predictive densities. In the BNP model

5.1 Categorical Responses Without Covariates

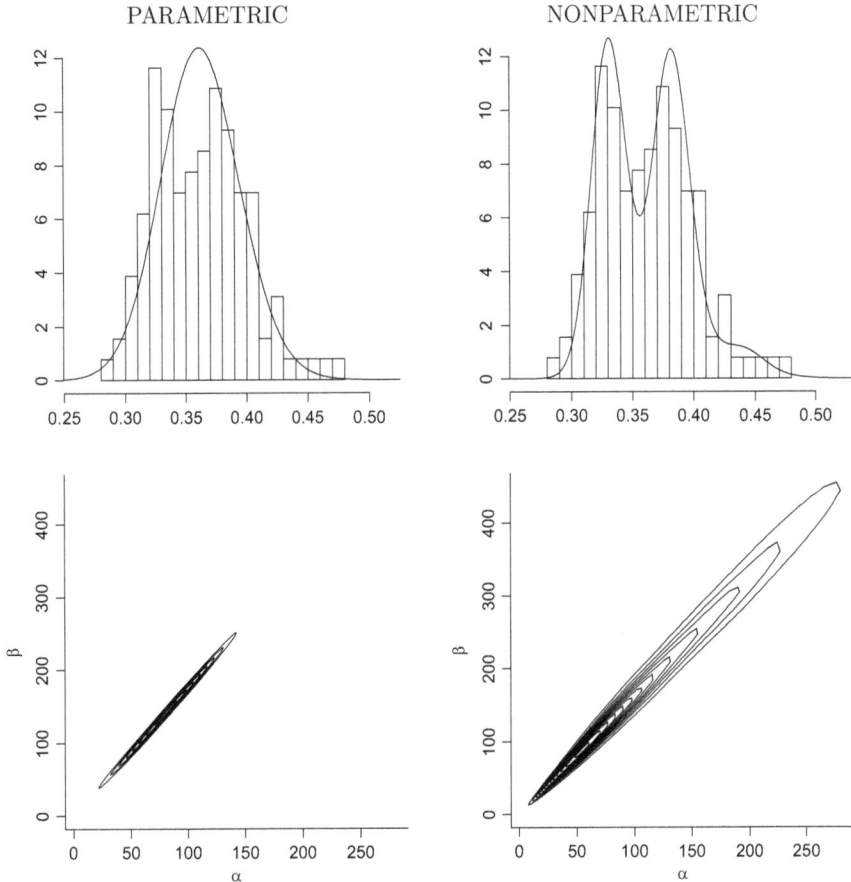

Fig. 5.1 Example 9. At bat performance of 1987 season players. The *top panel* shows histograms of the proportion of successes for the $n = 129$ players overlayed with the posterior predictive density $p(\theta_{n+1} \mid y)$ for the parametric (*left*) and nonparametric (*right*) models. Note that for the nonparametric model, $p(\theta_{n+1} \mid y) = E(F \mid y)$. The *bottom panel* shows contours of the posterior distribution $p(a, b \mid y)$ for the same models

$p(\theta_{n+1} \mid y) = E(F \mid y)$. That is, the posterior predictive equals the posterior estimated random effects distribution.

Considering the large sample size, the histograms provide substantial evidence for a multimodal distribution for the true at-bat success rates. Of course, the parametric model fails at recognizing this multimodality, as it only supports unimodality. Inference under the nonparametric model includes a trimodal density estimate that better reflects the multimodality in the empirical distribution.

Similar inference can be implemented when replacing the DP prior with any other random probability measure, for example any of the models discussed in Chap. 3. Any discrete prior random probability measures would maintain the notion of clustering of experimental units, that is, players in the case of Example 9. The main computational challenge in the implementation is the updating of the configurations s.

5.1.2 Categorical Responses

We introduced the DP mixture of binomial model (5.2) for binary data. Many problems involve categorical responses with $c \geq 2$ possible outcomes. The model can easily be extended to accommodate such more general outcomes. Assume that for the ith experimental unit, $i = 1, \ldots, n$, we record ℓ_i trials with $c \geq 2$ possible outcomes each. Let $m_{ij}, j = 1, \ldots, c$, denote the number of these trials that resulted in category j being observed. Let $y_i = (m_{i1}, \ldots, m_{ic})$ be the vector of counts for the ith experimental unit, and denote the entire collection of responses by $y = (y_1, \ldots, y_n)$. Let Multin($y; \ell, \theta$) denote a multinomial distribution with sample size ℓ and classification probabilities $\theta_1, \ldots, \theta_c$. We generalize model (5.2) to this data structure, by assuming

$$y_i \mid \theta_i \overset{ind}{\sim} \text{Multin}(y_i; \ell_i, \theta_i), \quad \theta_i \mid F \overset{iid}{\sim} F, \quad F \sim \text{DP}(M, F_0), \quad (5.3)$$

where $i = 1, \ldots, n$, $F_0 \equiv \text{Dir}(c, \alpha)$, the Dirichlet distribution on the $(c-1)$-dimensional simplex $\Delta_{c-1} = \{(x_1, \ldots, x_c) : \sum_{j=1}^{c} x_j = 1, \text{ and } x_j \geq 0 \text{ for all } j\}$, and $\alpha \in (\mathbb{R}^+)^c$. Model (5.3) reduces to (5.2) when $c = 2$ and $\alpha = (a, b)$.

Test of Homogeneity Data with such structure are often represented in a contingency table with n rows and c columns. When n is a small number it is even possible to carry out exact analytical posterior calculations under model (5.3). Quintana (1998) uses such results to propose a test for homogeneity (of classification probabilities) in contingency tables with fixed (right) margins. In this context homogeneity means that $\theta_1 = \cdots = \theta_n$, and therefore, the probability of being classified into any of the c categories is the same for all rows in the contingency table. Because the DP total mass parameter M plays a key role in the derivation of the test, Quintana (1998) assumed additionally a prior distribution $\pi(M) = \text{Ga}(a_1, b_1)$ which allows for a better control of the prior structure, as explained below.

Recall the discussion in Sect. 2.3, about the random partition of experimental units that is implied by a DP mixture model as in (5.3). Recall our earlier notation for a random partition $\rho = (S_1, \ldots, S_k)$ of $S = \{1, \ldots, n\}$ into k nonempty and disjoint subsets. The contingency table is homogeneous if $\rho = \{S\}$, i.e., if there is a single cluster and the partition has exactly one subset (of size n), namely, S. The number of clusters in a given partition ρ of S will be denoted by $|\rho|$.

5.1 Categorical Responses Without Covariates

We develop now the calculations to implement the test of homogeneity that is proposed in Quintana (1998). For a vector of positive entries $\boldsymbol{\alpha} \in (\mathbb{R}^+)^c$ let

$$D(\boldsymbol{\alpha}) = \Gamma\left(\sum_{j=1}^{c} \alpha_j\right) \bigg/ \prod_{j=1}^{c} \Gamma(\alpha_j),$$

be the normalization constant of a Dirichlet distribution with parameter vector $\boldsymbol{\alpha}$. Let $n_\ell = |S_\ell|$ denote the size of the ℓ-th subset in the partition ρ, and let $\boldsymbol{y}_\ell^\star = \sum_{i \in S_\ell} \boldsymbol{y}_i$ denote the counts aggregated by clusters. Write also for $r = 1, \ldots, n$

$$\gamma_r = \int_0^\infty \left(\frac{M^r}{\prod_{j=1}^{n}(M+j-1)}\right) \pi(M)\, dM \text{ and } \mathcal{L}_r(\boldsymbol{y}) = \sum_{\rho:|\rho|=r} \left\{\prod_{\ell=1}^{r} \frac{(n_\ell - 1)! D(\boldsymbol{\alpha})}{D(\boldsymbol{\alpha} + \boldsymbol{y}_\ell^\star)}\right\},$$

where the summation in the right-hand side of the last expression is over all size r partitions $\rho = (S_1, \ldots, S_r)$ (i.e., with exactly r nonempty subsets). It can be shown (Quintana 1998) that the posterior distribution of the number of clusters is given by

$$p(|\rho| = r \mid \boldsymbol{y}) = \frac{\gamma_r \mathcal{L}_r(\boldsymbol{y})}{\sum_{q=1}^{n} \gamma_q \mathcal{L}_q(\boldsymbol{y})}, \quad r = 1, 2, \ldots, n.$$

It is also easy to find that the posterior probability of a given partition ρ with exactly $r = |\rho|$ subsets can be written as

$$p(\rho \mid \boldsymbol{y}) = \frac{1}{\sum_{s=1}^{n} \gamma_s \mathcal{L}_s(\boldsymbol{y})} \left\{\gamma_r \prod_{\ell=1}^{r}(n_\ell - 1)! \frac{D(\boldsymbol{\alpha})}{D(\boldsymbol{\alpha} + \boldsymbol{y}_\ell^\star)}\right\}. \tag{5.4}$$

To carry out the test of homogeneity we compare the prior and posterior odds of homogeneity. The above results imply that the Bayes factor (BF) in favor of homogeneity is given by

$$BF = \frac{\mathcal{L}_1(\boldsymbol{y})(1 - (n-1)!\gamma_1)}{(n-1)! \sum_{r=2}^{n} \gamma_r \mathcal{L}_r(\boldsymbol{y})}, \tag{5.5}$$

which follows from the fact that the prior probability of a single cluster is simply $\gamma_1(n-1)!$. Of special interest is the case of $n = 2$ rows in the table, in which case (5.5) reduces, after some algebra, to $BF = \mathcal{L}_1(\boldsymbol{y})/\mathcal{L}_2(\boldsymbol{y})$.

Table 5.1 Example 10. Word counts from books by Jane Austen, including part of *Sanditon*, as completed by an admirer

Novel	Word						Total
	a	an	this	that	with	without	
Sense and sensibility	147	25	32	94	59	18	375
Emma	186	26	39	105	74	10	440
Sanditon (Chaps. 1 and 3)	101	11	15	37	28	10	202
Sanditon (Chaps. 12 and 24)	83	29	15	22	43	4	196

Example 10 (Jane Austen Word Counts) Rice (1995) analyzes a dataset on literary style, using data from Morton (1978). The data consist of counts of different words used by Jane Austen in some of her books, including the novel *Sanditon*, which was left unfinished at her death. An admirer completed the novel trying to imitate the writer's style, and the mixed result was later published. Comparing word counts between authenticated and disputed works is a traditional way to settle disputes on authorship. Morton presented results on counts for certain words in Chaps. 1 and 3 of *Sense and Sensibility*, Chaps. 1–3 of *Emma*, Chaps. 1 and 6 of *Sanditon*, which were written by Austen, and Chaps. 12 and 24 of *Sanditon*, written by the admirer. The data, as presented in Rice (1995) are reproduced in Table 5.1.

To analyze these data, we treat the rows in Table 5.1 as samples from multinomial distributions, with categories defined by the words and considering the right margin totals to be fixed. Homogeneity would then mean that the usage of these words occurs with the same proportions across books, in particular, implying that the admirer truly emulated Austen's style, at least as far as the usage of the chosen words is concerned.

Following the analysis in Rice (1995), we first consider the top three rows of Table 5.1, the authenticated output by Austen. The idea is to analyze the writer's own consistency in the use of these words across the selected novels. Thus, we take $n = 3$ and $c = 6$. Choosing an exponential with mean 1 as prior for M, we find numerically $(\gamma_1, \gamma_2, \gamma_3) = (0.24, 0.13, 0.15)$ and $(\log(\mathcal{L}_1(y)), \ldots, \log(\mathcal{L}_3(y))) = (-1535.5, -1541.9, -1550.0)$, and the Bayes factor in favor of homogeneity (5.5) is $BF = 1265.099$. This is strong evidence that Austen used the chosen words consistently across the three authenticated novels.

Next, we consider the analysis of the complete table, i.e. $n = 4$ and $c = 6$, using the same prior as before. With this, we find $(\gamma_1, \ldots, \gamma_4) = (.068, .031, .032, .054)$ and $(\mathcal{L}_1(y), \ldots, \mathcal{L}_4(y)) = (-1844.8, -1830.0, -1846.4, -1854.4)$, so that the Bayes factor for homogeneity becomes $BF = 0.0248$. This is evidence in favor of the non-homogeneity of the word usage distribution. In fact, using (5.4) we find posterior odds

$$\frac{p(\rho = \{\{1,2,3\},\{4\}\} \mid y)}{p(\rho = \{\{1,2,3,4\}\} \mid y)} = 58.63,$$

which explains the result of the homogeneity test. The evidence thus points to the fact that the admirer used the selected words in different proportion than Jane Austen did in her books.

Software note: In the software appendix for this chapter we show R code to implement the test of homogeneity in Example 10.

We note here that any discrete random probability measure implies a distribution on partitions and could therefore be potentially used to induce a prior probability on homogeneity, along the lines discussed here for the DP. In fact, most of the calculations developed above, such as Eq. (5.5), can be readily generalized, provided there is an analytical expression for the prior probability of a single cluster.

5.1.3 Multivariate Ordinal Data

A variation of the above example arises when data can still be accommodated in a contingency table but without margins that are fixed by design. In problems with data in this format a common inference goal is to study associations between the categorical variables.

Kottas et al. (2005) proposed a nonparametric approach for the case of multiple categorical variables of ordinal type. Consider a total of k ordinal categorical variables $V = (V_1, \ldots, V_k)$, with corresponding numbers of categories $C_1, \ldots, C_k$. For each of n experimental units, the values of the k variables are recorded, and the results are stored as cell counts $m_{\ell_1, \cdots, \ell_k}$, which record the number of observations with $V = (\ell_1, \ldots, \ell_k)$. Data of this type can be arranged in a multidimensional contingency table with $C = \prod_{j=1}^{k} C_j$ cells, and frequencies $\{m_{\ell_1 \cdots \ell_k}\}$, now constrained only by $\sum_{\ell_1 \cdots \ell_k} m_{\ell_1 \cdots \ell_k} = n$. Denote by $p_{\ell_1 \cdots \ell_k} = p(V_1 = \ell_1, \ldots, V_k = \ell_k)$ the classification probability for cell $(\ell_1, \ldots, \ell_k)$. A popular probability model for such multivariate ordinal data structure is based on latent variables. See, for instance, Albert and Chib (1993), and Johnson and Albert (1999). Introducing cutoffs $-\infty = \gamma_{j,0} < \gamma_{j,1} < \cdots < \gamma_{j,C_j-1} < \gamma_{j,C_j} = \infty$, for each variable, $j = 1, \ldots, k$, and a k-dimensional latent vector $Z = (Z_1, \ldots, Z_k)$, a latent variable model assumes

$$p_{\ell_1 \cdots \ell_k} = p\left(\gamma_{1,\ell_1-1} < Z_1 \leq \gamma_{1,\ell_1}, \ldots, \gamma_{k,\ell_k-1} < Z_k \leq \gamma_{k,\ell_k}\right). \tag{5.6}$$

In other words, variable V_j takes on the value ℓ if the corresponding latent variable Z_j lies on the interval $(\gamma_{j,\ell-1}, \gamma_{j,\ell}]$. The classification probabilities are then completely determined by the cutoffs and latent variables.

A standard assumption is that the latent vector Z has a multivariate normal distribution. As a consequence, if any two of the latent vector components are uncorrelated, the corresponding ordinal categorical variables are independent. The correlation coefficients $r_{u,w} = \text{Cor}(Z_u, Z_w)$ are called polychoric correlations and are widely used in the social sciences as a measure of association among ordinal variables. See further discussion about this and related concepts in Olsson (1979), Ronning and Kukuk (1996) and references therein.

Despite its popularity, there are serious limitations to this multivariate probit model. One practical concern is that the use of cutoffs complicates posterior simulation. This is because of the high posterior correlation of the cutoffs $\gamma_{j,\ell}$ and the latent variables $\mathbf{Z}$. And secondly, a multivariate normal assumption for $\mathbf{Z}$ concentrates most of the probability mass in cells that are located in one portion of the table. But this is inappropriate for cases where substantial mass is placed at or near the (multiple) corners. Motivated by these considerations, Kottas et al. (2005) proposed a flexible DPM-based approach to replace the multivariate normal assumption. An important feature of the proposed model is that the flexible distribution for the latent variables removes the need for variable cutoffs. Cutoffs can be fixed and arbitrarily chosen.

Kottas et al. (2005) propose the following model. Denote by $\mathbf{V}_i = (V_{i1}, \ldots, V_{ik})$, the vector of ordinal responses for the ith experimental unit, $i = 1, \ldots, n$, and let $\mathbf{Z}_i = (Z_{i1}, \ldots, Z_{ik})$ represent the vector of corresponding latent variables, so that $V_{ij} = \ell \in \{1, \ldots, C_j\}$ if and only if $Z_{ij} \in (\gamma_{j,\ell-1}, \gamma_{j,\ell}]$. That is, $V_{ij} = V_{ij}(Z_{ij})$, is a deterministic function of the latent variables. The joint likelihood function is therefore entirely determined by whatever probability model we choose for $\mathbf{Z}_i$. Let $\phi_k(\mathbf{x} \mid \mathbf{m}, \mathbf{S})$ denote the p.d.f. of a k-variate normal distribution with moments $\mathbf{m}$ and $\mathbf{S}$. Kottas et al. (2005) use a DP mixture model

$$\mathbf{Z}_i \mid F \sim \int \phi_k(\mathbf{Z}_i \mid \mathbf{m}, \mathbf{S})\, dF(\mathbf{m}, \mathbf{S}), \tag{5.7}$$

and $F \mid M, F_0 \sim \mathsf{DP}(MF_0)$, with centering distribution F_0 defined as the joint distribution of independent multivariate normal and inverse Wishart random variables, $F_0(\mathbf{m}, \mathbf{S}) = \mathsf{N}(\mathbf{m} \mid \boldsymbol{\lambda}, \boldsymbol{\Sigma}) \times \mathsf{IWis}_k(\mathbf{S} \mid \nu, \mathbf{D})$. The model replaces the standard multivariate normal model by a DP location-scale mixture of normals. A practical consequence of this assumption is that now the distribution of the latent $\mathbf{Z}_i$'s can place mass in arbitrary ways. In particular, probability mass can be centered around multiple modes spread across the table. Tables with arbitrary classification probabilities can be represented as (5.7). The model is completed with

$$M \sim \mathsf{Ga}(a_0, b_0), \quad \boldsymbol{\lambda} \sim \mathsf{N}(\mathbf{q}, \mathbf{Q}),$$
$$\boldsymbol{\Sigma} \sim \mathsf{IWis}(b, \mathbf{B}), \text{ and } \mathbf{D} \sim \mathsf{IWis}(c, \mathbf{C}),$$

with fixed scalar hyperparameters ν, a_0, b_0, b, c, a k-dimensional vector $\mathbf{q}$, and $k \times k$ positive definite matrices $\mathbf{B}$, $\mathbf{C}$ and $\mathbf{Q}$. The hyper-priors are chosen to be of conjugate-style to simplify posterior simulation.

Example 11 (Teacher Evaluations) Bishop et al. (1975) discuss data arising from two different supervisors rating the classroom style of 72 student teachers. Specifically, they were asked to classify each teacher by degree of strictness as permissive,

5.1 Categorical Responses Without Covariates

Table 5.2 Example 11. Classification of student teachers as rated by two supervisors

Ratings by supervisor 1	Ratings by supervisor 2			
	Permissive	Democratic	Authoritarian	Total
Permissive	13	3	10	26
Democratic	0	12	5	17
Authoritarian	8	4	17	29
Total	21	19	32	72

democratic or authoritarian. The data originally appeared in Gross (1971) and are reproduced here in Table 5.2.

Kottas et al. (2005) propose default choices for the hyperparameters. In Example 11 with $k = 2$ ordinal variables, and $C_1 = C_2 = 3$ categories each, the default choices amount to $\gamma_{j,1} = -1$ and $\gamma_{j,2} = 0$, for $j = 1, 2$. The choice of the hyperparameters is guided by considering the limiting case $M \to 0$, when the model for the latent variables becomes parametric, with $Z_i \mid m, S \overset{iid}{\sim} N(m, S)$. Fixing m, B, C and Q we aim to specify a distribution for Z that is centered around the chosen cutoffs and covers the range of cutoffs. Note that the cutoffs γ_{jk} are centered around $m_\gamma = -0.5$, and their range can be characterized as $s_\gamma = 4$, which is four times $\gamma_{j,2} - \gamma_{j,1}$. Define $H = (s_\gamma/4)^2 I$ which reduces to the identity matrix I. We define the prior for m by matching its prior moments to the center and range previously defined, so that $q = (m_\gamma, m_\gamma)$ and $(b-k-1)^{-1}B + Q = 2H$, where an extra inflation factor of 2 was introduced in the right-hand side. For simplicity, we assume $(b-k-1)^{-1}B = Q = H$, and $b = k + 2 = 4$, the smallest integer value giving a finite mean. Also, since $E(S) = (\nu - k - 1)^{-1}cC$, we set $E(S) = H$, $\nu = 4$ and $c = k = 2$, which implies $C = \frac{1}{2}I$.

Posterior simulation is based on the usual MCMC posterior simulation methods for DP mixture models, as we discussed in Sect. 2.4. The only nonstandard transition probability is the resampling of the latent vector Z. For $V_i = (\ell_1, \ldots, \ell_k)$ the corresponding full conditional for Z_i is a multivariate normal truncated to the set $(\gamma_{1,\ell_1-1}, \gamma_{1,\ell_1}] \times \cdots \times (\gamma_{k,\ell_k-1}, \gamma_{k,\ell_k}]$. We can define a set of Gibbs sampling transition probabilities by noting that the distribution of each coordinate conditional on the others is a univariate normal, truncated to the corresponding interval. See further details in Kottas et al. (2005).

Example 11 (Teacher Evaluations, ctd.) We used the described default hyperparameter choices and implemented posterior simulation. We find that the posterior mode of the number of clusters was $k = 4$ (with posterior probability 0.256) and most of the mass concentrated between $k = 3$ and 6 clusters (0.8226). Table 5.3 summarizes the estimated cell probabilities for all possible combinations, including the observed relative frequencies to facilitate comparison.

Table 5.3 Example 11. Observed and fitted (in boldface) frequencies for students teachers example, including 95 % credibility intervals (in parentheses)

Ratings by supervisor 1	Ratings by supervisor 2		
	Permissive	Democratic	Authoritarian
Permissive	0.1806 **0.1816**	0.0417 **0.0414**	0.1389 **0.1356**
	(0.1709,0.1923)	(0.0359,0.0469)	(0.1261,0.1451)
Democratic	0.0000 **0.0018**	0.1667 **0.1672**	0.0694 **0.0652**
	(0.0006,0.0030)	(0.1569,0.1775)	(0.0584,0.0720)
Authoritarian	0.1111 **0.1168**	0.0556 **0.0600**	0.2361 **0.2308**
	(0.1079,0.1257)	(0.0534,0.0666)	(0.2191,0.2425)

One limitation of the model can be seen in Table 5.3: structural zeroes can not be accurately predicted in the sense that the model assigns positive albeit possibly very low probability to any cell. See, for example, the combination of categorical variables $(V_1, V_2) = (2, 1)$. Of course, this is only a concern if a particular combination were judged impossible. If a zero count could arise by sampling variation, then the shrinkage towards a positive prior mean is more appropriate. In this example, the estimated cell probability of 0.0018 is more reasonable than the exact zero maximum likelihood estimate.

5.2 Categorical Responses with Covariates

Many statistical inference problems involving categorical responses include covariates. In that case the sampling model for the categorical responses y_i should include a regression on these covariates. Assume then that for each of n experimental units, categorical responses $y_1, \ldots, y_n$ are recorded, together with a corresponding set of covariates $x_i = (x_{i1}, \ldots, x_{iq})$, $i = 1, \ldots, n$. We include here the possibility that $x_{i1} = 1$ for all i for an intercept term as in the usual regression-like models.

In a parametric context, a standard approach is to relate responses and covariates by means of a generalized linear model (GLM) (McCullagh and Nelder 1983). The distribution of responses y_i is assumed to be a member of the exponential family, and the mean responses $\mu_i = E(y_i)$ are related to a linear combination $x_i'\beta$ by means of

$$g(\mu_i) = \eta_i(\beta) = x_i'\beta. \tag{5.8}$$

Here, g is referred to as the *link function*, and it is defined in a possibly bounded space Ω, depending on the nature of the y_i. For example, for binary y_i we use $\Omega = [0, 1]$. In addition, we assume that g is a strictly increasing differentiable function.

Several approaches to introduce a semiparametric component into GLMs have been considered in the literature. The two most common ones involve a

5.2.1 Nonparametric Link Function: A Semiparametric GLM

Centrally Standardized DP Link Function Newton et al. (1996) consider the particular case of binary responses. They model the inverse link function as the c.d.f. of a random probability measure. This is possible, since the inverse link function for a binary response and under the usual monotonicity and smoothness assumptions can be interpreted as a c.d.f. We therefore denote g^{-1} simply as F and consider models of the form $p(y_i = 1 \mid \boldsymbol{\beta}) = F(\boldsymbol{x}_i'\boldsymbol{\beta})$. This can be rewritten equivalently in terms of a latent random variable V_i as

$$y_i = I\{V_i \leq \boldsymbol{x}_i'\boldsymbol{\beta}\} \quad \text{with} \quad V_i \sim F. \tag{5.9}$$

To verify, note that $p(y_i = 1 \mid \boldsymbol{\beta}) = p(V_i \leq \boldsymbol{x}_i'\boldsymbol{\beta}) = F(\boldsymbol{x}_i'\boldsymbol{\beta})$, as claimed. In the usual parametric case, F is assumed to be a known and fixed c.d.f. For instance, logistic regression arises when $F(t) = \exp(t)/(1 + \exp(t))$, probit regression corresponds to $F(t) = \Phi(t)$, the standard normal c.d.f. etc. Assume $\boldsymbol{x}_i'\boldsymbol{\beta}$ includes an intercept term. Then a nonparametric approach where F is an arbitrary c.d.f. would suffer from a double confounding. First, the intercept will be confounded with the location of F. Second, the overall scale of the elements of $\boldsymbol{\beta}$ will be confounded with the scale of F. Motivated by these considerations, Newton et al. (1996) proposed a nonparametric model for F subject to identifiability constraints. They restrict F to have median $F^{-1}(0.5) = 0$ and a central probability-p interval of length d. Using $p = 0.5$ the latter becomes a constraint on the inter-quartile range. In general

$$F^{-1}(0.5) = 0, \quad F^{-1}(0.5 - p/2) = \theta - d \quad \text{and} \quad F^{-1}(0.5 + p/2) = \theta,$$

for some fixed values $0 < p < 1$, $d > 0$ and $0 < \theta < d$. They modify the DP to generate distributions that satisfy these requirements, resulting in the *centrally standardized DP* (CSDP). For instance, when $p = 1/2$, every distribution F that satisfies the above restrictions would have zero median and inter-quartile range d. To do so, they start with a c.d.f. F_0 on the real line that has some positive mass outside $(-d, d)$, a positive constant M, and a probability density function h supported on $(0, d)$, e.g., the Uni$(0, d)$ distribution. Next, draw $\theta \sim h$ and partition $\mathbb{R}$ into four intervals

$$A_1(\theta) = (-\infty, \theta - d], \quad A_2(\theta) = (\theta - d, 0], \quad A_3(\theta) = (0, \theta], \quad A_4(\theta) = (\theta, \infty).$$

Define now four measures by restricting $m = M \times F_0$ to each of the A_j subsets, i.e., $m_j(B) = m(B \cap A_j(\theta))$, $j = 1, \ldots, 4$, and for any Borel set B. Note that the total mass of m_j is $M_j = M \times F_0(A_j(\theta))$ and that $F_{0j} = m_j/M_j$ is a c.d.f. on $A_j(\theta)$. With the above settings, define four independent DPs, $F_j \sim \mathsf{DP}(M_j, F_{0j})$. By construction the support of F_j is restricted to A_j. Finally, we paste them together to get a CSDP as

$$F(\cdot) = \frac{1-p}{2}(F_1(\cdot) + F_4(\cdot)) + \frac{p}{2}(F_2(\cdot) + F_3(\cdot)). \tag{5.10}$$

We denote this by $F \sim \mathsf{CSDP}(m, p, d, h)$. It follows (Newton et al. 1996) that any $F \sim \mathsf{CSDP}(m, p, d, h)$ satisfies the desired constrains and will therefore be suitable for a random link function model.

Example 12 (Unemployment Data) We consider unemployment data from the R package `catdata`. The data are discussed in Tutz (2012). We use the complete set of $n = 982$ observations and two variables: age of the person in years (from 16 to 61, AGE) and a binary indicator of short-term (0) or long-term (1) unemployment (UNEMP). We are interested in studying the effect of $x_i = $ AGE on $y_i = $ UNEMP. Using the previous notation, we take $q = 2$ and $\eta_i(\boldsymbol{\beta}) = \beta_0 + \beta_1 x_i$.

The model proposed in Newton et al. (1996) is implemented in `DPpackage` as the function `CSDPbinary`. The function implements inference in the model

$$y_i = I\{V_i \leq x_i^t \boldsymbol{\beta}\} \quad \text{with} \quad V_i \mid F \stackrel{\text{iid}}{\sim} F, \tag{5.11}$$

and prior $F \sim \mathsf{CSDP}(m, p, d, h)$. The model specification is completed with

$$\boldsymbol{\beta} \mid \boldsymbol{\beta}_0, S \sim \mathsf{N}(\boldsymbol{\beta}_0, S).$$

A prior on M, e.g, $M \sim \mathsf{Ga}(a_0, b_0)$ could be also adopted.

Example 12 (Unemployment Data, ctd.) We implement inference using the R function `CSDPbinary`. We fix $F_0(t)$ to be the logistic distribution and use $d = 2\log(3)$. Under F_0 the mass outside the interval $[-d, d]$ is $1 - (F_0(d) - F_0(-d)) = 0.2$. Next we let h be the uniform distribution on $(0, d)$. We set $p = 0.5$, that is, the centralization is on the median and interquartile range, and $\boldsymbol{\beta}_0 = (0, 0)$ and $S = \mathrm{diag}(100, 100)$.

Figure 5.2 summarizes the resulting inference for the unemployment data. Most of the marginal posterior mass of β_0 is on the negative numbers, which is explained by the fact that most of the cases reported short-term unemployment, that is, $y_i = 0$ (640 out of 982, or 34.83%). Most of the posterior marginal mass for β_1 is on the positive numbers, suggesting that long-term unemployment tends to increase with age. Panel (c) shows the estimated random link function (solid line), including 95% pointwise credible bands. For comparison, also the centering logistic distribution function (dashed line) is shown. The two curves are similar, but model (5.11) allows inference on the uncertainty of the link function (shown as light grey margins). Finally, panel (d) shows the mean posterior predictive probabilities of long-term unemployment for all available individuals in the sample (solid line). For comparison, the figure also includes the m.l.e. in a simple parametric

5.2 Categorical Responses with Covariates

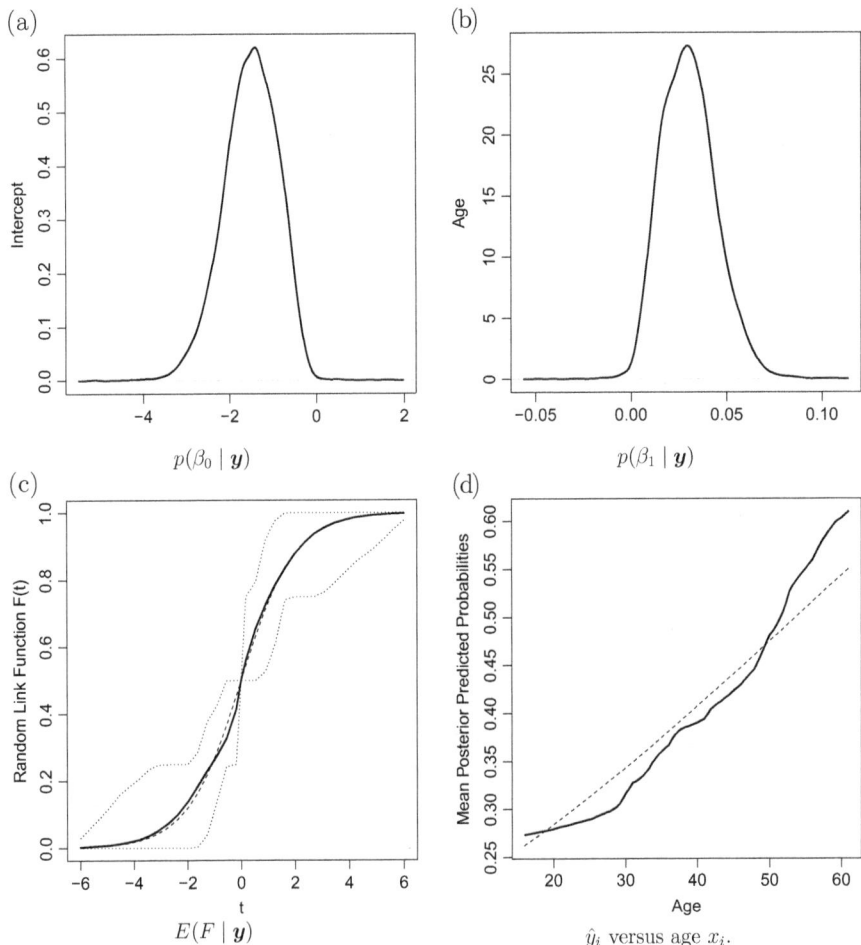

Fig. 5.2 Example 12. Panels (**a**) and (**b**) show the marginal posterior densities $p(\beta_0 \mid y)$ (*left*) and $p(\beta_1 \mid y)$ (*right*). Panel (**c**) shows the estimated random link function $E(F \mid y)$ with 95 % (point wise) posterior credible bands. Panel (**d**) shows the fitted posterior predictive probabilities of long-term unemployment for all individuals in the sample, plotted against age

logistic regression model (dashed line). The CSDP-based model captures substantial deviations from the simple logistic regression. The largest differences occur around the median age (27 years) and around the maximum age (61 years).

Software note: See the software appendix to this chapter for R code for Example 12.

A Mixture of Beta Link Function Mallick and Gelfand (1994) discuss an interesting alternative to a BNP prior on the link function. They consider a model for the *inverse link function*, that is, the function g^{-1} based on a (transformed) finite mixture of beta c.d.f.'s. Their approach is defined for general Ω, using an additional mapping T to map from a general Ω into $[0, 1]$ if needed. Let $J(\eta) = T(g^{-1}(\eta))$ denote the inverse link function with the possibly additional mapping T. They model $J(\cdot)$ as a mixture of r beta c.d.f.'s. The construction is centered around a baseline link function $g_0(\cdot)$. Letting $J_0(\eta) = T(g_0^{-1}(\eta))$, Mallick and Gelfand (1994) propose the model

$$J(\eta) = \sum_{\ell=1}^{r} w_\ell \mathsf{IB}(J_0(\eta); a_\ell, b_\ell), \qquad (5.12)$$

where $w_1, \ldots, w_r$ are nonnegative weights such that $\sum_{\ell=1}^{r} w_\ell = 1$, and $\mathsf{IB}(u; a, b)$ is the incomplete beta function associated to the beta density $\mathsf{Be}(u; a, b)$, that is, $\mathsf{IB}(u; a, b) = \int_0^u \mathsf{Be}(t; a, b) \, dt$ for $a, b > 0$, and $0 \le u \le 1$.

The representation as a finite mixture of beta functions is motivated by Diaconis and Ylvisaker (1985), who argue that discrete mixtures of beta densities form a dense class of models for densities on the unit interval. Following this argument, the proposal in (5.12) constructs a semiparametric model by treating a transformed inverse link function as part of the rich class of mixtures of incomplete beta functions.

Generalized Additive Models An alternative to random links is the use of generalized additive models (GAM), described in Sect. 4.3.2. A GAM essentially considers a transformation of each of the p predictors $\mathbf{x}_i = (x_{i1}, \ldots, x_{ip})'$ in a GLM simultaneously. Such models can be fit in the `gam` function in `DPpackage` or the freely-available `BayesX` package.

5.2.2 Models for Latent Scores

In Sect. 5.2.1 we introduced a regression on covariates in the linear predictor of a GLM and then proceeded with nonparametric extensions of the link function. We discuss an alternative interpretation of the same nonparametric model that arises from the following construction. Instead of targeting the link function we now focus on the distribution of the latent scores. Of course, the two are mathematically equivalent, as can be seen from (5.9). Jara et al. (2006) considered the following model formulation

$$y_i = I\{Z_i \le \mathbf{x}_i'\boldsymbol{\beta}\} \quad \text{with} \quad Z_i \mid F \overset{\text{iid}}{\sim} F, \quad F \sim \mathsf{DP}(M, F_0), \qquad (5.13)$$

$i = 1, \ldots, n$, and where F_0 may be taken to be the standard normal, logistic or Cauchy distributions. Similarly, Hanson (2006) considers a PT for the random link F, with first and second quartiles fixed; this model can be fit via FPTbinary in DPpackage. Again, the idea in these constructions is to center the nonparametric model on the usual parametric models. The CSDP process and the PT-based approach of Hanson (2006) address the confounding issue related to location and scale of the random probability measure F.

Example 12 (Unemployment Data ctd.) We consider again the data from Example 12, this time under model (5.13). The model is completed with priors

$$\boldsymbol{\beta} \mid \boldsymbol{\beta}_0, \boldsymbol{S} \sim \mathsf{N}(\boldsymbol{\beta}_0, \boldsymbol{S}) \quad \text{and} \quad M \sim \mathsf{Ga}(a_0, b_0).$$

Figure 5.3 shows the marginal posterior distribution of the regression coefficients β_0 and β_1 and the estimated link function $F(t)$. The plot shows results under three different choices for the centering distribution F_0, including a logistic (solid line), normal (dashed line) or Cauchy (dotted line) distribution. For more comparison, we also include the earlier results under the CSDP model (semi-dotted line). Table 5.4 shows some posterior summaries of the regression coefficients for the four models considered here. The centering distribution F_0 plays a key role in the reported inferences. Comparing the effect of different F_0 choices we see non-negligible shifts in the posterior distributions. A more concentrated F_0 tends to produce more concentrated posterior distributions, specially for the intercept coefficient β_0. This concentration is also notable when comparing models (5.13) and (5.10) with a logistic F_0. A possible explanation is the confounding problem mentioned above, which is addressed by the CSDP construction, but not by the DP-based model.

Model (5.13) can be extended in many possible ways. Jara et al. (2007), for example, considered the case of multiple binary responses for each individual. The

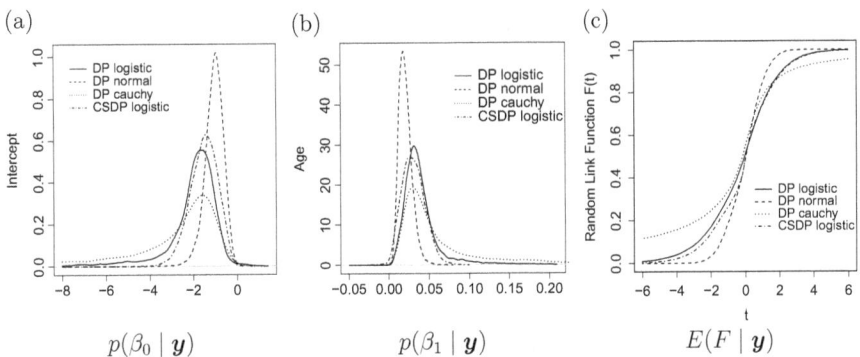

Fig. 5.3 Example 12. Panels (**a**) and (**b**) show the posterior marginal distributions of intercept β_0 and slope β_1. Panel (**c**) shows the estimated link function. Each plot shows inference under model (5.13), with F_0 equal to a logistic (*solid line*), normal (*dashed line*) or Cauchy (*dotted line*) distributions. For comparison, we also include the corresponding earlier results, under model (5.10) (*semi-dotted line*)

Table 5.4 Example 12. Posterior summaries for unemployment data

Model	β_0			β_1		
	Mean	C.I.	SD	Mean	C.I.	SD
DP logistic	−2.076	(−6.082,−0.608)	1.325	0.039	(0.012,0.103)	0.022
DP normal	−1.045	(−1.986,−0.331)	0.423	0.021	(0.008,0.039)	0.008
DP Cauchy	−3.366	(−11.716,−0.658)	2.880	0.060	(0.014,0.207)	0.051
CSDP	−1.525	(−2.877,−0.445)	0.632	0.030	(0.006,0.059)	0.014

For each of the models indicated in the rows, we show the posterior mean, 95 % credibility interval and standard deviation of each of the two regression coefficients β_0 and β_1

approach involves a matching vector $\mathbf{Z} = (Z_{i1}, \ldots, Z_{ik})$ of latent scores from which the binary responses $\mathbf{y}_i = (y_{i1}, \ldots, y_{ik})$ are obtained as $y_{ij} = I\{Z_{ij} \leq 0\}$ for all $j = 1, \ldots, k$ and $i = 1, \ldots, n$. Their proposal considers a flexible model for the latent score vectors $\mathbf{Z}_1, \ldots, \mathbf{Z}_n$, which may be thought of as a multivariate extension of model (5.13).

5.2.3 Nonparametric Random Effects Model

A traditional and very common use of nonparametric models involves the modeling of random effects in various settings. Later, in Chap. 7, we will discuss nonparametric random effects models as an example of hierarchical models. Below we briefly consider the special case of random effects models that arise as a generalization of GLM's. Consider a GLM with data that are arranged in groups, in the sense that groups of outcomes are related to each other, e.g. as in longitudinal studies or in experiments with multiple measurements on a given group of individuals. To account for correlation within each group, Zeger and Karim (1991) considered a *generalized linear mixed model* (GLMM), where cluster-specific random effects induce the desired correlation among responses in each group. Let $\mu_{ij} = E(y_{ij})$, let g denote a link function, and let $\mathbf{x}_{ij}$ and $\mathbf{z}_{ij}$ denote design vectors for fixed and random effects, respectively. Zeger and Karim (1991) assume

$$g(\mu_{ij}) = \mathbf{x}'_{ij}\boldsymbol{\beta} + \mathbf{z}'_{ij}\mathbf{b}_i, \quad j = 1, \ldots, n_i, \quad i = 1, \ldots, n \quad (5.14)$$

with group-specific random effects $\mathbf{b}_i$. Here i indexes groups of data, e.g., all repeat measurements on patient i, and j indexes observations within each group. A standard distributional assumption for the random effects $\mathbf{b}_i$ is a multivariate normal model. The assumption is usually motivated only by computational convenience. Many applications involve heterogeneous populations of experimental units, such as heterogeneous patient populations, that would more appropriately be modeled with multimodal random effects distributions. Similarly, outliers are better accommodated with more general random effects distributions. These considerations led many investigators to propose semi-parametric generalizations of GLMMs.

A standard approach is to replace the multivariate normal distribution assumptions by a nonparametric alternative. Kleinman and Ibrahim (1998) considered a DP-based approach with

$$b_i \mid F \stackrel{iid}{\sim} F, \quad F \sim \mathsf{DP}(M, F_0), \qquad (5.15)$$

where F_0 is the $\mathsf{N}(0, D)$ multivariate normal distribution in the appropriate space, i.e., the nonparametric model is a priori centered at the parametric proposal in Zeger and Karim (1991). It is straightforward to generalize F_0 to a $\mathsf{N}(\mu, D)$ distribution, with an additional hyperprior on both μ and D, like in (2.8).

Model (5.14) and (5.15) gives rise to identifiability problems when some random effects are paired with corresponding fixed effects, that is, $z_{ijk} = x_{ij\ell}$ for some k, ℓ (Li et al. 2011). The problem originates in the fact that the DP prior implies a non-zero mean for the random effects distribution. For a more detailed description of the mean of a DP, see Hjort and Ongaro (2005). This creates an interpretation problem, and complicates inference. Li et al. (2011) solve the problem by adjusting inference using a post-processing technique based on an analytic evaluation of the moments of the random moments of the DP. Jara et al. (2009) propose an alternative approach modeling the random effects distribution with a PT prior. They also consider a simple extension of the Kleinman and Ibrahim (1998) model which consists of replacing the DP by a DP mixture, based in turn on an earlier proposal by Müller and Rosner (1997) in the context of random effects models.

Example 13 (Epilepsy Trial) Thall and Vail (1990) consider data from a clinical trial on epilepsy. The data consist of sequences of seizure counts in each of the 2 week intervals between four consecutive occasions, $j = 1, \ldots, 3$, for $n = 59$ epileptic patients, randomly assigned to treatment with progabide or to placebo. These data have been considered by many authors, including Breslow and Clayton (1993), Diggle et al. (1994) and Jara et al. (2009). Let y_{ij} denote the number of epileptic seizures for the ith patient in the jth period. Additional baseline covariates include the seizure counts in the 8-week period prior to the trial (CT8), and age at the beginning of the trial (AGE). We introduce a binary indicator x_{i1} for treatment assignment (TRT) with $x_{i1} = 1$ if patient i was assigned to progabide and 0 otherwise. Let $x_{i2} = \log(CT8_i/4)$ and $x_{i3} = \log(AGE_i)$. Finally, let $x_{j4} = 1$ if $j = 4$ and 0 otherwise be an indicator of the fourth visit. We consider here a variation of model III in Breslow and Clayton (1993). We start by assuming Poisson-distributed responses y_{ij} with

$$\log[E(y_{ij})] = \beta_0 + \beta_1 x_{i1} + \beta_2 x_{i2} + \beta_3 x_{i3} + \beta_4 x_{j4} + \beta_5 x_{i1} x_{i2} + b_i. \qquad (5.16)$$

The model includes main effects for the covariates, plus an interaction of treatment and previous number of seizures. Also, the indicator for the fourth visit was added to account for the notable decay of counts in the 2 weeks prior to the fourth visit. The model also includes a subject-specific random effect b_i which introduces correlation across the repeated measurements for each patient. The data are given in Thall and

Vail (1990) and are also available as part of the Examples Guide in OpenBUGS software (Lunn et al. 2009).

Software note: Inference for model (5.15) is implemented in the function DPglmm in DPpackage. The function assumes model (5.16) and (5.15) where in this case, F_0 is a univariate normal distribution with mean μ and variance D. To complete the model specification, DPglmm assumes

$$M \sim \text{Ga}(a_0, b_0), \quad \boldsymbol{\beta} \sim \text{N}(\boldsymbol{\beta}_0, S_0),$$
$$\mu \sim \text{N}(\mu_b, S_b), \quad D \sim \text{IWis}(\nu_0, T),$$

where the inverse Wishart distribution is parametrized in such a way that $E(D) = T^{-1}/(\nu_0 - 2)$.

Figure 5.4b–f shows the marginal posterior distribution for the fixed effects specified in model (5.16) (solid line). For comparison, we also include results under a

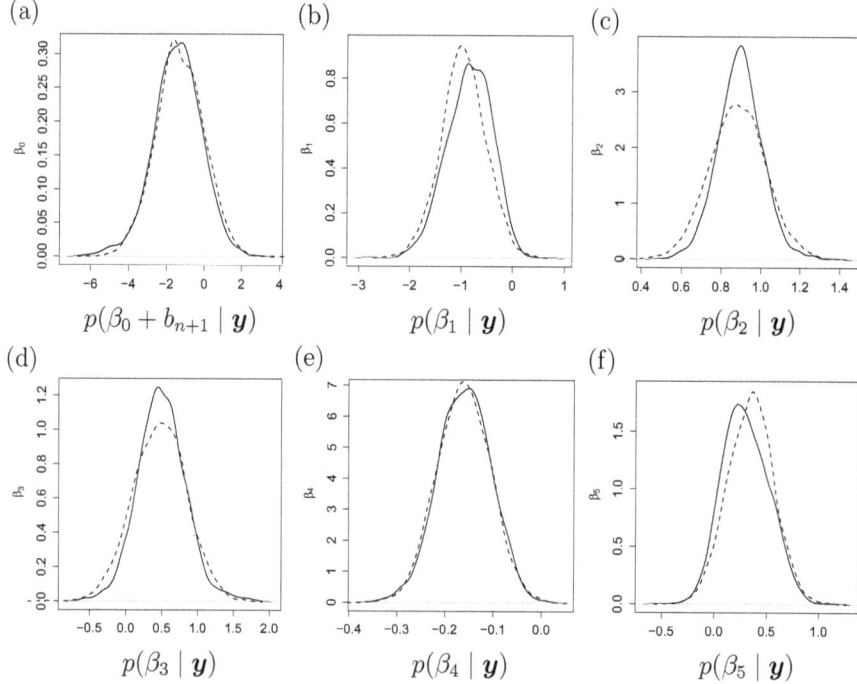

Fig. 5.4 Example 13. Panels (**b**)–(**f**) show the marginal posterior distribution $p(\beta_j \mid \boldsymbol{y})$ for the fixed effects $\beta_1, \ldots, \beta_5$ for the nonparametric model (*solid line*), together with the corresponding results for a parametric model (*dashed line*). Panel (**a**) shows the posterior predictive distribution of random effects (*solid line*), together with the intercept term for the parametric model (*dashed line*)

corresponding parametric model (dashed line) that uses the multivariate normal baseline F_0 of (5.15) as a random effects distribution. Panel (a) in the same figure shows the posterior predictive distribution of a new random effect, $p(b_{n+1} \mid y)$ together with the intercept term in the parametric model. Generally speaking, inference for $\beta_1, \ldots, \beta_5$ is similar under the two models. The non-parametric model (5.16) tends to produce slightly less dispersed distributions. Inference in both models agrees in finding a treatment effect. Treated patients have a lower expected number of seizure counts than placebo patients, as determined by the fact that most of the posterior mass in $p(\beta_1 \mid y)$ is on $\beta_1 < 0$. Finally, we use log-pseudo marginal likelihood statistics (LPML) (Geisser and Eddy 1979) for an overall model comparison of model (5.16) versus the corresponding parametric model. We find only a minor difference in LPML scores, with -669.9741 for the parametric case and -669.9499 for the nonparametric version.

Software note: The software appendix to this chapter shows R code with the call to the `DPglmm` function of `DPpackage`.

5.2.4 Multivariate Ordinal Regression

Recall the DP mixture of multivariate ordinal probit model (5.7). Bao and Hanson (2015) generalize the model to accommodate predictors. The data are $\{(x_i, V_i)\}_{i=1}^n$ where $x_i = (x_{i1}, \ldots, x_{ip})'$ are the predictors for subject i. Bao and Hanson (2015) replace the normal kernel in (5.7) by a normal linear regression,

$$Z_i \mid x_i, F \sim \int \phi_k(Z_i \mid X_i\beta, S) \, dF(\beta, S) \quad (5.17)$$

Here, $X_i = \text{block-diag}(x'_{i1}, \ldots, x'_{ik})$ is a design matrix allowing for different predictors to affect each of the k ordinal responses. The hyperpriors are largely the same as before. Model (5.17) is a multivariate version of the LDDP model (4.12) that we already saw in Sect. 4.4.2.

Example 14 (New Mexican DWI Offenders) McMillan et al. (2005) consider bivariate ordinal data on drinking behavior. The Lovelace Comprehensive Screening Instrument (LCSI) was given to over 2000 driving-while-intoxicated (DWI) offenders mandated by the court to undergo screening. Among other topics, the LCSI asks offenders questions about psychological issues, drug and alcohol use, and sexual abuse history. The study sample includes $n = 1964$ offenders who completed the LCSI and were self-reported beer drinkers. Subjects were asked "*How many times each month do you drink beer?*" and could reply that they drank beer "*up to 1–2 times per month,*" "*a few times per month,*" "*a few times per week,*" or "*almost daily;*" these correspond to $V_{i1} = 1, 2, 3, 4$ respectively. Respondents also were asked, "*How much beer do you drink?*" and specified the quantity of beer consumed per drinking occasion as "*1,*" "*2–3,*" "*4–5*" or "*6 or more*" beers, corresponding to $V_{i2} = 1, 2, 3, 4$ respectively. In addition, subjects were asked, *"When you were growing up, were you ever sexually abused or molested by anyone?"* ($x_{i1} = 0$ for no and $x_{i1} = 1$ for yes). Because beer is the primary source of alcohol intoxication among DWI offenders, interest is in how history of sexual abuse as a child, along with gender ($x_{i2} = 0$ for female and $x_{i2} = 1$ male) and age ($x_{i3} = 0$ for ≤ 30 years old and $x_{i3} = 1$ for > 30), is associated with current beer-drinking patterns.

Model (5.17) was fit to these data; Fig. 5.5 shows the fitted densities $p(Z_{n+1} \mid x_{n+1})$ on frequency and quantity. The fitted density is obtained by averaging (5.17) with respect to the posterior on F. Note that having been abused places more mass into frequency 4 (almost daily) across all four levels of age and gender. The nonparametric models were grossly preferred over parametric models, judging by the log pseudo marginal likelihood criterion of Geisser and Eddy (1979).

5.3 ROC Curve Estimation

A widely-used application of binary regression models is diagnostic screening: the classification of individuals y based on predictors x into one of two mutually exclusive categories, often "diseased" ($y = 1$) or "non-diseased" ($y = 0$). Initially consider univariate $x = x$. Each individual has an associated biomarker x (e.g. ELISA test, cholesterol level, age, etc.) such that increased values of x increase the probability of disease, yielding data $\{(x_i, y_i)\}_{i=1}^n$. These can be viewed as training data for classification, with the ultimate goal to accurately choose between $\hat{y}_{n+1} = 0$ and $\hat{y}_{n+1} = 1$ based on a new biomarker value x_{n+1}. Assume that the biomarker x has c.d.f. F_1 among the diseased and c.d.f. F_0 among the non-diseased. A threshold t is used to classify disease via the biomarker value x through $y = I\{x > t\}$. The sensitivity of the test is $se(t) = p(x > t \mid y = 1) = 1 - F_1(t)$, the probability of a true positive. The specificity of the test is the probability of a true negative $sp(t) = p(x < t \mid y = 0) = F_0(t)$.

A receiver-operator characteristic (ROC) curve plots the probability of a true positive $se(t)$ versus the probability of a false positive $1 - sp(t)$ across all t. The area under the ROC curve (AUC) can be shown to be the probability that a randomly selected diseased individual will have a value of x larger than a randomly selected non-diseased individual. The AUC is unity when the supports of F_0 and F_1 do not overlap, i.e. diseased and non-diseased scores x are perfectly separated; this yields an ROC curve of 1 across $(0, 1)$. The closer an ROC curve is to 1, the better the discriminatory ability of the biomarker. ROC curves and associated AUC summarize the diagnostic utility of a biomarker x for discriminating among diseased and non-diseased across all decision rules, independent of the prevalence of the disease in the general population. Empirical estimates are often used to estimate F_0 and F_1 as $\hat{F}_0 = \frac{1}{n_0} \sum_{i:y_i=0} I\{x_i \leq t\}$ and $\hat{F}_1 = \frac{1}{n_1} \sum_{i:y_i=1} I\{x_i \leq t\}$ where $n_0 = \sum_{i=1}^n I\{y_i = 0\}$ and $n_1 = \sum_{i=1}^n I\{y_i = 1\}$ are the number of non-diseased and diseased in the

5.3 ROC Curve Estimation

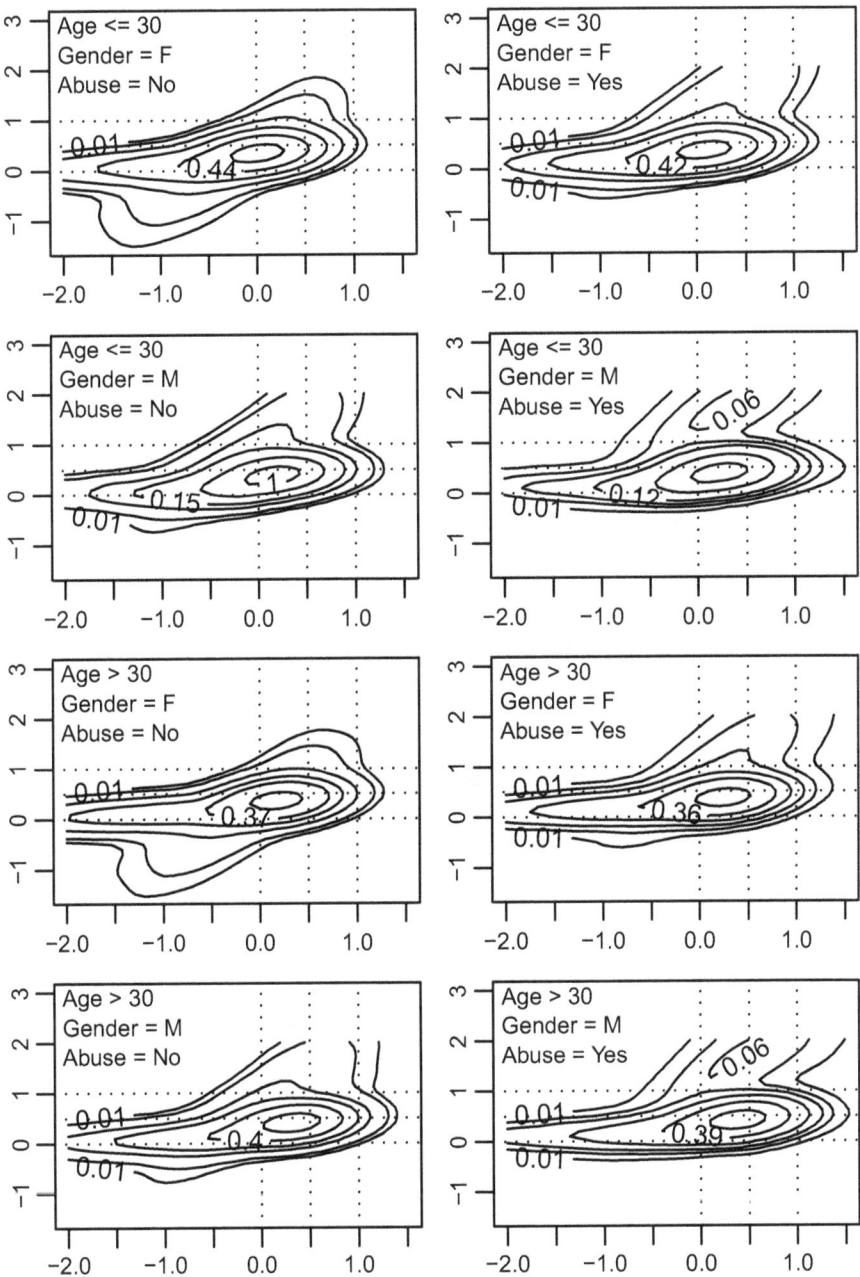

Fig. 5.5 Latent bivariate traits underlying drinking frequency (x-axis) and frequency (y-axis) for different groups

sample, respectively. This defines the empirical ROC curve $(1 - \hat{F}_0(t), 1 - \hat{F}_1(t))$ plotted for all t.

Model-based approaches to ROC curve estimation posit independent probability models for F_0 and F_1, for example MPT or DPM. Branscum et al. (2008) consider MPT models for F_0 and F_1 under various scenarios; Hanson et al. (2008) generalize a single biomarker to multiple, i.e. multivariate F_0 and F_1; and Hanson et al. (2008) compare MPT to DPM models for ROC estimation enforcing a stochastic ordering constraint on the diseased and non-diseased subpopulations. DPpackage includes DProc for simple ROC estimation using DPM of normals.

Example 15 (Sperm Deformity Index) This example follows the DPpackage documentation for DProc. The sperm deformity index (SDI) was recorded from $n = 158$ men who took part in an infertility study. The event of interest is whether each male's partner *did not* become pregnant. Greater values of the SDI increase the likelihood of pregnancy not being achieved.

DProc provides posterior p.d.f. and c.d.f. estimates for F_0 and F_1, an optimal threshold t_o suggested by Kraemer (1992), as well as the estimated ROC curve with the error rates cleanly illustrated at the optimal threshold $(1 - \hat{F}_0(t_o), 1 - \hat{F}_1(t_o))$. Figure 5.6 shows the estimated ROC curve from DPpackage's DProc function following the DPpackage documentation. Superimposed is the nonparametric estimate; this is also the estimate from a logistic regression fit from regressing pregnancy outcome onto SDI.

Software note: See the on-line software page for this chapter for R code.

So far we assumed a univariate predictor x_i. In general, let z_i denote a covariate vector (reserving x_i in anticipation of the upcoming argument). A simple trick reduces the general case again to the same univariate setting. Let $\hat{\pi}_i = 1/\{1 + \exp(-\hat{\boldsymbol{\beta}}' z_i)\}$ denote a logistic regression of y_i on z_i and use $x_i = \hat{\pi}_i$ as a composite

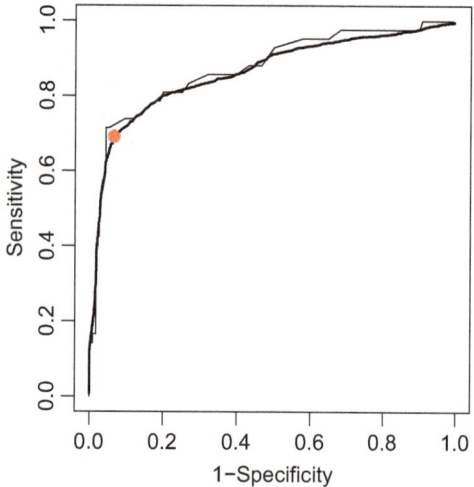

Fig. 5.6 DProc function ROC curve for evaluating the use of SDI in predicting pregnancy

"biomarker" and proceed as before. Thresholds $t \in (0, 1)$ are then introduced to classify subjects as diseased or non-diseased as before. That is, $\hat{\pi} > t$ implies diseased and $\hat{\pi} < t$ implies non-diseased. Then the empirical sensitivity and specificity is $\widehat{se}(t) = \frac{1}{n_1}\sum_{i:y_i=1} I\{\hat{\pi}_i > t\}$ and $\widehat{sp}(t) = \frac{1}{n_0}\sum_{i:y_i=0} I\{\hat{\pi}_i < t\}$. Note that any monotone transformation of x_i gives the same ROC curve, including $x_i = \boldsymbol{\beta}'\boldsymbol{z}_i$. These types of ROC curves are automatically provided by standard statistical software.

Also model-based estimation of ROC curves can use covariates beyond a univariate biomarker. The prior on F_0 and F_1 can be defined to depend on additional covariates, producing so-called covariate-adjusted ROC curves; these ROC curves exhibit how a biomarker's ability to discriminate changes with predictors. The DPpackage function LDDProc nicely ties together separate LDDPdensity fits to the diseased and non-diseased subpopulations, allowing for easy estimation, evaluation of covariate-dependent ROC curves, etc. This function was developed and illustrated in de Carvalho et al. (2013).

References

Albert JH, Chib S (1993) Bayesian analysis of binary and polychotomous response data. J Am Stat Assoc 88:669–679

Albright SC (1993) A statistical analysis of hitting streaks in baseball. J Am Stat Assoc 88:1175–1183

Bao J, Hanson T (2015) Bayesian nonparametric multivariate ordinal regression. Can J Stat (in press)

Bishop YMM, Fienberg SE, Holland PW (1975) Discrete multivariate analyses: theory and practice. MIT Press, Cambridge

Branscum A, Johnson W, Hanson T, Gardner I (2008) Bayesian semiparametric ROC curve estimation and disease risk assessment. Stat Med 27:2474–2496

Breslow NE, Clayton D (1993) Approximate inference in generealized linear models. J Am Stat Assoc 88:9–25

de Carvalho V, Jara A, Hanson T, de Carvalho M (2013) Bayesian nonparametric ROC regression modeling. Bayesian Anal 8:623–646

Diaconis P, Ylvisaker D (1985) Quantifying prior opinion. In: Bayesian statistics, vol 2 (Valencia, 1983). North-Holland, Amsterdam, pp 133–156 (with discussion and a reply by Diaconis)

Diggle PJ, Liang KY, Zeger SL (1994) Analysis of longitudinal data. Oxford University Press, Oxford

Geisser S, Eddy W (1979) A predictive approach to model selection. J Am Stat Assoc 74:153–160

Gross P (1971) A study of supervisor reliability. Mimeograph, Laboratory of Human Development. Harvard Graduate School of Education, Cambridge

Hanson T, Kottas A, Branscum A (2008) Modelling stochastic order in the analysis of receiver operating characteristic data: Bayesian nonparametric approaches. J R Stat Soc Ser C 57:207–225

Hanson TE (2006) Inference for mixtures of finite Polya tree models. J Am Stat Assoc 101(476):1548–1565

Hjort NL, Ongaro A (2005) Exact inference for random Dirichlet means. Stat Infer Stoch Process (An International Journal Devoted to Time Series Analysis and the Statistics of Continuous Time Processes and Dynamical Systems) 8(3):227–254

Jara A, García-Zattera MJ, Lesaffre E (2006) Semiparametric Bayesian analysis of misclassified binary data. In: XXIII international biometric conference, July 16–21, Montréal, Canada

Jara A, García-Zattera MJ, Lesaffre E (2007) A Dirichlet process mixture model for the analysis of correlated binary responses. Comput Stat Data Anal 51:5402–5415

Jara A, Hanson T, Lesaffre E (2009) Robustifying generalized linear mixed models using a new class of mixture of multivariate Polya trees. J Comput Graph Stat 18:838–860

Johnson VE, Albert JH (1999) Ordinal data modeling. Springer, New York

Kleinman KP, Ibrahim JG (1998) A semi-parametric Bayesian approach to generalized linear mixed models. Stat Med 17:2579–2596

Kottas A, Müller P, Quintana FA (2005) Nonparametric Bayesian modeling for multivariate ordinal data. J Comput Graph Stat 14:610–625

Kraemer HC (1992) Evaluating medical tests. Sage Publications, Newbury Park

Li Y, Müller P, Lin X (2011) Center-adjusted inference for a nonparametric Bayesian random effect distribution. Stat Sin 21(3):1201–1223

Liu JS (1996) Nonparametric hierarchical Bayes via sequential imputations. Ann Stat 24:911–930

Lunn D, Spiegelhalter D, Thomas A, Best N (2009) The BUGS project: Evolution, critique and future directions (Pkg: P3049–3082). Stat Med 28(25):3049–3067

Mallick BK, Gelfand AE (1994) Generalized linear models with unknown link functions. Biometrika 81(2):237–245

McCullagh P, Nelder JA (1983) Generalized linear models. Monographs on statistics and applied probability. Chapman & Hall, London

McMillan G, Hanson T, Bedrick E, Lapham S (2005) Using the bivariate Dale model to jointly estimate predictors of frequency and quantity of alcohol use. J Stud Alcohol 65:643–650

Morton AQ (1978) Literary detection. Scribner's, New York

Müller P, Rosner G (1997) A Bayesian population model with hierarchical mixture priors applied to blood count data. J Am Stat Assoc 92:1279–1292

Newton MA, Czado C, Chapell R (1996) Bayesian inference for semiparametric binary regression. J Am Stat Assoc 91:142–153

Olsson U (1979) Maximum likelihood estimation of the polychoric correlation coefficient. Psychometrika 44:443–460

Quintana FA (1998) Nonparametric Bayesian analysis for assessing homogeneity in $k \times l$ contingency tables with fixed right margin totals. J Am Stat Assoc 93:1140–1149

Rice JA (1995) Mathematical statistics and data analysis, 2nd edn. Duxbury Press, Belmont

Ronning G, Kukuk M (1996) Efficient estimation of ordered probit models. J Am Stat Assoc 91:1120–1129

Thall PF, Vail SC (1990) Some covariance models for longitudinal count data with overdispersion. Biometrics 46:657–671

Tutz G (2012) Regression for categorical data. Cambridge series in statistical and probabilistic mathematics, vol 34. Cambridge University Press, Cambridge

Zeger SL, Karim MR (1991) Generalized linear models with random effects: a Gibbs sampling approach. J Am Stat Assoc 86:79–86

Chapter 6
Survival Analysis

Abstract Inference for event time data is one of the most traditional applications of nonparametric Bayesian inference. For survival data, especially in biomedical applications, it is natural to focus on inference for detailed features of the survival function rather than only summaries like mean and variance. We extensively discuss semi- and nonparametric Bayesian methods for survival regression. Inference for such data has been traditionally dominated by the proportional hazards model. We review in detail nonparametric Bayesian alternatives which we introduce as natural generalizations of a parametric accelerated failure time model. We conclude with a discussion of three case studies.

6.1 Distribution Estimation for Event Times

A special case of density estimation arises in survival analysis as density estimation with event time data, usually involving censoring. Survival analysis is a very traditional application of BNP in the early literature. Any of the earlier discussed models for density estimation can be used for event time data, including DP, DP mixtures, PT, etc. In the following example we use a mixture of finite PTs (MPT) and a DP prior to estimate an event time distribution.

Example 2 (Oral Cancer, ctd.) Let F denote the unknown distribution of survival times for patients with aneuploid cancers, that is, we assume $T_i \mid F \sim F$, $i = 1, \ldots, n_0$. We consider a mixture of finite PT prior, $F \sim \mathsf{MPT}$ (see Sect. 3.2.1) with $c = 0.1$ and $J = 4$ levels (Hanson 2006a). Let $S(t) = p(T \leq t)$ denote the survival function. Figure 6.1a shows the estimated survival curve $E\{S(t) \mid data\}$, together with pointwise approximate 80 % CIs. The model is fit via the MCMC algorithm described in Hanson (2006a). Alternatively, we fit a DP model, $F \sim \mathsf{DP}(M, F^\star)$. The centering distribution $F^\star$ is fixed as an exponential model with m.l.e. rate and the DP mass parameter is $M = 1$. Figure 6.1b shows the estimated survival curves under the DP prior.

Software note: R code for the fit under the DP prior is available at this chapter's software page on-line.

Besides the PT and DP models, many other priors for baseline hazard, cumulative hazard, or survival functions have been successfully employed over the last 20

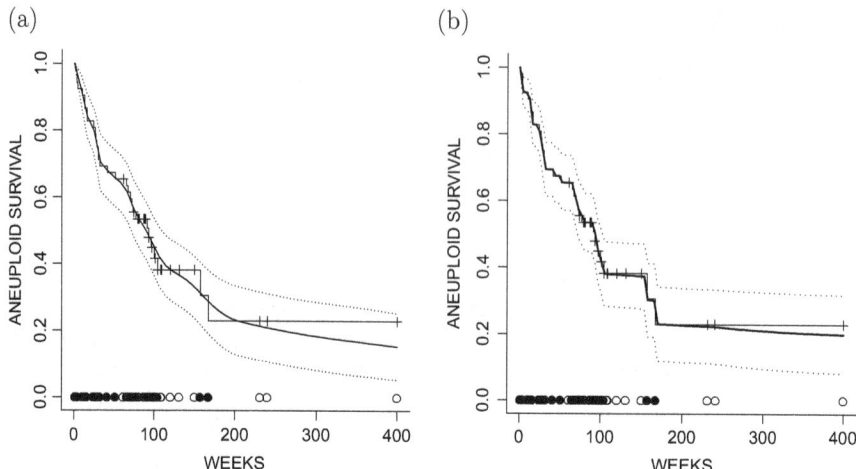

Fig. 6.1 Example 2. Estimated survival curve $E[S(t) \mid data]$ for the aneuploid group assuming a finite MPT (*left panel*) and assuming a DP prior (*right panel*) as prior for the unknown distribution F of survival times. The *two dotted curves* show pointwise 80 % credible intervals. For comparison the figures also show a Kaplan-Meier plot of the observed event times. The event (censoring) times are also shown as filled (open) *circles* along the x-axis. (**a**) $F \sim$ MPT. (**b**) $F \sim$ DP

years. Recent reviews appear in Sinha and Dey (1997), Ibrahim et al. (2001), and Hanson et al. (2005). Historically the DP (Susarla and Van Ryzin 1976), gamma process (Kalbfleisch 1978), and beta process (Hjort 1990) were some of the earlier proposals. An important family of priors that includes all three of these as special cases is the class of neutral to the right priors.

6.1.1 Neutral to the Right Processes

Many stochastic process priors that have been proposed as nonparametric prior distributions for survival data analysis belong to the class of neutral to the right (NTR) processes. A random probability measure F on the real line is an NTR process if $1 - F(t_1)$, $(1 - F(t_2))/(1 - F(t_1))$, ..., $(1 - F(t_m))/(1 - F(t_m))$ are independent for any m and $t_1 < t_2 \cdots < t_m$, (assuming that the denominators are non-zero) (Ferguson 1974). Equivalently, F is NTR if and only if it can be expressed as $F(t) = 1 - \exp\{-Y(t)\}$, where $Y(t)$ is a stochastic process with independent increments, almost surely right-continuous and non-decreasing with $P\{Y(0) = 0\} = 1$ and $P\{\lim_{t \to \infty} Y(t) = \infty\} = 1$ (Doksum 1974). Walker et al. (1999) call $Y(t)$ an NTR Lévy process. The posterior under a NTR prior and i.i.d. sampling is again a NTR process (Doksum 1974). This remains true under right censoring (Ferguson and Phadia 1979).

6.1 Distribution Estimation for Event Times

Recall from Chap. 1 the definition of the hazard rate $\lambda(t) = \lim_{h \to 0} \frac{1}{h} p(t \leq T < t + h \mid T \geq t)$ and let $\Lambda(t) = \int_0^t \lambda(s)\, ds$ denote the cumulative hazard function. Independent increment processes are used in many approaches that construct probability models for λ or Λ, rather than directly for F. Dykstra and Laud (1981) define the extended gamma process, generalizing the gamma process studied in Ferguson (1973). The idea is to consider first a gamma process process $\{Y(t)\}$ such that $Y(t) - Y(s) \sim \mathsf{Ga}(\alpha(t) - \alpha(s), 1)$ for all $t > s \geq 0$, where α is a nondecreasing left-continuous function on $[0, \infty)$. A new process is defined as $\int_0^t \beta(s)\, dY(s)$ for a positive right-continuous function β. Dykstra and Laud (1981) consider such processes as a prior probability model for the hazard function λ, studying their properties and obtaining estimates of the posterior hazard function without censoring and with right-censoring. In particular, the resulting function λ is monotone.

An alternative model was proposed by Hjort (1990), by placing a beta process prior on Λ. To understand this construction, let us look at a discrete version of the process first. Following Nieto-Barajas and Walker (2002), consider a partition of the time axis $0 = \tau_0 < \tau_1 < \tau_2 \cdots$, and failures occurring at times chosen from the set $\{\tau_1, \tau_2, \ldots\}$. Let λ_j denote the hazard at time τ_j, $\lambda_j = p(T = \tau_j \mid T \geq \tau_j)$. Hjort (1990) assumes independent beta priors for $\{\lambda_j\}$. This generates a discrete process with independent increments for the cumulative hazard function $\Lambda(\tau_j) = \sum_{i=0}^{j} \lambda_i$. The class is closed under prior to posterior updating as the posterior process is again of the same type. The continuous version of this discrete beta process is derived by a limit argument as the interval lengths $\tau_j - \tau_{j-1}$ approach zero (Hjort 1990). Full Bayesian inference for a model with a beta process prior for the cumulative hazard function using Gibbs sampling can be found in Damien et al. (1996). A variation of this idea was used by Walker and Mallick (1997). They assumed λ to be constant at $\lambda_1, \lambda_2, \ldots$ over the intervals $[0, \tau_1], (\tau_1, \tau_2], \ldots$ with independent gamma priors on $\{\lambda_j\}$. As pointed out in Nieto-Barajas and Walker (2002), there is no limit version of this process.

6.1.2 Dependent Increments Models

We have already discussed independent increments models for the cumulative hazard function Λ. In the discrete version this implies independence for the hazards $\{\lambda_j\}$. A different modeling perspective is obtained by assuming dependence. A convenient way to introduce dependence is a Markov process prior on $\{\lambda_k\}$. Gamerman (1991) proposes the following model: $\log(\lambda_j) = \log(\lambda_{j-1}) + \epsilon_j$ for $j \geq 2$, where $\{\epsilon_j\}$ are independent with $E(\epsilon_j) = 0$ and $Var(\epsilon_j) = \sigma^2 < \infty$. In the linear Bayesian method of Gamerman (1991) only a partial specification of the $\{\epsilon_j\}$ is required.

Later, Gray (1994) used a similar prior process but directly on the hazards $\{\lambda_j\}$, without the log transformation. A further generalization involving a martingale process was proposed in Arjas and Gasbarra (1994). More recently, Nieto-Barajas and Walker (2002) proposed a model based on a latent process $\{u_k\}$ such that $\{\lambda_j\}$ is included as

$$\lambda_1 \to u_1 \to \lambda_2 \to u_2 \to \cdots$$

and the pairs (u, λ) are generated from conditional densities $f(u|\lambda)$ and $f(\lambda|u)$ implied by a specified joint density $f(u, \lambda)$. The main idea is to ensure linearity in the conditional expectation: $E(\lambda_{k+1}|\lambda_k) = a_k + b_k \lambda_k$. Nieto-Barajas and Walker (2002) show that both the gamma process of Walker and Mallick (1997) and the discrete beta process of Hjort (1990) are obtained as special cases of their construction, under appropriate choices of $f(u, \lambda)$.

In the continuous case, Nieto-Barajas and Walker (2002) proposed a Markovian model where the hazard rate function is modeled as

$$\lambda(t) = \int_0^t \exp\{-a(t-u)\}\, dL(u), \tag{6.1}$$

for $a > 0$, and where L is a pure jump process, i.e., an independent increments process on $[0, \infty)$ without Gaussian components (Ferguson and Klass 1972; Walker and Damien 2000). This model, called Lévy driven Markov process, extends Dykstra and Laud's (1981) proposal by allowing non-monotone sample paths for λ. In addition, the sample paths are piece-wise continuous functions. Nieto-Barajas and Walker (2002) obtain posterior distributions under (6.1) for different types of censoring and discuss applications in several special cases, including the Markov-gamma process.

6.2 Semiparametric Survival Regression

A common starting point in the specification of a regression model for time-to-event data is the definition of a baseline survival function, S_0, that is modified (either directly or indirectly) by subject-specific covariates x_i. Let T_0 be a random survival time from the baseline group (with all covariates equal to zero). The baseline survival function is defined as $S_0(t) = p(T_0 > t)$. Continuous survival is assumed throughout. Thus, the baseline density and hazard functions are defined by $f_0(t) = -\frac{d}{dt} S_0(t)$ and $h_0(t) = f_0(t)/S_0(t)$, respectively. The survival, density and hazard functions for a member of the population with covariates x will be denoted by $S_x(t), f_x(t)$, and $h_x(t)$, respectively.

6.2.1 Proportional Hazards

The proportional hazards (PH) model (Cox 1972), for continuous data, is obtained by expressing the covariate-dependent survival function $S_x(t)$ as

$$S_x(t) = S_0(t)^{\exp(x'\beta)}.$$

In terms of hazards, this model reduces to

$$h_x(t) = \exp(x'\beta)h_0(t). \tag{6.2}$$

Note then that for two individuals with covariates x_1 and x_2, the ratio of hazard curves is constant, equal to $h_{x_1}(t)/h_{x_2}(t) = \exp\{(x_1 - x_2)'\beta\}$, hence the name "proportional hazards." Cox (1972) is the second most cited statistics paper of all time (Ryan and Woodall 2005), and the proportional hazards model is easily the most popular semiparametric survival model in statistics, to the point where medical researchers tend to compare different populations' survival in terms of instantaneous risk (hazard) rather than mean or median survival as in common regression models. Part of the popularity of the model has to do with the incredible momentum the model has gained from how easy it is to fit the model through partial likelihood (Cox 1975) and its implementation in SAS in the procedure `proc phreg`. The use of partial likelihood and subsequent counting process formulation (Andersen and Gill 1982) of the model has allowed ready extension to stratified analysis, proportional intensity models, frailty models, and so on (Therneau and Grambsch 2000).

Full Bayesian inference under (6.2) requires a prior for the baseline hazard (or survival function). This is where BNP comes in. By adding a BNP prior for S_0, model (6.2) becomes a semiparametric Bayesian model. The first Bayesian semiparametric approach to PH models posits a gamma process as a prior on the baseline cumulative hazard $H_0(t) = \int_0^s h_0(s)ds$ (Kalbfleisch 1978); partial likelihood emerges as a limiting case (of the marginal likelihood as the precision approaches zero). The use of the gamma process prior in PH models, as well as the beta process prior (Hjort 1990), piecewise exponential priors, and correlated increments priors are covered in Ibrahim et al. (2001) (pp. 47–94) and Sinha and Dey (1997). Other approaches include what are essentially Bernstein polynomials (Gelfand and Mallick 1995; Carlin and Hodges 1999) and penalized B-splines (Hennerfeind et al. 2006; Kneib and Fahrmeir 2007). The last two models are available in a public domain program called `BayesX` (Belitz et al. 2009), which can be called from the R package `R2BayesX`.

Example 2 (Oral Cancer, ctd.) Recall that data comprised of $n = 80$ survival times for mouth cancer patients, some right-censored. Samples are recorded as aneuploid (abnormal number of chromosomes) versus diploid (two copies of each chromosome) tumors. We define $x_i \in \{0, 1\}$ as an indicator for aneuploid tumors and carry out inference under model (6.2) with a BNP prior on $h_0(\cdot)$. Figure 6.2a shows the estimated hazard curves under $x = 0$ and $x = 1$. The log-baseline hazard is

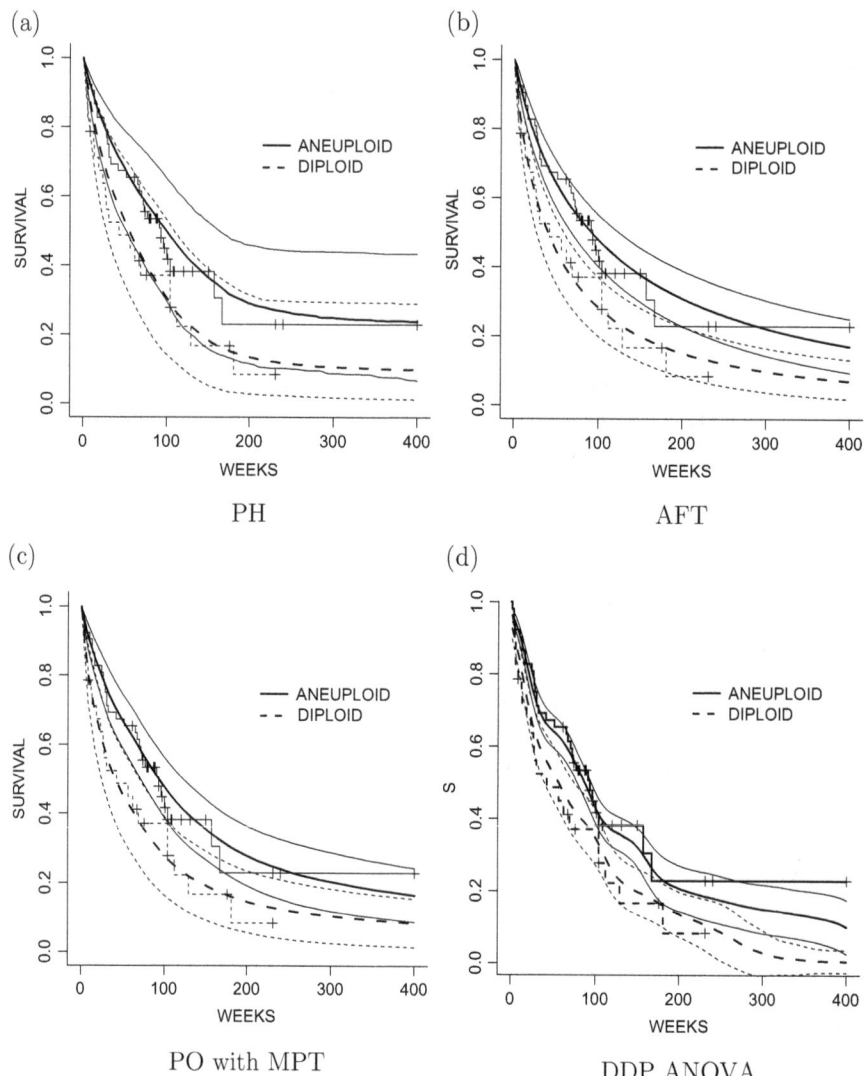

Fig. 6.2 Example 2 (ctd.). Survival curves for aneuploid (*solid lines*) and diploid (*dashed lines*) groups under the proportional hazard model (**a**), an AFT model with penalized B-spline (**b**), a PO model with a MPT prior (**c**), and under a DDP ANOVA model (**d**). In all figures the *thin (solid and dashed) lines* centered around each of the survival curves show pointwise 80 % CIs. The piecewise constant lines plot Kaplan-Meier estimates for each group independently

modeled as a penalized B-spline (Hennerfeind et al. 2006), described in Sect. 4.3.2. The model is fit through the R2BayesX package. Use the function bayesx(..., family="cox").

6.2.2 Accelerated Failure Time

The accelerated failure time (AFT) model is obtained by expressing the covariate-dependent survival function $S_x(t)$ as

$$S_x(t) = S_0\{\exp(-x'\beta)t\}. \tag{6.3}$$

This is equivalent to a linear model for the log time-to-event T,

$$\log T = x'\beta + \epsilon, \tag{6.4}$$

where $p(\epsilon > \log t) = S_0(t)$. The mean, median, and any quantile of survival for an individual with covariates x_1 is changed by a factor of $\exp\{(x_1 - x_2)'\beta\}$ relative to those with covariates x_2.

The first nonparametric Bayesian AFT model was introduced by Christensen and Johnson (1988). Based on a DP prior they derive approximate marginal inferences under the AFT model. A fully Bayesian treatment using the DP is not practically possible (Johnson and Christensen 1989). Approaches based on DPM models have been considered by Kuo and Mallick (1997), Kottas and Gelfand (2001) and Hanson (2006b). The DPM "fixes" the discrete nature of the DP, as do other discrete mixtures of continuous kernels. Alternatively, continuous densities for the residuals ϵ in (6.4) can directly be modeled with tail-free priors (Walker and Mallick 1999; Hanson and Johnson 2002; Hanson 2006a; Zhao et al. 2009). In the example below we use an approach from Komárek et al. (2007), which models the ϵ density directly as an approximate penalized B-spline.

Example 2 (Oral Cancer, ctd.) Here we consider an AFT model where the baseline error density on ϵ is modeled as a penalized B-spline (Komárek et al. 2007). Figure 6.2b shows the estimated survival curves under $x = 0$ and $x = 1$, fitted using the function bayessurvreg2 (·) from R package bayesSurv.

Although the PH model is by far the most commonly-used semiparametric survival model, several studies have shown vastly superior fit and interpretation from AFT models (Hanson 2006a; Hanson and Yang 2007; Kay and Kinnersley 2002; Orbe et al. 2002; Hutton and Monaghan 2002; Portnoy 2003). Cox pointed out himself (Reid 1994) "*... the physical or substantive basis for ... proportional hazards models ... is one of its weaknesses ... accelerated failure time models are in many ways more appealing because of their quite direct physical interpretation ...*".

Since the AFT model is a log-linear model, one can obtain a point estimate of survival for covariates x as simply $\exp(x'\hat{\beta})$, where $\hat{\beta}$ is an estimate of β. Prediction is impossible within the PH model framework without an estimate of the baseline hazard function. So reporting only coefficients—which is common—disallows others to predict survival.

6.2.3 Proportional Odds

The proportional odds (PO) model has recently gained attention as an alternative to the PH and AFT models. The PO model defines the survival function $S_x(t)$ for an individual with covariate vector x through the relation

$$\frac{S_x(t)}{1-S_x(t)} = \exp\{-x'\beta\} \frac{S_0(t)}{1-S_0(t)}. \tag{6.5}$$

The odds of dying before any time t are $\exp\{(x_2-x_1)'\beta\}$ times greater for those with covariates x_1 versus x_2. Bayesian nonparametric approaches for the PO model have been based on Bernstein polynomials (Banerjee and Dey 2005), B-splines (Wang and Dunson 2011), and Polya trees (Hanson 2006a; Hanson and Yang 2007; Zhao et al. 2009; Hanson et al. 2011).

Example 2 (Oral Cancer, ctd.) Here we consider a PO model where S_0 is modeled as a finite MPT with $c = 1$ and $J = 4$ levels (Hanson 2006a; Hanson and Yang 2007). A flat prior is assumed for the regression effect. Figure 6.2c shows estimated survival curves for $x = 0$ and $x = 1$, with approximate 80 % CIs, fit via MCMC Algorithm 3 in Hanson and Yang (2007). The implementation was hand-coded in R. The posterior median and 95 % CI for the type effect is 0.986 (0.318, 1.737). The odds of surviving past any time t is estimated to be $e^{0.986} \approx 2.7$ times greater for the aneuploid group.

The PH, AFT, and PO models all make overarching assumptions about the data generating mechanism for the sake of obtaining succinct data summaries. An important aspect associated with the BNP formulation of these models is that, by assuming the *same, flexible model* for the baseline survival function, they can be placed on a common ground (Hanson 2006a; Hanson and Yang 2007; Zhang and Davidian 2008; Zhao et al. 2009; Hanson et al. 2011). Compare Fig. 6.2, panels (a), (b), and (c).

Hanson (2006a), Hanson and Yang (2007), Zhao et al. (2009) and Hanson et al. (2011) considered several variations of PT-based BNP models for survival regression. Of these models, the PO model was chosen over the PH and AFT models on the basis of the LPML criterion (Geisser and Eddy 1979). In three of these references, the parametric log-logistic model, a special case of PO that also has the AFT property, was chosen. This may be due to the fact that the PO assumption implies that $\lim_{t\to\infty} \frac{h_{x_1}(t)}{h_{x_2}(t)} = 1$, that is, eventually everyone has the same risk of dying tomorrow. These authors also found that, everything else being equal, the actual semiparametric model chosen (PO, PH or AFT) affects prediction far more than whether the baseline is modeled nonparametrically. Remarkably, none of these papers favored the semiparametric PH model in actual applications.

6.2.4 Other Semiparametric Models and Extensions

PH, AFT, and PO are the three most widely-used semiparametric survival models in practice. There are a few more hazard-based models including the additive hazards model (Aalen 1980), given by

$$h_x(t) = h_0(t) + x'\beta.$$

An empirical Bayes approach to this model based on the gamma process was implemented by Sinha et al. (2009). Fully Bayesian approaches require elaborate model specification to incorporate the rather awkward constraint $h_0(t) + x'\beta \geq 0$ for $t > 0$, e.g. Yin and Ibrahim (2005). Recently, there has been some interest in the accelerated hazards (AH) model (Chen and Wang 2000), given by

$$h_x(t) = h_0\{\exp(-x'\beta)t\}.$$

This model allows hazard and survival curves to cross. A Bayesian treatment of the AH model can be found in Chen et al. (2014) where baseline is modeled as a transformed Bernstein polynomial. Li et al. (2015) consider a extended hazard model that includes PH, AFT, and AH as formally nested special cases, generalized to areal spatial data that models the baseline using a parametric family-centered B-spline.

There are several generalizations for the models of Sect. 6.2.1–6.2.3. A standard approach for accomodating correlated data has been the introduction of frailty terms to the linear predictor, e.g., $x'_{ij}\beta + \gamma_i$ for the jth subject in cluster i. Frailties can be assumed exchangeable (either parametric or nonparametric) or have some additional structure. Banerjee et al. (2004) broadly discuss both georeferenced (e.g. latitude/longitude) and areal (e.g. county-level) frailties γ_i. Zhao et al. (2009) compare PH, AFT, and PO models with exchangeable parametric, nonparametric MPT, and spatially-smoothed intrinsic conditionally autoregressive (ICAR) frailties. Spatially smoothing frailties can improve the estimation of fixed effects as well as improve the prediction of survival for new patients. Both georeferenced as well as areal spatial frailties can be fit via R2BayesX for the PH model; general additive predictor effects (see Sect. 4.3.2) can also be included (Belitz et al. 2009). The recently contributed R package spBayesSurv, written by Haiming Zhou, has compiled functions to fit areal and georeferenced PO, AFT, and PH survival models for general interval-censored data using a MPT baseline. Other spBayesSurv functions allow for copula-based marginal spatial analysis using a generalization of the ANOVA DDP AFT discussed in Sect. 6.3.2 and spatial-frailty generalizations of the LDTFP survival model in Sect. 6.3.3.

Hazard-based models (proportional, additive, and accelerated) naturally accommodate time-dependent covariates; the linear predictor is simply generalized to be $x(t)'\beta$. Similarly, hazard-based models can also include time-dependent regression effects via $x'\boldsymbol{\beta}(t)$ or even $\boldsymbol{x}(t)'\boldsymbol{\beta}(t)$. All of these are possible for the PH model in BayesX.

Other model modifications include cure rate models, joint longitudinal/survival models, recurrent events models, multistate models, competing risks models, and multivariate models that incorporate dependence more flexibly than frailty models.

6.3 Fully Nonparametric Survival Regression

6.3.1 Extensions of the AFT model

In earlier chapters we introduced fully nonparametric regression or density regression. Two of these models are easily generalized to accommodate censored data: (i) the ANOVA DDP (De Iorio et al. 2009) (Definition 5), the related LDDP (Definition 6) and (ii) the linear dependent tail-free process (LDTFP) (Jara and Hanson 2011) (Sect. 4.4.3). As we show below, both can be viewed as natural heteroscedastic generalizations of the AFT model, allowing for crossing hazard and/or survival curves. Later, in Sect. 6.4, both approaches are compared on three survival data sets. The two models provide roughly the same inferences, although the DDP gives slightly better prediction according to the LPML criterion. However, the LDTFP has the advantage that regression parameters retain the same simple interpretation as in standard accelerated failure time models, describing how median survival changes with covariates.

Data analysis for event time data naturally includes inference on the entire density, in contrast to traditional linear models that focus on the trend (mean or median) only. Perhaps this is one of the reasons why inference for event time data has been a traditional focus of BNP applications. In what follows, consider standard interval-censored failure time data $\{(l_i, u_i, \tilde{\boldsymbol{x}}_i)\}_{i=1}^n$, where the responses are known up to an interval, $T_i \in (l_i, u_i]$, and $\tilde{\boldsymbol{x}}_i$ are covariates for subject i, *without the intercept term*. Recall the AFT model (6.4) as $y_i = \log(T_i) = \tilde{\boldsymbol{x}}_i'\boldsymbol{\beta} + \epsilon_i$.

6.3.2 ANCOVA-DDP: Linear Dependent DP Mixture

In Sect. 4.4.2 we introduced the ANOVA DDP for a family of dependent probability measures $\{G_x, x \in X\}$. Recall Definition 5. Let $y_i = \log(T_i)$. We use the ANOVA DDP model to generalize (6.4) to

$$y_i \mid x_i, G_{x_i} \overset{\text{ind}}{\sim} \int N(\mu, \sigma^2) \, dG_{x_i}(\mu, \sigma^2) \quad \text{and} \quad \{G_x; x \in X\} \sim \text{ANOVA DDP}. \tag{6.6}$$

6.3 Fully Nonparametric Survival Regression

This is exactly (4.12), that is, the ANOVA DDP with an additional normal kernel. See De Iorio et al. (2009) and Jara et al. (2010) for more discussion. We refer to (6.6) as ANOVA DDP AFT model.

Software note: Inference under model (6.6) is implemented as `LDDPsurvival` in the R package `DPpackage` (Jara et al. 2011).

The model can be characterized as a natural nonparametric extension of the AFT model (6.4), and the name of the `DPpackage` function is based on another characterization of the model that was introduced as a separate definition as the LDDP. Both characterizations arise by the following alternative construction of the model. We start with the AFT model (6.4). In a first step consider a DPM of normals for the residual distribution in (6.4). That is, assume $\epsilon_i \stackrel{ind}{\sim} N(\mu_i, \sigma^2), \mu_1, \ldots, \mu_n \mid G \stackrel{iid}{\sim} G$, and $G \mid M, G_0 \sim \mathsf{DP}(M\, G_0)$. This model is proposed and discussed in Kuo and Mallick (1997). Writing $\tilde{x}_i$ for the covariate vector without intercept, we get

$$y_i \mid \boldsymbol{\beta}, G \stackrel{ind}{\sim} \sum_{h=1}^{\infty} w_h \mathsf{N}(\mu_h + \tilde{x}_i' \boldsymbol{\beta}, \sigma_h^2), \tag{6.7}$$

with the stick-breaking prior for w_h and $\mu_h \stackrel{iid}{\sim} G_0$, for some base measure G_0. The interpretation of the components of $\boldsymbol{\beta}$ remains as usual and the model can be fit using standard algorithms for DPM models. See Kuo and Mallick (1997) for more discussion.

Now consider additional mixing over the regression coefficients. Let $x_i = (1, \tilde{x}_i')'$. We get

$$y_i \mid G \stackrel{ind}{\sim} \sum_{h=1}^{\infty} w_h \mathsf{N}(x_i' \boldsymbol{\beta}_h, \sigma_h^2).$$

We complete the model with the stick-breaking prior on $w_h = v_h \prod_{\ell < h}(1 - v_\ell)$ for $v_h \stackrel{iid}{\sim} \mathsf{Be}(1, M)$, and independent priors $\boldsymbol{\beta}_h \stackrel{iid}{\sim} \mathsf{N}(m_0, V_0)$ and $\sigma_h^2 \stackrel{iid}{\sim} \mathsf{IGamma}(a, b)$. But this is exactly (6.6).

Example 16 (Columbian Children Mortality) Somoza (1980) considers data on childhood mortality in Columbia. The data report overall survival for $n = 1437$ children. Covariates $\tilde{x}_i = (u_i, v_i, w_i)$ include sex (u_i), birth cohort (3 levels, v_i), and an indicator for urban versus rural home (w_i). Let G_x denote the distribution of overall survival times y_i for children with covariates $\tilde{x}_i = x$. We use the ANOVA-DDP model (6.6) to define a dependent prior for the $12 = 2 \times 3 \times 2$ distributions G_x. Figure 6.3 shows $E(G_x \mid y)$ for three covariate combinations corresponding to urban male children and the three birth cohorts.

The model trades easy interpretability offered by a single $\boldsymbol{\beta}$ for greatly increased flexibility. In particular, the ANOVA-DDP model does not stochastically order

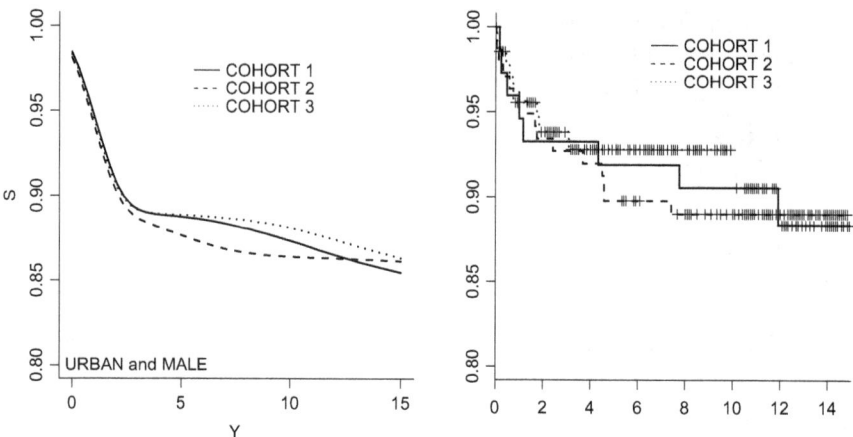

Fig. 6.3 Example 16. $E(G_x \mid y)$ (as survival function) for urban male children from the three birth cohorts, under a fully nonparametric regression model. (**a**) $E(S_x \mid y)$. (**b**) Data as KM plot

survival curves from different predictors x_{i_1} and x_{i_2}, and both the survival and hazard curves can cross.

If the data warrant only a few weights from $\{w_1, w_2, \ldots\}$ with non-negligible mass, the model can be re-fit using simple, finite mixture of log-normal distributions. The number of components J in the finite mixture can be estimated from the posterior number of components from a fit of (6.6) yielding

$$y_i \mid w, \beta, \tau \overset{ind.}{\sim} \sum_{j=1}^{J} w_j N(x_i' \beta_j, \sigma_j^2), \qquad (6.8)$$

where $w = (w_1, \ldots, w_J)$, $\beta = (\beta_1, \ldots, \beta_J)$ and $\tau = (\sigma_1^2, \ldots, \sigma_J^2)$. This model defines J homogeneous subpopulations with simple *unimodal* survival densities $LN(\beta_{j1}, \tau_j)$ and accompanying acceleration factors given through $(\beta_{j2}, \ldots, \beta_{jp})$. These can be viewed as homogeneous subpopulations corresponding to an omitted variable with J levels. Generalization of this model, where weights also depend on covariates naturally lead again to conditional density regression models, as in Sect. 4.4.4, can be found in, for instance, Müller et al. (1996) and Chung and Dunson (2009).

Example 2 (Oral Cancer, ctd.) Earlier in this section we reported inference using the PH, PO and AFT models. As a final comparison we add inference under the DDP ANOVA AFT model (6.6). Figure 6.2d shows estimated survival curves for $x = 0$ and $x = 1$, with approximate 80 % CIs.

6.3.3 Linear Dependent Tail-Free Process (LDTFP)

Recall the definition of the Polya tree (PT) prior in Sect. 3.1. We construct a survival regression based on a variation of the PT prior to define another semi-parametric generalization of the AFT model (6.4). We have already briefly introduced the model earlier as the LDTFP, in Sect. 4.4.3, but deferred the formal definition until now, simply because the model was originally proposed in the context of survival regression.

Recall that the PT defines the conditional probabilities Y_e in (3.1) as beta random variables. We use $e = \varepsilon_1 \cdots \varepsilon_m$ to denote the binary sequence that indexes the partitioning subsets (we use e instead of ϵ, as in Sect. 3.1, to avoid confusion with the residual ϵ in the AFT model). Maintaining the same structure of independent splitting probabilities in a nested sequence of partitions Π, we can replace the beta prior with a logistic regression for each of these probabilities Y_e, allowing the *entire* shape of the density to change with predictors. This is the approach considered by Jara and Hanson (2011). Recall that $Y_{e1} = 1 - Y_{e0}$. Given covariates x, we model (Y_{e0}, Y_{e1}) as a logistic regression

$$\log\{Y_{e0}(x)/Y_{e1}(x)\} = x'\tau_e.$$

If $e = \varepsilon_1 \cdots \varepsilon_m$ is a length m binary vector, then there are $2^m - 1$ vectors of regression coefficients, $T = \{\tau_e\}$. For instance, for $m = 3$, $T = \{\tau_\bullet, \tau_0, \tau_1, \tau_{00}, \tau_{01}, \tau_{10}, \tau_{1,1}, \tau_{2,4}\}$. Let $X = [x_1 \cdots x_n]'$ be the $n \times p$ design matrix. Let $m(e)$ denote the number of binary digits in e. Following Jara and Hanson (2011), each τ_e is assigned an independent normal prior,

$$\tau_e \sim \mathsf{N}\left(0, \frac{2}{c(m(e)+1)^2}\Psi\right), \tag{6.9}$$

independently across e, and scaled by the depth in the nested partition tree Π. Several options could be considered for Ψ. Jara and Hanson (2011) discussed in detail the case where $\Psi = n(X'X)^{-1}$, that is, a g-prior (Zellner 1983) for the regression coefficients.

In the previous construction, the beta random variables in the PT definition from Sect. 3.1 are replaced by $Y_e(x)$. Also, we truncate the PT at a finite level, say level J. We also assume the PT to be centered at a standard normal distribution, by using standard normal quantiles to define the nested partition boundaries, that is we use the nested partition sequence Π of a $\mathsf{PT}(G^\star, \mathcal{A})$ with a standard normal $G^\star = \mathsf{N}(0, 1)$. In summary,

Definition 7 (Linear Dependent Tail-Free Process, LDTFP) Let $\Pi = \{B_e, e \in \bigcup_{j=1}^{J}\{0,1\}^j\}$ denote a nested partition sequence defined by the dyadic quantiles of a fixed distribution $G^\star$. Let $Y_{e0}(x) = G_x(B_{e0} \mid B_e)$ and $Y_{e1}(x) = 1 - Y_{e0}(x)$. A family of random probability measures $\mathcal{G} = \{G_x, x \in \mathcal{X}\}$ has an LDTFP prior if (i) $\log\{Y_{e0}(x)/Y_{e1}(x)\} = x'\tau_e$; (ii) $\tau_e \sim N_p\left(\mathbf{0}, 2/[c(m(e)+1)^2]\mathbf{\Psi}\right)$. We write

$$\{G_x, x \in X\} \sim \text{LDTFP}(c, \mathbf{\Psi}, G^\star, J).$$

We use $g_x(\cdot)$ to denote the corresponding p.d.f. The parameter $c \in \mathbb{R}^+$ is the coefficient in (6.9). It controls how non-normal $g_x(e)$ is, and can be interpreted as a measure of the random L_1 distance $||g_x - \phi||$ (Hanson et al. 2008).

Software note: Inference under the LDDTFP is implemented as LDTFPsurvival in the R package DPpackage (Jara et al. 2011).

We now use the LDTFP as a prior for the residual distribution in (6.4) and add a restriction to a zero median. This defines the LDTFP AFT model

$$y_i = x_i'\beta + \sigma\epsilon_i, \quad \epsilon_i \mid \tau \stackrel{\text{ind}}{\sim} g_{x_i}.$$

Unlike the ANOVA DDP, the LDTFP separates survival into one distinct trend $x'\beta$ and an evolving log-baseline survival density g_x. By setting g_x to have median-zero, e^{β_j} gives a factor by which the median survival changes when x_j is increased *just as in standard AFT models*. This convenient interpretability in terms of median-regression in the presence of heteroscedastic error allows a fit of the LDTFP model to easily relate covariates x to median survival.

The LDTFP models the probability of falling above or below quantiles of the $N(x'\beta, \sigma^2)$ distribution, but in terms of conditional probabilities. This model can be viewed as a particular kind of quantile regression model. By augmenting a median-zero tail-free process with a general trend $x'\beta$ we accomplish the objective of nesting the ubiquitous normal-errors linear model within a highly flexible median regression model, but with heteroscedastic error that changes shape with covariate levels $x \in \mathcal{X}$.

6.4 More Examples

The two generalizations of the AFT model described in Sect. 6.3 are illustrated now in three data sets. The generalized AFT models were fit using the R functions LDDPsurvival and LDTFPsurvival in DPpackage (Jara et al. 2011).

6.4.1 Example 17: Breast Retraction Data

We consider a dataset involving time to cosmetic deterioration of the breast for women with stage 1 breast cancer who have undergone a lumpectomy (Beadle et al. 1984). The data come from a retrospective study designed to compare the cosmetic

6.4 More Examples

effects of radiotherapy versus radiotherapy plus chemotherapy on women with early breast cancer. Both treatments are alternatives to a mastectomy that preserve (and thus enhance the appearance of) the breast. It is postulated that chemotherapy in addition to radiotherapy (treatment A) reduces the cosmetic effect of the procedure by inducing breast retraction more quickly than radiotherapy alone (treatment B).

There are $n_B = 46$ radiation only and $n_A = 48$ radiation plus chemotherapy patients. Patients were typically observed every 4–6 months, at which point a clinician graded the level of breast retraction as none, moderate, or severe. We compare time to moderate or severe retraction across treatments. That is, the event of interest is moderate or severe breast retraction. Event times are interval censored, with interval endpoints occurring at clinic visits. Hanson and Johnson (2004) analyzed the same data using the (homoscedastic) AFT model (6.7) with a mixture of DPs as a prior for the baseline distribution F_0.

We fit the same data using the ANOVA DDP and the LDTFP models. The only predictor is the treatment indicator. For the LDTFP model we set $J = 4$ and $\Psi = n(X'X)^{-1}$, where n is the sample size. The median function parameters $\boldsymbol{\beta} = (\beta_0, \beta_1)$ were given a Zellner's g-prior (Zellner 1983), $\boldsymbol{\beta} \sim \mathsf{N}(0, g(X'X)^{-1})$, with $g = 2n$. For the LDTFP parameters, we assume $\sigma^{-2} \sim \mathsf{Ga}(5.01, 2.01)$ and $c \sim \mathsf{Ga}(10, 1)$.

For the ANOVA DDP model, we assume $\boldsymbol{m}_0 \sim \mathsf{N}(\boldsymbol{0}_2, 100 \times \boldsymbol{I}_2)$, $\boldsymbol{V}_0^{-1} \sim \mathsf{Wis}(4, \boldsymbol{I}_2)$, $a = 3.01$, $b \sim \mathsf{Ga}(3.01, 1.01)$ and $M \sim \mathsf{Ga}(10, 1)$. For all models, a burn-in of 20,000 iterates was followed by a run of 100,000 thinned down to 10,000 iterates.

The two models based on dependent process priors outperformed a classical semiparametric analysis based on the AFT assumption. Rounded to the nearest integer, the LPML values for the ANOVA DDP and LDTFP model were -147 and -149, respectively. For comparison we consider as a third alternative inference under the DP mixture model (6.7) of Hanson and Johnson (2004). Fixing the total mass parameter $\alpha = 5$ and using a centering distribution, $G_0 = \mathsf{N}(\gamma, \theta^2)$, we find a LPML of -159. Figure 6.4 shows the estimated survival curves for the two treatment

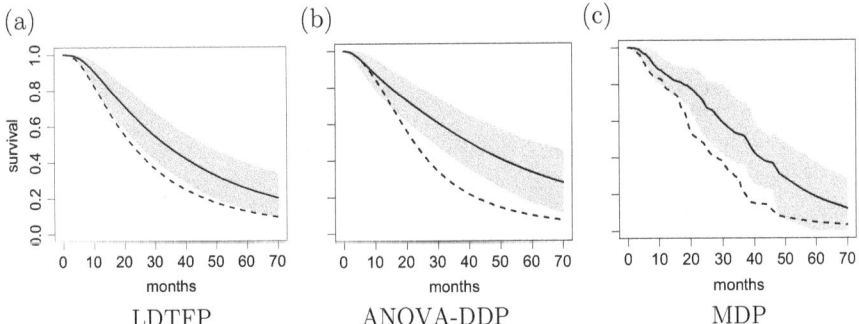

Fig. 6.4 Example 17. Panels (**a**), (**b**) and (**c**) show estimated survival curves for treatments A (*continuous line*) and B (*dashed line*) under the LDTFP, ANOVA-DDP and mixture of DP model, respectively. In all cases, the pointwise 95 % credible bands are also displayed as a *grey* area for treatment A. The widths of the pointwise 95 % CIs for the treatment B are of comparable size in all cases

groups under the three different models, evaluated on a grid of 200 equally-spaced points. The survival curves under the two fully nonparametric survival regressions are similar to the ones reported by Hanson and Johnson (2004), with the exception that the estimated survival curves under the ANOVA DDP and LDTFP model are initially indistinguishable up to 15 months after treatment; the AFT model forces a more pronounced stochastic ordering of the survival curves. Although the ANOVA DDP model shows marginally better predictive performance than the LDTFP model for these data, the survival point estimates obtained under the two models are qualitatively similar. The better predictive performance of the ANOVA DDP models is explained by its lower posterior variability.

Under the LDTFP model, the estimated treatment effect was $\hat{\beta}_1 = 0.30$ and non-significant with a 95 % highest posterior density (HPD) interval of $(-0.07, 0.68)$. The median time to retraction under treatment B is estimated to be $e^{0.30} \approx 1.38$ times longer than under treatment A with 95 % HPD interval $(0.90, 1.91)$. Priors favoring smaller values of c yielded qualitatively similar inferences, although estimated point estimates of the survival curves cross at about 15 months.

The results of the AFT analyses with homoscedastic error show a significant regression effect, indicating lower times to retraction under treatment A as expected, somewhat contradicting the LDTFP analysis where no significant difference in median survival was found. However, a glance at Fig. 6.4 shows marginal evidence of different median lifetimes given the large variability of the survival curves across the groups. Under the homoscedastic AFT model the regression parameter affects all quantiles simultaneously and indicates a net scale shift in probability; under the LDTFP model the conditional probabilities change beyond the median function. The significant effect under the homoscedastic model can be viewed as an averaging of the overall warping of the density across treatment levels, embodied in the parameters $\{\tau_{j,k}\}$ in the LDTFP.

6.4.2 Example 8 (ctd.): Breast Cancer Trial

We consider data from a cancer clinical trial described in Rosner (2005), and analyzed by De Iorio et al. (2009) using a ANOVA DDP mixture of normals model. The data record the event-free survival time in months for 761 women. That is, the response of interest is time until death, relapse or treatment-related cancer. Researchers are interested in determining whether high doses of the treatment are more effective for treating the cancer compared to lower doses. High doses of the treatment are known to be associated with a high risk of treatment-related mortality. The clinicians hope that this initial risk is offset by a substantial reduction in mortality and disease recurrence or relapse, consequently justifying more aggressive therapy. Thus the primary reason for carrying out the clinical trial was to compare low versus high dose. Following De Iorio et al. (2009), we consider two categorical covariates, one continuous covariate, and one interaction term: treatment dose—low (LO) or high (HI), estrogen receptor status—negative (ER−) or positive (ER+), tumor size (TS, standardized to zero mean and unit variance), and the treatment dose and ER status interaction (HI*ER).

The ANOVA DDP and LDTFP models were fit to the data. For the LDTFP, we set $J = 5$ and $\Psi = 10^3 I_5$, and the median function parameters were assigned independent normal priors $\beta \sim N(\mathbf{0}_5, 10^3 I_5)$, $\sigma^{-2} \sim \text{Ga}(1.5, 6.0)$, and $c \sim \text{Ga}(7.0, 0.1)$. For the ANOVA DDP model, we assume $m_0 \sim N(\mathbf{0}_5, 100 \times I_5)$, $V_0^{-1} \sim \text{Wis}(7, I_5)$, $a = 1.01$, $b \sim \text{Ga}(1.51, 3.01)$ and $M \sim \text{Ga}(5, 1)$. For both models, a burn-in of 20,000 iterates was followed by a run of 100,000 thinned down to 10,000 iterates.

Qualitatively similar inference was obtained under the two models. Figures 6.5 and 6.6 show the estimated survival curves, and corresponding posterior uncertainty, under the LDTFP and ANOVA DDP model, respectively. The two models based on dependent process priors outperformed a classical semiparametric analysis based on the AFT assumption. Rounded to the nearest integer, the LPML for the ANOVA DDP and LDTFP model was -2048 and -2052, respectively, better than -2063 obtained under a parametric AFT log-normal regression model.

An advantage of the LDTFP model over the ANOVA DDP model is that direct inference can be made on the median survival time. In order to evaluate the posterior evidence against the hypothesis of null effect of the covariates on the median survival function, the pseudo contour probability (PsCP) was evaluated for each hypothesis. The PsCP is defined as one minus the smallest credible level for which the null hypothesis is contained in the corresponding HDP.

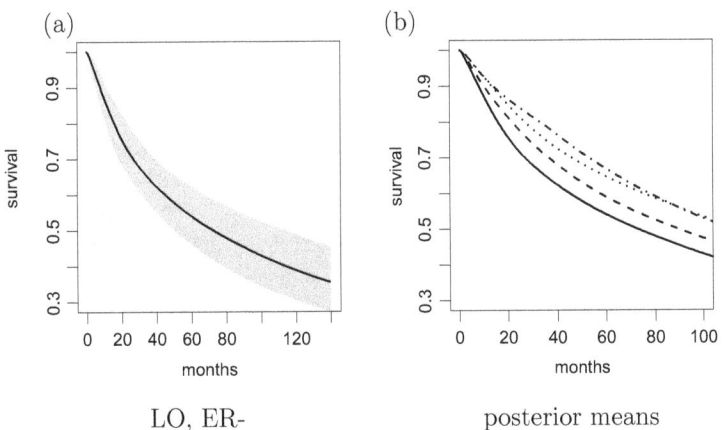

Fig. 6.5 Example 8: LDTFP model. In both panels the results are displayed for TS 2.0 cm (first quartile) under the LDTFP model. Panel (**a**) shows the posterior mean (and pointwise 95 % HPD band in *grey*) for the survival curve for patients with low dose treatment and ER- status. Panel (**b**) shows the posterior mean for all four combinations of treatment dose and ER status, including LO, ER- (*solid line*); HI, ER- (*dashed*); LO, ER+ (*dotted*); and HI, ER+ (*dotdash*). The widths of the 95 % HPD bands in the other cases are all comparable to the length of the pointwise C.I.'s in (**a**)

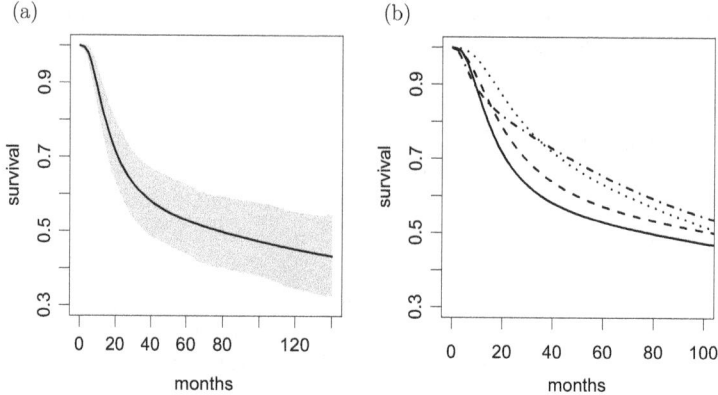

Fig. 6.6 Example 8: ANOVA DDP model. Same as Fig. 6.5, but now under the ANOVA DDP model. (**a**) LO, ER- (**b**) posterior means

The PsCP was computed based on the highest posterior density (HPD) intervals, which were estimated using the method proposed by Chen and Shao (1999). The results suggest a non-important effect of the treatment dose (PsCP = 0.55) and its interaction with ER status (PsCP = 0.5), and an important effect of the ER status (PsCP < 0.01) and a negative effect of the tumor size (PsCP < 0.01) on the median survival time.

6.4.3 Example 18: Lung Cancer Data

We consider data from Maksymiuk et al. (1994) on the treatment of limited-stage small-cell lung cancer in $n = 121$ patients. The data have been analyzed in the literature using median-regression models (Ying et al. 1995; Walker and Mallick 1999; Yang 1999; Kottas and Gelfand 2001; Hanson 2006a). In the study, it was of interest to determine which sequencing of the drugs cisplaten and etoposide increased the lifetime from time of diagnosis, measured in days, for patients with limited-stage small-cell lung cancer. Treatment A applied cisplaten followed by etoposide, whereas treatment B applied etoposide followed by cisplaten. The patients' ages in years at entry into the study was also included as a concomitant variable. The LDTFP model was fit to the data using $J = 5$ and $\Psi = 10^3 I_3$. The median function parameters were assigned independent priors $\beta \sim N(0_3, 10^3 I_3)$, $\sigma^{-2} \sim Ga(3, 1.5)$, and $c \sim Ga(1.0, 1.0)$. For the ANOVA DDP model, we assume $m_0 \sim N(0_3, 100 I_3)$, $V_0^{-1} \sim Wis(5, I_3)$, $a = 3.01$, $b \sim Ga(3.01, 3.01)$ and $M \sim Ga(5, 1)$. For both models, a burn-in of 20,000 iterates was followed by a run of 100,000 thinned down to 10,000 samples.

The LPML measures for the ANOVA DDP and LDTFP models were −732 and −733, respectively. These results suggest that both dependent models slightly outperform from a predictive point of view alternative parametric and semiparametric survival models. In fact, the LPML for the Weibull, log-logistic, and PO, PH, and AFT models, using a MPT prior for the baseline survival function, were −747, −735, −734, −737, and −734, respectively (Hanson 2006a). The ANOVA DDP and LDTFP models in some sense predict the data "best", but there is little real predictive difference among the ANOVA DDP, LDTFP, PO and AFT models. The Weibull model is clearly inferior, whereas the ANOVA DDP and LDTFP models have a pseudo Bayes factor of about 50 relative to the PH model. The similar predictive behavior of the dependent model is confirmed by the density plots in Figs. 6.7 and 6.8. Table 6.1 presents posterior inference for the regression parameter under the MPT AFT, PO, and PH models and under the LDTFP model. Holding age fixed, patients typically survive $e^{0.345} \approx 1.4$ times longer under treatment A versus

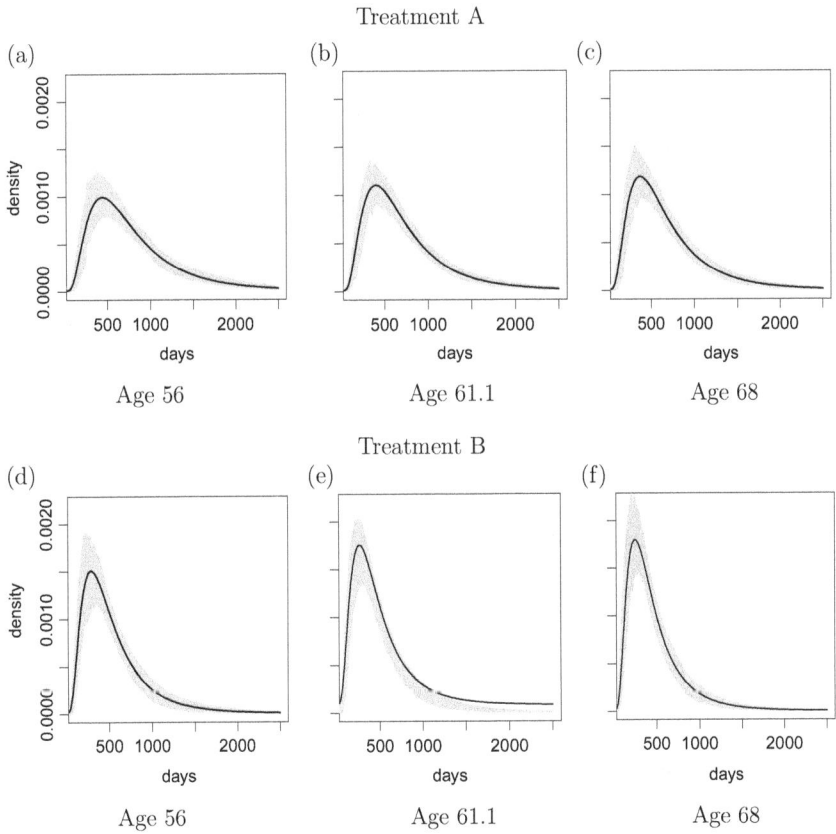

Fig. 6.7 Example 18. Posterior mean (and pointwise 95 % HPD band in *grey*) for the densities at age 56, 61.1 and 68 for treatments A and B under the ANOVA-DDP model

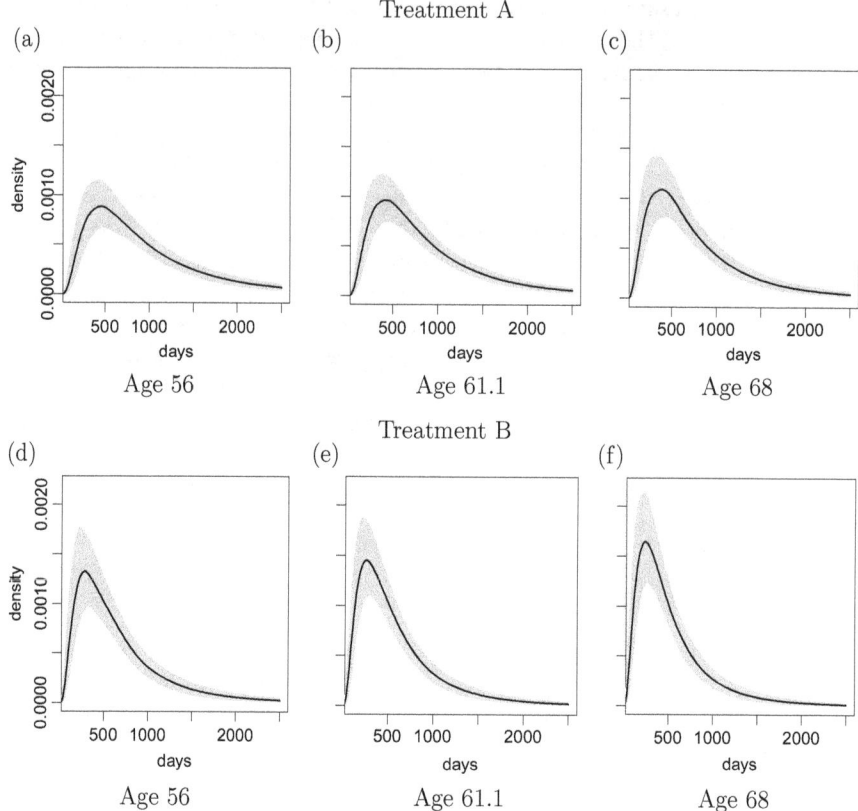

Fig. 6.8 Example 18. Posterior mean (and pointwise 95 % HPD band in *grey*) for the densities at age 56, 61.1 and 68 for treatments A and B under the LDTFP model

Table 6.1 Example 18. Posterior mean (95 % credible interval) for the regression coefficients

Coefficient	MPT AFT	MPT PO	MPT PH	LDTFP
β_1 (Age)	0.007	0.034	0.028	−0.019
	(−0.004, 0.036)	(−0.001, 0.071)	(0.003, 0.054)	(−0.037, −0.001)
β_2 (Treatment)	0.345	0.930	0.533	0.407
	(0.157, 0.533)	(0.292, 1.568)	(0.130, 0.926)	(0.130, 0.691)

treatment B under the AFT assumption. The PO model indicates that the odds of surviving past any time t is $e^{0.93} \approx 2.5$ greater for treatment A versus treatment B. Similarly to the inference under the MPT AFT model, the results of the LDTFP suggest that the median survival time for patients under treatment A is $e^{0.407} \approx 1.5$ times the median survival time for patients under treatment B.

References

Aalen OO (1980) A model for nonparametric regression analysis of counting processes. In: Lecture notes in statistics, vol 2. Springer, New York, pp 1–25

Andersen PK, Gill RD (1982) Cox's regression model for counting processes: a large sample study. Ann Stat 10(4):1100–1120

Arjas E, Gasbarra D (1994) Nonparametric Bayesian inference from right censored survival data, using the Gibbs sampler. Stat Sin 4:505–524

Banerjee S, Dey DK (2005) Semi-parametric proportional odds models for spatially correlated survival data. Lifetime Data Anal 11:175–191

Banerjee S, Carlin BP, Gelfand AE (2004) Hierarchical modeling and analysis for spatial data. Chapman & Hall/CRC, Boca Raton

Beadle G, Harris J, Silver B, Botnick L, Hellman S (1984) Cosmetic results following primary radiation therapy for early breast cancer. Cancer 54:2911–2918

Belitz C, Brezger A, Kneib T, Lang S (2009) BayesX—software for Bayesian inference in structured additive regression models. Version 2.00. Available from http://www.stat.uni-muenchen.de/~bayesx

Carlin BP, Hodges JS (1999) Hierarchical proportional hazards regression models for highly stratified data. Biometrics 55:1162–1170

Chen MH, Shao QM (1999) Monte Carlo estimation of Bayesian credible and HPD intervals. J Comput Graph Stat 8(1):69–92

Chen Y, Hanson T, Zhang J (2014) Accelerated hazards model based on parametric families generalized with Bernstein polynomials. Biometrics 70:192–201

Chen YQ, Wang MC (2000) Analysis of accelerated hazards models. J Am Stat Assoc 95:608–618

Christensen R, Johnson WO (1988) Modeling accelerated failure time with a Dirichlet process. Biometrika 75:693–704

Chung Y, Dunson DB (2009) Nonparametric Bayes conditional distribution modeling with variable selection. J Am Stat Assoc 104:1646–1660

Cox DR (1972) Regression models and life-tables (with discussion). J R Stat Soc Ser B 34:187–220

Cox DR (1975) Partial likelihood. Biometrika 62(2):269–276

Damien P, Laud P, Smith A (1996) Implementation of Bayesian nonparametric inference using beta processes. Scand J Stat 23:27–36

De Iorio M, Johnson WO, Müller P, Rosner GL (2009) Bayesian nonparametric non-proportional hazards survival modelling. Biometrics 65:762–771

Doksum K (1974) Tailfree and neutral random probabilities and their posterior distributions. Ann Probab 2:183–201

Dykstra RL, Laud P (1981) A Bayesian nonparametric approach to reliability. Ann Stat 9:356–367

Ferguson TS (1973) A Bayesian analysis of some nonparametric problems. Ann Stat 1:209–230

Ferguson TS (1974) Prior distribution on the spaces of probability measures. Ann Stat 2:615–629

Ferguson TS, Klass MJ (1972) A representation of independent increment processes without Gaussian components. Ann Math Stat 43:1634–1643

Ferguson TS, Phadia EG (1979) Bayesian nonparametric estimation based on censored data. Ann Stat 7:163–186

Gamerman D (1991) Dynamic Bayesian models for survival data. Appl Stat 40:63–79

Geisser S, Eddy W (1979) A predictive approach to model selection. J Am Stat Assoc 74:153–160

Gelfand AE, Mallick BK (1995) Bayesian analysis of proportional hazards models built from monotone functions. Biometrics 51:843–852

Gray RJ (1994) A Bayesian analysis of institutional effects in a multicenter cancer clinical trial. Biometrics 50:244–253

Hanson T, Johnson WO (2002) Modeling regression error with a mixture of Polya trees. J Am Stat Assoc 97:1020–1033

Hanson T, Johnson WO (2004) A Bayesian semiparametric AFT model for interval-censored data. J Comput Graph Stat 13:341–361

Hanson T, Kottas A, Branscum A (2008) Modelling stochastic order in the analysis of receiver operating characteristic data: Bayesian nonparametric approaches. J R Stat Soc Ser C 57:207–225

Hanson TE (2006a) Inference for mixtures of finite Polya tree models. J Am Stat Assoc 101(476):1548–1565

Hanson TE (2006b) Modeling censored lifetime data using a mixture of gammas baseline. Bayesian Anal 1:575–594

Hanson TE, Yang M (2007) Bayesian semiparametric proportional odds models. Biometrics 63(1):88–95

Hanson TE, Branscum A, Johnson WO (2005) Bayesian nonparametric modeling and data analysis: an introduction. In: Dey D, Rao C (eds) Bayesian thinking: modeling and computation. Handbook of statistics, vol 25. Elsevier, Amsterdam, pp 245–278

Hanson TE, Branscum A, Johnson WO (2011) Predictive comparison of joint longitudinal-survival modeling: a case study illustrating competing approaches. Lifetime Data Anal 17:3–28

Hennerfeind A, Brezger A, Fahrmeir L (2006) Geoadditive survival models. J Am Stat Assoc 101(475):1065–1075

Hjort NL (1990) Nonparametric Bayes estimators based on beta processes in models for life history data. Ann Stat 18:1259–1294

Hutton JL, Monaghan PF (2002) Choice of parametric accelerated life and proportional hazards models for survival data: asymptotic results. Lifetime Data Anal 8:375–393

Ibrahim JG, Chen MH, Sinha D (2001) Bayesian survival analysis. Springer, New York

Jara A, Hanson TE (2011) A class of mixtures of dependent tailfree processes. Biometrika 98:553–566

Jara A, Lesaffre E, De Iorio M, Quintana FA (2010) Bayesian semiparametric inference for multivariate doubly-interval-censored data. Ann Appl Stat 4:2126–2149

Jara A, Hanson TE, Quintana FA, Müller P, Rosner GL (2011) DPpackage: Bayesian semi- and nonparametric modeling in R. J Stat Softw 40(5):1–30

Johnson WO, Christensen R (1989) Nonparametric Bayesian analysis of the accelerated failure time model. Stat Probab Lett 8:179–184

Kalbfleisch JD (1978) Nonparametric Bayesian analysis of survival time data. J R Stat Soc Ser B Methodol 40:214–221

Kay R, Kinnersley N (2002) On the use of the accelerated failure time model as an alternative to the proportional hazards model in the treatment of time to event data: a case study in influenza. Drug Inform J 36:571–579

Kneib T, Fahrmeir L (2007) A mixed model approach for geoadditive hazard regression. Scand J Stat 34(1):207–228

Komárek A, Lesaffre E, Legrand C (2007) Baseline and treatment effect heterogeneity for survival times between centers using a random effects accelerated failure time model with flexible error distribution. Stat Med 26:5457–5472

Kottas A, Gelfand AE (2001) Bayesian semiparametric median regression modeling. J Am Stat Assoc 96:1458–1468

Kuo L, Mallick B (1997) Bayesian semiparametric inference for the accelerated failure-time model. Can J Stat 25:457–472

Li L, Hanson T, Zhang J (2015) Spatial extended hazard model with application to prostate cancer survival. Biometrics (in press)

Maksymiuk AW, Jett JR, Earle JD, Su JQ, Diegert FA, Mailliard JA, Kardinal CG, Krook JE, Veeder MH, Wiesenfeld M, Tschetter, LK, Levitt R (1994) Sequencing and schedule effects of cisplatin plus etoposide in small cell lung cancer results of a north central cancer treatment group randomized clinical trial. J Clin Oncol 12:70–76

Müller P, Erkanli A, West M (1996) Bayesian curve fitting using multivariate normal mixtures. Biometrika 83:67–79

Nieto-Barajas L, Walker SG (2002) Markov beta and gamma processes for modelling hazard rates. Scand J Stat 29:413–424

References

Orbe J, Ferreira E, Núñez Antón V (2002) Comparing proportional hazards and accelerated failure time models for survival analysis. Stat Med 21(22):3493–3510

Portnoy S (2003) Censored regression quantiles. J Am Stat Assoc 98:1001–1012

Reid N (1994) A conversation with Sir David Cox. Stat Sci 9:439–455

Rosner GL (2005) Bayesian monitoring of clinical trials with failure-time endpoints. Biometrics 61:239–245

Ryan T, Woodall W (2005) The most-cited statistical papers. J Appl Stat 32(5):461–474

Sinha D, Dey DK (1997) Semiparametric Bayesian analysis of survival data. J Am Stat Assoc 92:1195–1212

Sinha D, McHenry MB, Lipsitz SR, Ghosh M (2009) Empirical Bayes estimation for additive hazards regression models. Biometrika 96(3):545–558

Somoza JL (1980) Illustrative analysis: infant and child mortality in Colombia. World Fertility Survey Scientific Reports 10

Susarla V, Van Ryzin J (1976) Nonparametric Bayesian estimation of survival curves from incomplete observations. J Am Stat Assoc 71:897–902

Therneau TM, Grambsch PM (2000) Modeling survival data: extending the Cox model. Springer, New York

Walker SG, Damien P (2000) Representation of Lévy processes without Gaussian components. Biometrika 87:447–483

Walker SG, Mallick BK (1997) Hierarchical generalized linear models and frailty models with Bayesian nonparametric mixing. J R Stat Soc Ser B 59:845–860

Walker SG, Mallick BK (1999) A Bayesian semiparametric accelerated failure time model. Biometrics 55(2):477–483

Walker SG, Damien P, Laud PW, Smith AFM (1999) Bayesian nonparametric inference for random distributions and related functions (with discussion). J R Stat Soc B 61:485–527

Wang L, Dunson DB (2011) Semiparametric Bayes' proportional odds models for current status data with underreporting. Biometrics 67(3):1111–1118

Yang S (1999) Censored median regression using weighted empirical survival and hazard functions. J Am Stat Assoc 94:137–145

Yin G, Ibrahim JG (2005) A class of Bayesian shared gamma frailty models with multivariate failure time data. Biometrics 61:208–216

Ying Z, Jung SH, Wei LJ (1995) Survival analysis with median regression models. J Am Stat Assoc 90:178–184

Zellner A (1983) Applications of Bayesian analysis in econometrics. Statistician 32:23–34

Zhang M, Davidian M (2008) "Smooth" semiparametric regression analysis for arbitrarily censored time-to-event data. Biometrics 64(2):567–576

Zhao L, Hanson TE, Carlin BP (2009) Mixtures of Polya trees for flexible spatial frailty survival modelling. Biometrika 96(2):263–276

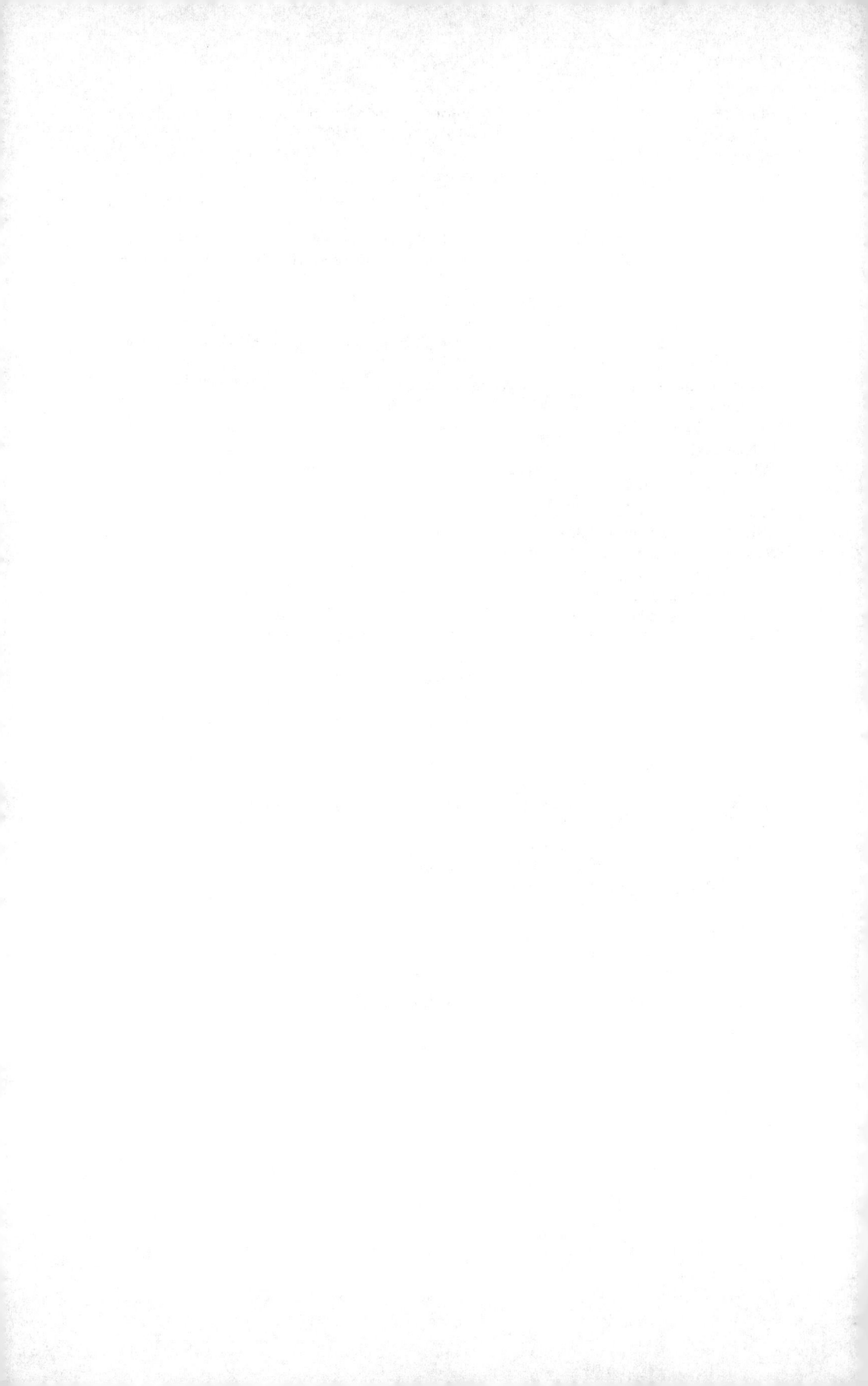

Chapter 7
Hierarchical Models

Abstract One of the great success stories of Bayesian methods in biostatistics is inference in hierarchical models. The model-based Bayesian approach allows for coherent propagation of uncertainties and borrowing of strength across submodels and more. In this chapter we discuss nonparametric Bayesian approaches in hierarchical models, including nonparametric priors on random effects distributions and extensions of such models across multiple related studies. Honest accounting for uncertainties becomes particularly important for applications to classification, when we use posterior predictive inference for a future experimental unit to estimate unknown membership in one of several subpopulations.

7.1 Nonparametric Random Effects Distributions

An important application of BNP approaches arises in modeling random effects distributions in hierarchical mixed effects models. We have already briefly discussed this use of BNP models before, in Sect. 5.2.3, in the context of GLM's. When modeling random effects distributions, often little is known about the specific form of the distribution. Assuming a specific parametric form is typically motivated by technical convenience rather than by genuine prior beliefs. Although inference about the random effects distribution itself is rarely of interest, it can have implications on the inference of interest. A typical example is the classification in the upcoming Example 23. Thus it is important to allow for population heterogeneity, outliers, skewness, etc.

In the context of a traditional randomized block ANOVA model with random effects θ_i a BNP can be used to allow for more general random effects distributions. Let

$$y_{ik} = \theta_i + \beta' x_{ik} + \epsilon_{ik}$$

denote a generic block ANOVA with residuals $\epsilon_{ij} \mid \sigma^2 \overset{iid}{\sim} N(0, \sigma^2)$, fixed effects β and random effects θ_i for blocks $i = 1, \ldots, I$. Let $\mathsf{Ga}(a, b)$ denote a gamma distribution with mean a/b. For technically convenient posterior analysis we often assume a normal random effects distribution $\theta_i \mid \tau^2 \overset{iid}{\sim} N(0, \tau^2)$, $i = 1, \ldots, I$, and conditionally conjugate priors $\boldsymbol{\beta} \sim \mathsf{N}(\mu, \Sigma)$, $\sigma^{-2} \sim \mathsf{Ga}(s/2, sS/2)$ and $\tau^{-2} \sim \mathsf{Ga}(r/2, rR/2)$ (see Gelman 2006 for a discussion of alternative priors on variance parameters in hierarchical models). While the prior for the fixed effects might be based on substantive prior information, the choice of the random effects distribution is rarely based on actual prior knowledge. The relaxation of the convenient, but often arbitrary distributional assumption for the random effects distribution is a typical application of BNP models. A BNP model allows us to relax the assumption without losing interpretability and without substantial loss of computational efficiency. We replace the normal random effects distribution by $\theta_i \mid G \stackrel{\text{iid}}{\sim} G$, with a BNP prior for the unknown G. The random effects distribution itself becomes an unknown quantity. For later reference we state the full mixed effects model

$$p(y_{ik} \mid \boldsymbol{\beta}, \theta_i), \qquad k = 1, \ldots, n_i$$

$$\theta_i \mid G \stackrel{\text{iid}}{\sim} G \quad \text{and} \quad G \mid \eta \sim \pi(\cdot \mid \eta). \tag{7.1}$$

Here $\boldsymbol{\beta}$ are additional parameters in the sampling model. The sampling model $p(\cdot \mid \boldsymbol{\beta}, \theta_i)$ could be, for example, the earlier mentioned ANOVA model. The BNP prior $\pi(\cdot \mid \eta)$ is a prior for density estimation for the random effects θ_i, indexed with possible hyper-parameters η. We could use any prior that was discussed in the earlier chapters on density estimation. The only difference is that now the latent θ_i replace the observed data in the earlier density estimation problem.

Many BNP models allow us to center the random probability measure G around some parametric model p_η, indexed by hyper-parameters η. For example, we could center G around a $\mathsf{N}(0, \eta^2)$ model. The construction allows us to think of the nonparametric model as a natural extension of the fully parametric model.

Bush and MacEachern (1996) propose a DP prior for G, $G \sim \mathsf{DP}(MG_0)$. Kleinman and Ibrahim (1998) propose the same approach in a more general framework for a linear model with random effects. They discuss an application to longitudinal random effects models. Müller and Rosner (1997) use DPM of normals to avoid the awkward discreteness of the implied random effects distribution. Also, the additional convolution with a normal kernel significantly simplifies posterior simulation for sampling distributions beyond the normal linear model. Mukhopadhyay and Gelfand (1997) implement the same approach in generalized linear models with linear predictor $\theta_i + x_i'\boldsymbol{\beta}$ and a DPM model for the random effect θ_i. In Wang and Taylor (2001) random effects W_i are entire longitudinal paths for each subject in the study. They use integrated Ornstein-Uhlenbeck stochastic process priors for W_i.

Example 19 (Example: Mammogram Usage) Malec and Müller (2008) model mammogram usage for counties across 50 states in the US. The data are reported in the National Health Interview Survey (NHIS). They use a semi-parametric mixed effects model with a logistic regression and a BNP prior on the random effects distribution to model the number of respondents in each county who have used a mammogram. The data are reported by six demographic domains. Each demographic domain is characterized by an age bracket and an ethnicity, including, for example, "non-black, age 30–39", etc. Let n_{id} denote the number of individuals interviewed in demographic domain d and county i and let $y_{id} \mid n_{id}, p_{id} \stackrel{\text{ind}}{\sim}$ $\text{Bin}(n_{id}, p_{id})$ denote the number of positive responses among these n_{id} individuals. Here p_{id} is the unknown mammography usage in county i and demographic group d. Counties are nested within strata, $s = 1, \ldots, S$. Strata are groups of between 1 and 23 counties (average of 4.8), that are defined for census purposes. For notational convenience we index the counties across strata $i = 1, \ldots, I$ and let $s(i)$ denote the stratum that contains county i. The aim of this study was inference on state level mammography usage. The state level mammography usage P_{state} is simply the weighted average of the p_{id}, weighted with the known total populations in each county and demographic group. Malec and Müller (2008) use a hierarchical logistic regression model with county specific random effects

$$\text{logit}(p_{id}) = x'_{id}\boldsymbol{\beta} + b_{id} + v_s,$$

with a regression on county and demographic domain level covariates x_{id} and county-specific random effects $\boldsymbol{b}_i = (b_{i1}, \ldots, b_{iD})$. In this analysis, the domain level covariates included the proportion of persons aged 25+, with less than ninth grade education (x_{id1}) and the proportion of persons in the work-force, 16+ with white-collar job (x_{id2}). The model is completed with a random effects distribution

$$\boldsymbol{b}_i \mid G \stackrel{\text{iid}}{\sim} G,$$

and priors $v_s \sim \text{N}(0, \delta)$ and $\boldsymbol{\beta} \sim \text{N}(\boldsymbol{m}, \boldsymbol{V})$.

The choice of the random effects distribution G is determined by several considerations. First, the random effects b_{id} across demographic groups $d = 1, \ldots, D$ within the same county i are different but highly correlated. That is why we consider a multivariate random effects distribution G for the D-dimensional vector of county specific random effects. Second, the recorded covariates only account for some of the population heterogeneity. The random effects distribution needs to allow for considerable remaining heterogeneity. Finally, the model needs to accommodate outliers without unduly influencing inference. These considerations lead us to use a DPM of normals prior for G. Figure 7.1 shows some summaries of the estimate $E(G \mid data)$. The figure shows two bivariate marginals of the 6-dimensional random effects distribution. A traditional parametric random mixed effects model would use a multivariate normal distribution and miss the skewed nature of G.

Figure 7.2 shows posterior estimated rates for each state (as a percentage of total population for each state). For comparison the figure also shows the empirical fractions for each state and the synthetic estimates. The latter are based on estimating mammogram usage for each demographic group and using the known composition of demographic groups in each state.

There are many examples in the recent literature that develop and use BNP priors for random effects distributions. We mention a few more that use models similar

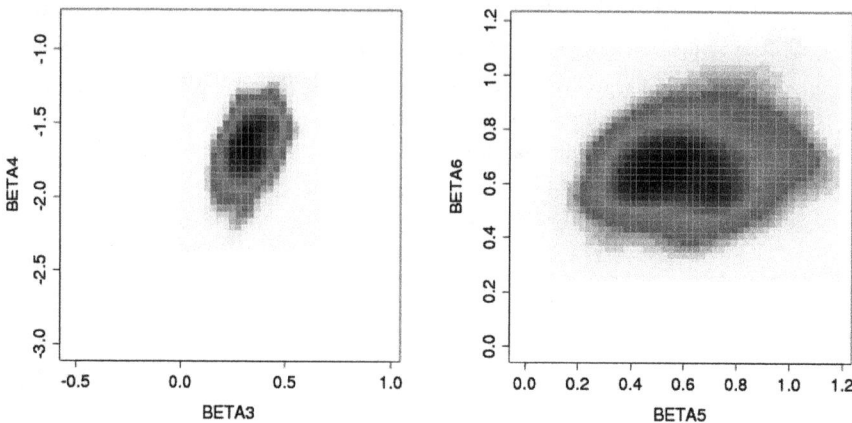

Fig. 7.1 Example 19. Estimated by random effects distribution

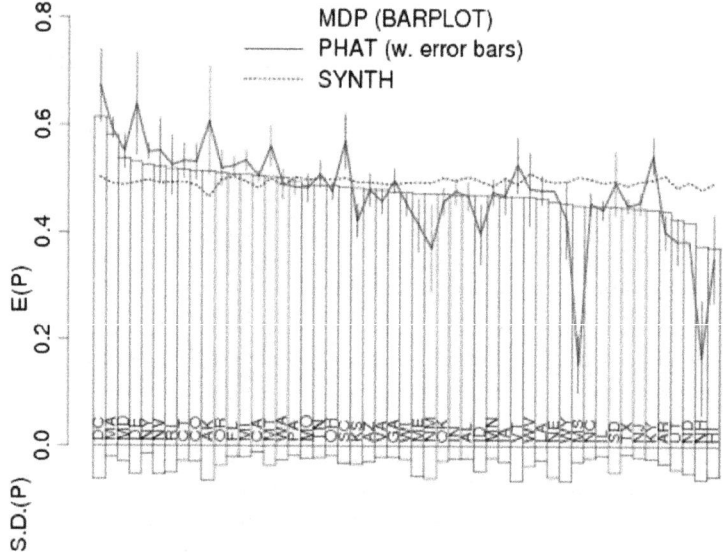

Fig. 7.2 Example 19. Estimated rates P_{state} of mammogram usage per state under the proposed model (*bar plot*), the synthetic method (*dashed line*) and as sample averages over observed samples in each state (*dotted line*). The short bars below the horizontal axis show one posterior standard deviation $SD(P_{\text{state}} \mid y)$ for the state totals. Error bars at each sample average estimate indicate corresponding sampling errors (assuming that all observations in a given state were independent). The sample did not include any data for NE and ND. Thus, there is no "sample estimate" for these states

to those that we introduced in earlier sections. As noted before, in Sect. 5.2.3, Jara et al. (2009) propose a smoothed multivariate MPT prior for the random effects distribution $G \sim \text{PT}(G_0 = \text{N}(\mathbf{0}, \mathbf{S}), \mathcal{A}_c)$. The model compares favorably to both the DP and DPM models. The density of G is further smoothed through the use of a novel decomposition of the centering covariance matrix $S = MLM'$ via the usual spectral decomposition. The covariance matrix is written as $S = [ML^{1/2}O][ML^{1/2}O]'$, using random orthogonal matrices O with a Haar prior. These models are implemented in DPpackage using the PTglmm function. This MPT prior on G was used in Ghosh and Hanson (2010) for the analysis of bivariate longitudinal outcomes.

An interesting generalization of random intercept models within the context of a GLMM is developed by Jara and Hanson (2011). They consider standard GLMMs with univariate-random effects admitting cluster-specific predictors. Restated in other words, model (7.1) is generalized to $\theta_i \mid G_{z_i}$ where G_{z_i} is a median-zero LDTFP that changes smoothly with covariates z_i. This model is implemented in DPpackage as the function LDTFPglmm. Similarly, Zhou et al. (2015) generalize a static nonparametric MPT random effects distribution G to a covariate-adjusted version through the use of a LDTFP to analyze time to death of breast cancer patients in Iowa; they consider a particular proportional hazards model which leads to a Poisson GLMM. Instead of the spatially smoothed county-level random effects $\theta_1, \ldots, \theta_{99}$ considered by Zhao et al. (2009), the random effects instead follow a LDTFP that smoothly changes with two measures: a score from 1 to 9 indicating how rural/urban each county is, and median household income, both obtained from census data. The model provides unique insight into the effect of ruralness (which serves as a proxy for healthcare access), showing much greater variability, including bimodality, in random effect densities for more rural counties. The inclusion of county-level covariates into the random effects density obviates the need for a spatially-smoothed version and also enhances interpretation.

7.2 Population PK/PD Models

Mixed effects models find use in many diverse application areas. As a typical example we consider in some more detail models for population pharmacokinetic and population pharmacodynamic studies. The pharmacokinetics (PK) of a drug relate to what happens to the drug once it enters the body. The time course of the drug and its metabolites in the body reflect each patient's individual PK. Pharmacodynamics (PD) concerns the reaction of the body to the drug. Toxic side effects, tumor shrinkage, reduced nausea and vomiting are all examples of PD effects. In short, PK is what the body does to the drug, and PD is what the drug does to the body. Researchers study PK and PD of drugs in a population of patients to learn about variation in response or reaction to therapy. The slower a drug clears from the body, the greater the systemic exposure (PK). The greater the systemic exposure to the active agent, the greater the chance of effect (PD), both good (e.g., tumor shrinkage) and bad (e.g., toxicity). Statistical models that implement the desired inference on the variation of PK and PD parameters over a population of interest are known as population PK/PD models.

From the perspective of statistical modeling, the analysis of population PK/PD data is inference for repeated measurement data. Let y_{ik} denote the kth measurement on the ith patient, and let x_i denote patient-specific covariates. A traditional mechanism to induce dependence across repeated measurements for the same patient is the use of mixed-effects models with patient-specific random effects. Let θ_i denote a random-effects vector for patient i. The common structure of population PK or PD models is

$$p(y_{ik} \mid \theta_i), \quad p(\theta_i \mid x_i, \phi), \quad \pi(\phi). \tag{7.2}$$

Here $p(y_{ik} \mid \theta_i)$ is typically a parametric nonlinear regression for response over time, such as a compartmental PK model for drug concentrations. The second level of the model (called the population model) specifies the prior for the random-effects vectors θ_i, possibly including a regression on patient-specific covariates, x_i; ϕ denotes the hyper-parameters. Bayesian models similar to (7.2) have been considered in Zeger and Karim (1991) for generalized linear mixed models and Wakefield et al. (1994) for the general population model assuming a multivariate normal population distribution. Wakefield et al. (1999) review popular Bayesian approaches. Davidian and Giltinan (1995) provide an extensive treatment of the analysis of repeated measurements with nonlinear models.

Heterogeneity in the patient population, outliers, and over-dispersion make a strict parametric model for the population distribution $p(\theta_i \mid x_i, \phi)$ unrealistic. Concerns about the effects of such aberrations led to research into nonparametric extensions. In maximum likelihood-based inference, two popular approaches to nonparametric extensions are the nonparametric maximum likelihood estimator (Mallet et al. 1988; Schumitzky 1993) and the so called semi-nonparametric family (SNP) of Davidian and Gallant (1993). BNP extensions are described in Walker and Wakefield (1998), Rosner and Müller (1997), Müller and Rosner (1997), and Kleinman and Ibrahim (1998), all with DP and DPM priors. The DPM prior model is specified as

$$\theta_i \mid S, G \overset{\text{iid}}{\sim} \int N(\theta_i \mid \mu, S) \, G(d\mu), \quad G \mid M, G^\star \sim \text{DP}(MG^\star).$$

Here S, M and the parameters defining $G^\star$ are all part of the generic hyper-parameter vector ϕ in (7.2). To include an additional regression on patient-specific covariates x_i in (7.2) we can use the same approach as in density regression (compare Sect. 4.4.4) and replace the DPM for θ_i by a DPM prior for the distribution of $\tilde{\theta}_i \equiv (x_i, \theta_i)$,

$$(x_i, \theta_i) \mid \mu_i \overset{\text{ind}}{\sim} N(\mu_i, S) \quad \text{and} \quad \mu_i \mid G \overset{\text{iid}}{\sim} G, \tag{7.3}$$

with a DP prior for G, that is, $G \mid M, G^\star \sim \text{DP}(MG^\star)$. This approach is taken, for example, in Rosner and Müller (1997).

7.2 Population PK/PD Models

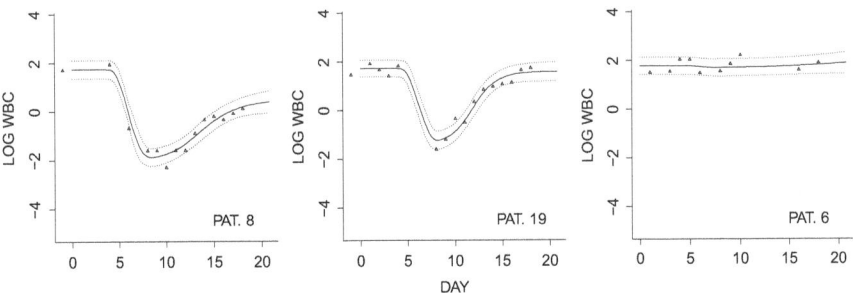

Fig. 7.3 Example 20. WBC profiles for three patients in study CALGB 8881. The sudden drop at the beginning of chemotherapy and the slow S-shaped recovery back to baseline are typical for most patients. Some patients are outliers

Example 20 (Population PD — CALGB 8881) In Müller and Rosner (1997) we consider data from a study carried out by the Cancer and Leukemia Group B (CALGB) (Lichtman et al. 1993). The trial was carried out to find the highest dose of cyclophosphamide that could be given every two weeks. The study enrolled $n = 52$ patients who were administered different doses of cyclophosphamide (CTX). Patients also received the drug GM-CSF to help reduce the ill effects of cyclophosphamide on the patients marrow. The measured outcome was white blood cell count (WBC) for each patient over time. Let y_{ik} denote the WBC for patient i at occasion $k = 1, \ldots, n_i$. WBC is recorded on a logarithmic scale. Figure 7.3 shows WBC profiles for three typical patients. Typical WBC profiles show an initial horizontal baseline, a sudden drop at the beginning of chemotherapy followed by a slow S-shaped recovery, and eventually leveling off close to the initial baseline. We define a sampling model for y_{ik} as a non-linear regression $E(y_{ik} \mid \theta_i) = f(t_{ik}; \theta_i)$ that fits these typical shapes. Here t_{ik} are the (known) sampling times. We use a piecewise linear, linear, logistic function. The function is described with a 7-dimensional parameter vector θ_i. The parameters include the level of the initial baseline, the change points before and after the sudden drop, and slope, intercept, offset and scale for a shifted and scaled logistic function to model the final recovery. We use patient-specific parameters, making θ_i patient-specific random effects.

The model construction continues with a random effects model $p(\theta_i \mid x_i)$, including a regression on baseline covariates x_i. The baseline covariates are the doses for CTX and GM-CSF. We implement the random effects model as a BNP regression $p(\theta_i \mid x_i = x) = G_x(\cdot)$. We use conditional regression as described in Sect. 4.4.4. That is, we define an augmented random effects vector $\tilde{\theta}_i = (\theta_i, x_i)$ and assume $\tilde{\theta}_i \mid G \stackrel{iid}{\sim} G$. The model is completed with a DPM of normals prior on G. The fitted lines in Fig. 7.3 show the estimated mean functions $E\{f(t_{ik}; \theta_i) \mid \text{data}\}$, together with pointwise posterior standard deviations. More importantly, the model allows us to report posterior predictive inference for a future $(n + 1)$-st patient. Figure 7.4 shows summaries of the posterior predictive distribution for a future patient.

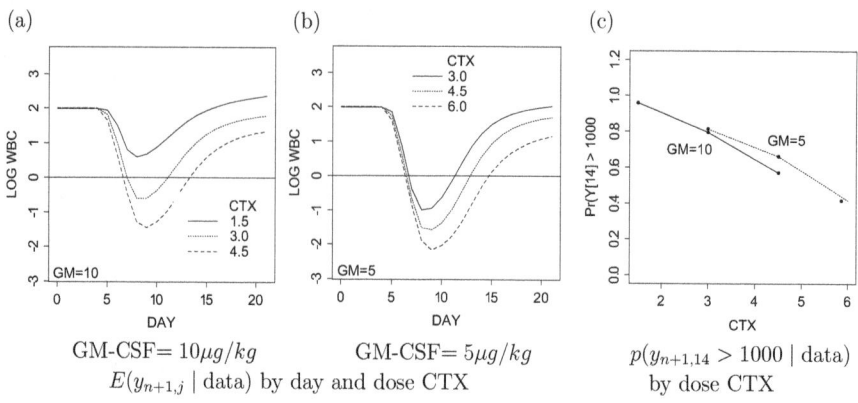

Fig. 7.4 Example 20. Predictive inference for a future $(n+1)$-st patient. Panels (**a**) and (**b**) show predictive WBC profiles. Panel (**c**) shows the probability of WBC beyond a critical threshold after 14 days plotted by dose CTX and GM-CSF

Yang et al. (2010) defined a variation of (7.2) for repeated measurement outcomes that are fractions. The need to include a positive probability for fractions of 0 or 1 introduces a minor complication in the desired inference. Such data often arise, for instance, in immunohistochemistry. Yang et al. (2010) use a DPM prior on random effects and latent continuous variables to define a sampling model for the fractional outcomes. The data are modeled as a mixture of point masses at 0 and 1, along with a normally-distributed random variable for values between 0 and 1. A regression model for the continuous component allows inclusion of covariates, as well as subject-specific random effects. These random effects were modeled with a PT prior (Lavine 1992, 1994). See further details in Yang et al. (2010).

7.3 Hierarchical Models of RPMs

7.3.1 Finite Mixtures of Random Probability Measures

If we want to analyze several related studies, $j = 1, \ldots, J$ we require a hierarchical extension of model (7.1) to multiple studies:

$$y_{jik} \mid \beta, \theta_{ji} \stackrel{\text{ind}}{\sim} p(\cdot \mid \beta, \theta_{ji}), \quad k = 1, \ldots, n_{ji}$$

$$\theta_{ji} \mid G_j \stackrel{\text{ind}}{\sim} G_j, \quad i = 1, \ldots, n_i, \quad \text{and} \quad G_1, \ldots, G_j \mid \eta \sim \pi(\cdot \mid \eta). \quad (7.4)$$

Let $\mathbf{y}_{ji} = (y_{jik}, k = 1, \ldots, n_{ji})$, denote the data vector for patient i in study j. After marginalization with respect to θ_{ji}, model (7.4) implies a marginal model

7.3 Hierarchical Models of RPMs

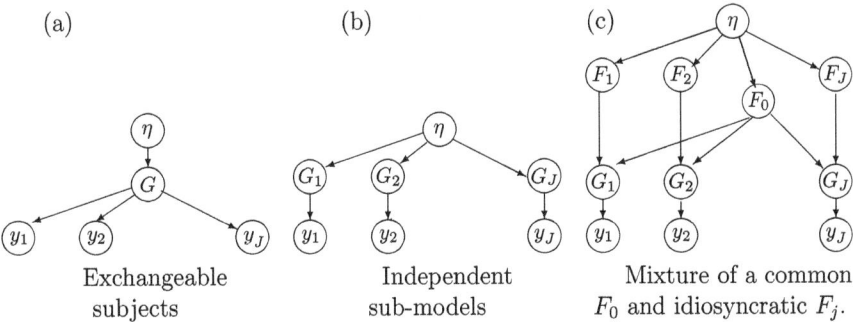

Fig. 7.5 Combining data from related studies assuming exchangeable subjects across studies (**a**) or independent sub-models (**b**). The desired level of borrowing strength across the sub-models is in-between these two extremes (**c**)

$p(y_{ji} \mid \beta, G_j) = \int p(y_{ji} \mid \theta_{ji}, \beta) \, dG_j(\theta_{ji})$. The use of fully parametric hierarchical models to "borrow strength" across different but related sub-models is a common theme in statistical modeling. For a hierarchical model over related studies where each sub-model $p(y_{ji} \mid G_j)$ is a nonparametric model, however, the nonparametric nature of G_j complicates modeling, except in two extreme cases shown in panels (a) and (b) of Fig. 7.5. If the sub-models G_j are independent given the hyper-parameters (panel b), then the problem reduces to analyzing J separate studies linked only by the finite dimensional hyper-parameter vector. At the other extreme, if the observations y_{ji} can be considered exchangeable across studies (panel a), then the problem reduces to estimating one random measure $G = G_1 = \cdots = G_J$. For many applications, the latter case enforces too much borrowing by assuming essentially one population, and the earlier allows too little borrowing of strength across studies. Lopes et al. (2003) and Müller et al. (2004) develop a model that allows one to link the sub-models at the desired intermediate level. A graphical representation is given in Fig. 7.5c. The model includes a common measure F_0, representing a baseline model that is common to all studies and random probability measures F_j that characterize any idiosyncratic behavior in study $j = 1, \ldots, J$. The split into a common effect and study-specific effects is akin to the setup of ANOVA models which include a similar distinction between overall means and study-specific offsets. When i indexes patients within studies, model (7.4) has an interpretation as modeling patient populations. The random probability measure G_j characterizes the j-th patient subpopulation.

We assume

$$G_j(\theta) = \epsilon \, F_0(\theta) + (1 - \epsilon) \, F_j(\theta), \quad j = 1, \ldots, J, \tag{7.5}$$

with random measures

$$F_0, \ldots, F_J \mid \eta \overset{iid}{\sim} p(\theta \mid \eta), \tag{7.6}$$

and a hyper-prior $\epsilon \sim \pi_0 \delta_0(\epsilon) + \pi_1 \delta_1(\epsilon) + (1 - \pi_0 - \pi_1) \text{Be}(\epsilon \mid a, b)$ that includes point masses at $\epsilon = 0$ and $\epsilon = 1$. The weight ϵ, $0 \leq \epsilon \leq 1$, represents the level of borrowing strength across studies. A fraction ϵ of the total mass is shared by all studies, and the rest $(1 - \epsilon)$ remains specific to each particular study. Thus, the data collected from each study contributes to the global learning about F_0, but learning on F_j can be accomplished only through $\{y_{ji}, \, i = 1, \ldots, n_j\}$. We decompose the distribution G_j into a common measure F_0 and a study-specific or idiosyncratic measure F_j. The common measure induces the desired dependence. The prior point masses at $\epsilon = 0$ and $\epsilon = 1$ allow for positive posterior probability of either of the two extreme models shown in Fig. 7.5a,b.

Lopes et al. (2003) implement model (7.5) with a finite mixture of normal prior for F_j in (7.6). That is, we write the common measure F_0 as a mixture of N multivariate normals $F_0(\theta_{ki}|\eta_0) = \sum_{m=1}^{N} \pi_m \text{N}(\mu + d_m, S)$, where π_m are the mixing weights, μ is the overall mean (location), and d_m are component-wise deviations or offsets from μ. We set $d_1 \equiv 0$ to ensure identifiability. Mengersen and Robert (1996) and Roeder and Wasserman (1997) discuss this parametrization for finite mixtures of normals. Similarly, the study-specific measures G_j are considered finite mixtures of multivariate normal densities, each with N' components.

In Müller et al. (2004) we developed an alternative approach, building a structure as in Fig. 7.5c with semi-parametric infinite mixtures of normals. The prior (7.6) is specified as a DPM of normals. Posterior inference in this model can be implemented with minimal changes to any posterior simulation algorithm that is used for DPM models. `DPpackage` refers to (7.5) with DPM prior as hierarchical Dirichlet process mixture (HDPM) and implements inference in the function `HDPMdensity`.

Example 21 (Two Related Studies — CALGB 8881 and 9160) Müller et al. (2004) use the hierarchical model (7.5)–(7.6) as a prior probability model for random effects distributions in two related studies. The data are log white blood cell counts over time for breast cancer patients in two related studies. Figure 7.3 showed some selected patients from the first study, CALGB 8881, $j = 1$. We discussed analysis of the data from CALGB 8881 before, in Example 20. Figure 7.6 shows data for a second similar study, CALGB 9160, $j = 2$. In CALGB 9160 patients received cyclophosphamide (CTX) and GM-CSF at the doses determined by CALGB 8881. That is, CTX= $3/m^2$ and GM-CSF= 5μg/kg. In CALGB 9160 some patients received an additional drug, amifostine (AMF). Patients were randomized to recieve AMF or not.

The model includes a non-linear regression mean curve $f(t; \theta_{ji})$ for blood count data for patient i, in study j, $i = 1, \ldots, n_i$ and $j = 1, 2$. The mean curve is indexed with patient-specific random effects θ_{ij}, similar to Example 20. The random effects θ_{ij} are assumed to arise from a study-specific random effects distribution G_j. The model is completed with the hierarchical prior in (7.5) for $\{G_1, G_2, G_3\}$, including a future third study $j = 3$. A future third study with $n_3 = 0$ patients is included to allow posterior predictive inference for a patient in the population at large, beyond

7.3 Hierarchical Models of RPMs

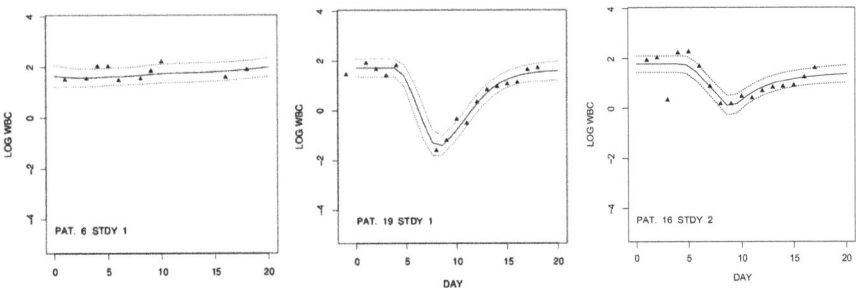

Fig. 7.6 Example 21. Some typical patients. The data show y_{ijk} for three arbitrarily selected patients from study $j = 2$. The triangles are the observed WBC. The *solid line* shows the posterior fitted mean curve, and the *dotted lines* show 95 % central HPD intervals for the mean curve

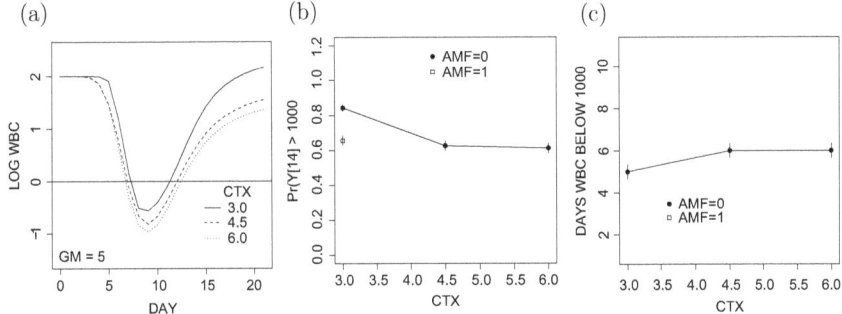

Fig. 7.7 Example 21. Posterior predictive inference for a hypothetical future patient in a future study $j = 3$ at CTX = 3, GM-CSF = 5 and with (AMF = 1) and without (AMF = 0) AMF. For AMF = 1, only CTX = 3.0 is shown (to avoid extrapolation beyond the range of the data). The point for (CTX = 3, AMF = 1) is overlaid with AMF = 0. The *short vertical bars* indicate one posterior predictive standard deviation. (**a**) Estimated WBC profile. (**b**) $Pr\{WBC > 1000\}$ on day 14. (**c**) $E(T_{14} \mid y)$ T_{14} = days WBC below 1000

the first two studies. Figure 7.7 shows posterior predictive inference for a patient from a future third study $j = 3$.

Kolossiatis et al. (2013) discuss an interesting variation of the model (7.5) and (7.6). They propose a specific choice of prior for ϵ that together with the DP priors for F_j ensures an implied DP prior for the linear combination G_j. In general, a linear combination (7.5) of DP random measures does not define a DP random measure.

7.3.2 Dependent Random Probability Measures

The problem of defining nonparametric dependent random effects distributions G_j for a set of studies can be considered to be a special case of BNP priors for families of dependent random probability measures. We ran into this problem already once before, when discussing fully nonparametric regression models in Sect. 4.4. First we generalize the hierarchical extension from $\{G_j, j = 1, \ldots, J\}$ to a more general family of subpopulations $\mathcal{G} = \{G_x : x \in \mathcal{X}\}$, where x could, for example, index different studies as well as different dose levels within studies. To be specific, without loss of generality, in the following discussion we assume $x = (j, w)$ with j indexing multiple studies and w indexing different doses of two drugs used in these studies. The goal is to borrow strength across different studies and doses.

In the presence of covariates it is now more convenient to include the study index j with the covariate vector, and use one running index for patients, $i = 1, \ldots, n$ for $n = \sum_j n_j$ and rewrite model (7.1) as

$$y_{ik} \mid \theta_i \overset{\text{ind}}{\sim} p(\cdot \mid \theta_i)$$

$$\theta_i \mid x_i \overset{\text{ind}}{\sim} G_{x_i}$$

$$\mathcal{G} = \{G_x : x \in \mathcal{X}\} \sim \pi. \tag{7.7}$$

Many alternative BNP prior models for $\{G_x : x \in \mathcal{X}\}$ have been proposed. The most popular is arguably the DDP prior.

Recall from Sect. 4.4.1 the DDP prior for $\mathcal{F} = \{F_x : x \in \mathcal{X}\}$ with $F_x(\cdot) = \sum_{h=1}^{\infty} \pi_h \delta_{\theta_{xh}}(\cdot)$ from Definition 4 (Sect. 4.4.1). The random probability measures $F_x \in \mathcal{F}$ are made dependent by introducing dependence on $(\theta_{xh}, x \in \mathcal{X})$ across x (maintaining independence across h). For categorical covariates, like the assumed $x = (j, w)$ here, the perhaps simplest method to induce dependence across θ_{xh} is through an ANOVA model

$$\theta_{xh} = m_h + A_{jh} + B_{wh}, \tag{7.8}$$

with a prior p^o on the terms m_h, A_{jh} and B_{wh}. We impose any of the usual ANOVA-type identifiability constraints, such as $A_{1h} = B_{1h} \equiv 0$. We denote the joint probability model as $\{F_x : x \in \mathcal{X}\} \sim$ ANOVA DDP(M, p^o), as in Definition 5 (Sect. 4.4.2). The model is parameterized by the total mass parameter M and the base measure p^o on the ANOVA effects in (7.8). Marginally, for each $x = (j, w)$, the random distribution F_x follows a DP with total mass M and centering measure F_x^o given by the convolution of p_m^o, p_{Aj}^o and p_{Bw}^o. In summary, Model (7.8) defines dependence across x by defining an ANOVA structure of the point masses θ_{xh} across the levels of x. Model (7.8) is not constrained to univariate distributions F_x. The point masses θ_{xh} and the ANOVA effects m_h, A_{jh}, B_{wh} can be q-dimensional vectors. This is important, for example, if the random distributions F_x are used for random

7.3 Hierarchical Models of RPMs

effects in a hierarchical model. Model specification and computation, however, are dimension independent.

The ANOVA DDP model can be used to model random effects' distributions $\mathcal{G}$ in related studies, in (7.7). We use an additional convolution with a normal kernel to avoid the discrete nature of the DP random measure. That is, we assume

$$G_x(\cdot) = \int N(\cdot \mid \mu, S) \, dF_x(\mu) \qquad (7.9)$$

with a DDP prior on $\mathcal{F}$, treating both, study index j and dose w as categorical factors. This is exactly the LDDP model (4.12) that is implemented as function LDDP in the R package DPpackage (Jara et al. 2011), with $\beta_h = (m_h, A_{jh}, B_{wh}; x = (j, h) \in \mathcal{X})$

Example 22 (Multiple Studies — CALGB 8881, 9160 and 8541) In the previous two examples we analyzed data from two clinical studies. In Example 20 we used a DPM for inference in one study, CALGB 8881. In Example 21 we extended the model and inference to jointly analyze data from two related early phase studies, CALGB 8881 and CALGB 9160 using a finite mixture of DPM models. We now extend the analysis one step further to joint inference for the two early phase studies, CALGB 8881 and 9160, and a large phase III study, CALGB 8541 (Wood et al. 1994). The large phase III study required collecting blood count measurements only once a week. There are between 1 and 4 WBC measurements per patient. These are too few data points to estimate with much precision summaries like nadir WBC or other measures of myelosuppression, as we did for the earlier studies. Compare Figs. 7.4 and 7.7. In Müller et al. (2005) we used the ANOVA DDP model (7.7) to borrow strength across all three studies, the small early phase studies with frequent blood count measurements on a small number of patients (Figs. 7.3 and 7.6) and the large phase III study with few repeat measurements on many patients.

The sample sizes of the three studies were $n_1 = 52$, $n_2 = 46$ and $n_3 = 513$, respectively (in CALCG 8541 we only use data on the group of women assigned to the most dose-intense regimen). Figure 7.8 compares posterior predictive mean profiles for a future patient in the large study under two models: the proposed hierarchical model and a model using data from only the large study. We used identical prior assumptions in both analyses. Without incorporating the information from the earlier studies, prediction is much more uncertain about the time of the nadir count and the start of the recovery, as would be expected for inference conditional on only the sparse phase III data. In contrast, the predicted WBC profile based on the hierarchical model is more consistent with what one would expect to see for patients receiving anticancer chemotherapy and has reasonable predictive precision.

Fig. 7.8 Example 22. Posterior estimated mean profile for a future patient from a large clinical trial. The figure shows the pointwise posterior quantiles of the WBC profile. The figure compares inference under the hierarchical model (*solid*) with inference using only data from the large randomized clinical trial (*dashed*)

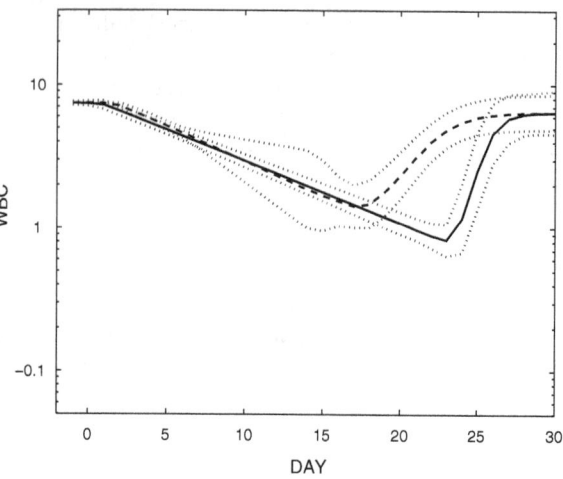

7.3.3 Classification

An interesting use of dependent random probability measures arises in classification. Consider data as in (7.7), and assume that responses y_{ik} and covariates x_i are observed for $i = 1, \ldots, n$. But now assume that we want to predict an unknown x_{n+1} for a new experimental unit with observed responses $y_{n+1,k}$, $k = 1, \ldots, n_{n+1}$. De la Cruz et al. (2007) propose a simple extension of (7.7) to implement the desired inference by augmenting (7.7) with a prior $p(x_i \mid \eta)$ on x_i. Let $\boldsymbol{y}$ and $\boldsymbol{x}$ denote the data for $i = 1, \ldots, n$. The desired classification is formalized as

$$p(x_{n+1} \mid y_{n+1}, \boldsymbol{y}, \boldsymbol{x}). \tag{7.10}$$

Example 23 (Classifying Pregnancies) De la Cruz et al. (2007) implement (7.10) to classify pregnancies as normal versus abnormal on the basis of hormone measurements y_{ik}. The data include longitudinal hormone measurement y_{ik} for women $i = 1, \ldots, n$, and the known status $x_i \in \{0, 1\}$ of their pregnancies, with $x_i = 0$ for a normal pregnancy. We could not obtain permission to use the original data for this example. We instead simulate similar data shown in Fig. 7.9. The data are simulated using as simulation truth an instance of model (7.7), including a sampling model

$$y_{ik} \mid x_i = x, \theta_i, b \stackrel{\text{ind}}{\sim} \text{N}(\mu_{ik}, \sigma^2) \quad \text{with} \quad \mu_{ik} = \frac{\theta_i}{1 + e^{-(t_{ik} - b_{x0})b_{x1}}}, \tag{7.11}$$

where $i = 1, \ldots, n$ and $k = 1, \ldots, K_i$. That is, a non-linear regression with subject-specific random effects θ_i and fixed effects $\boldsymbol{b}_x = (b_{x0}, b_{x1})$ for normal ($x = 0$) and abnormal ($x = 1$) pregnancies. As random effects distribution G_x we use the ANOVA DDP model of Sect. 4.4.2 with design vectors $d(0) = (1, 0)$ and $d(1) =$

7.4 Hierarchical, Nested and Enriched DP

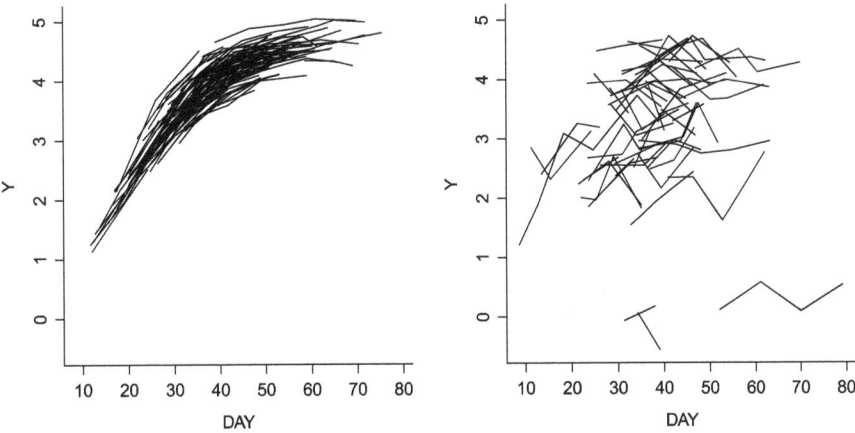

Fig. 7.9 Example 23. Simulated data for $n_0 = 124$ normal (*left panel*) and $n_1 = 49$ abnormal pregnancies. Repeat measurements y_{ik} for each woman are connected. (**a**) Data y_{ik} for $x_i = 0$ normal pregnancies. (**b**) Data y_{ik} for $x_i = 1$ abnormal pregnancies

(1, 1) for normal and abnormal pregnancies, respectively. We simulated hypothetical data for $n_0 = 124$ normal pregnancies and $n_1 = 49$ abnormal pregnancies, that is a total of $n = n_0 + n_1 = 173$ patients. The prior on x was then chosen to be $p(x = 0) = 124/173$ and $p(x = 1) = 49/173$, i.e. the empirical distribution of x. We generated between $K_i = 1$ and $K_i = 6$ repeat observations per patient, with an average of $1/n \sum K_i = 2.2$.

We then implemented inference under model (7.11) with the DDP mixture prior (4.12) on G_x. Figure 7.10a shows the estimated random effects distributions G_x, $x = 0, 1$, together with the simulation truth. Evaluating the reported inference, keep in mind that the data inform on G_x only indirectly through the latent random effects that have to be imputed on the basis of a small number of repeat measurements for a moderate number of patients. Considering this limitation the reported posterior inference is reasonable. More importantly, despite the limited information in the data about the underlying random effects distributions, posterior inference implies rather decisive posterior predictive classification (7.10), shown in Fig. 7.10b.

Software note: R code to implement inference in this example is included in the on-line software page for this chapter.

7.4 Hierarchical, Nested and Enriched DP

Many applications call for hierarchical priors on a set $\{G_j : j \in \mathcal{J}\}$ of random probability measures. Example 22 is typical for such applications. The nature of borrowing strength across the random probability measures G_j in (7.5) is appropriate

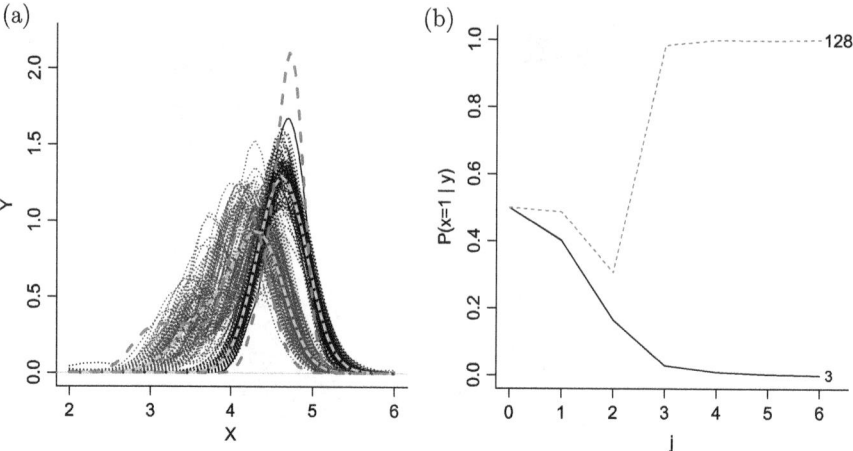

Fig. 7.10 Example 23. Panel (**a**) summarizes $p(G_x \mid y)$, $x = 0, 1$. The figure shows posterior estimated random effects distributions $E(G_x \mid y)$ (*dashed light grey curves*), posterior simulations $G_x \sim p(G_x \mid y)$ (*thin dotted curves*), and the simulation truth (*thick red dashed curves*). The curves peaked around 4.75 are for $x = 0$. The set of curves to the left are for $x = 1$. Panel (**b**) shows $p(x_{n+1} \mid y_{n+1,k}, k = 1, \ldots, j, y)$ as a function of j for two hypothetical future pregnancies (marked "3" and "128"). Measurements corresponding to the hypothetical future woman marked "3" were simulated assuming $x = 0$. The measurements marked "128" were simulated using $x = 1$

for that example, with different studies sharing a common subpopulation of patients in addition to study-specific subpopulations. The notion here is a subpopulation with a large number of experimental units (patients, in the case of Example 22) in each subpopulation. This is in contrast to applications of similar models for fully nonparametric regression. Recall also the related discussion in Sect. 4.4.1 when we introduced the DDP model for a family $\{G_x : x \in \mathcal{X}\}$ of random probability measures indexed by any set of covariates x. In general, many other forms of borrowing strength are possible. We discuss two more. A hierarchy of random probability measures defined by the hierarchical DP (HDP), and the closely related nested DP (NDP). Teh et al. (2006) propose the HDP as a prior for random probability measures $G_j, j = 1, \ldots, J$, with $G_j \mid M, G^0 \sim \mathsf{DP}(M, G^0)$, independently. By completing the model with a prior on the common base measure, $G^0 \mid B, G^{00} \sim \mathsf{DP}(B, G^{00})$, they define a joint probability model for $(G_1, \ldots, G_J)$. Importantly, the discrete nature of the G^0 as a DP random measure itself introduces positive probabilities for ties in the atoms of the random G_j, and thus the possibility of ties among samples $\theta_{ij} \sim G_j, i = 1, \ldots, n_j$, and $j = 1, \ldots, J$. We could again use these ties to define a random partition. Let $\{\theta_k^\star, k = 1, \ldots, K\}$ denote the unique values among the θ_{ij} and define clusters $S_k = \{(ji) : \theta_{ij} = \theta_k^\star\}$. This defines random clusters of experimental units across j. In summary, the HDP generates random probability measures G_j that share the same atoms across j. However, the random distributions G_j are different. The common atoms have different weights under each G_j.

This distinguishes the HDP from the related NDP of Rodríguez et al. (2008). The NDP allows for some of the G_j to be identical. While the HDP uses a common discrete base measure G^0 to generate the atoms in the G_j's, the NDP uses a common discrete prior

$$Q(\cdot) = \sum_{h=1}^{\infty} w_h \delta_{\tilde{G}_h}(\cdot)$$

for the distributions G_j themselves. In particular, under the HDP all G_j are distinct, but the HDP allows a positive prior probability for $G_{j_1} = G_{j_2}$. This is the case because Q is a (discrete) probability measure on probability measures. That is, with probability w_h a random distribution G_j is equal to $\tilde{G}_h$, thus allowing $p(G_j = G_{j'}) > 0$ for $j \neq j'$. The prior for Q is a DP prior whose base measure has to generate random probability measures which serve as the atoms of Q. Another instance of a DP prior is used for this purpose. In summary, $G_j \mid Q \stackrel{iid}{\sim} Q$ and $Q \mid M, \alpha, G^0 \sim \mathsf{DP}(M, \mathsf{DP}(\alpha, G^0))$. Other related extensions of the DP are the matrix stick-breaking of Dunson et al. (2008) and the enriched DP of Wade et al. (2011).

References

Bush CA, MacEachern SN (1996) A semiparametric Bayesian model for randomised block designs. Biometrika 83:275–285
Davidian M, Gallant A (1993) The nonlinear mixed effects model with a smooth random effects density. Biometrika 80:475–488
Davidian M, Giltinan D (1995) Nonlinear models for repeated measurement data. Chapman and Hall, London
De la Cruz R, Quintana FA, Müller P (2007) Semiparametric Bayesian classification with longitudinal markers. Appl Stat 56(2):119–137
Dunson DB, Xue Y, Carin L (2008) The matrix stick-breaking process: flexible Bayes meta-analysis. J Am Stat Assoc 103(481):317–327
Gelman A (2006) Prior distributions for variance parameters in hierarchical models. Bayesian Anal 1:515–533
Ghosh P, Hanson T (2010) A semiparametric Bayesian approach to multivariate longitudinal data. Aust N Z J Stat 52:275–288
Jara A, Hanson TE (2011) A class of mixtures of dependent tailfree processes. Biometrika 98:553–566
Jara A, Hanson T, Lesaffre E (2009) Robustifying generalized linear mixed models using a new class of mixture of multivariate Polya trees. J Comput Graph Stat 18:838–860
Jara A, Hanson TE, Quintana FA, Müller P, Rosner GL (2011) DPpackage: Bayesian semi- and nonparametric modeling in R. J Stat Softw 40(5):1–30
Kleinman K, Ibrahim J (1998) A semi-parametric Bayesian approach to the random effects model. Biometrics 54:921–938
Kolossiatis M, Griffin J, Steel M (2013) On Bayesian nonparametric modelling of two correlated distributions. Stat Comput 23(1):1–15. doi:10.1007/s11222-011-9283-7. http://dx.doi.org/10.1007/s11222-011-9283-7
Lavine M (1992) Some aspects of Polya tree distributions for statistical modeling. Ann Stat 20:1222–1235

Lavine M (1994) More aspects of Polya tree distributions for statistical modeling. Ann Stat 22:1161–1176

Lichtman SM, Ratain MJ, Van Echo DA, Rosner G, Egorin MJ, Budman DR, Vogelzang NJ, Norton L, Schilsky RL (1993) Phase i trial of granulocyte-macrophage colony-stimulating factor plus high-dose cyclophosphamide given every 2 weeks: a cancer and leukemia group b study. J Nat Cancer Inst 85(16):1319–1326

Lopes HF, Muller P, Rosner GL (2003) Bayesian meta-analysis for longitudinal data models using multivariate mixture priors. Biometrics 59(1):66–75

Malec D, Müller P (2008) A Bayesian semi-parametric model for small area estimation. In: Ghoshal S, Clarke B (eds) Festschrift in honor of J.K. Ghosh. IMS, Hayward, pp 223–236

Mallet A, Mentré F, Steimer JL, Lokiec F (1988) Nonparametric maximum likelihood estimation for population pharmacokinetics, with application to cyclosporine. J Pharmacokinet Biopharm 16:311–327

Mengersen KL, Robert CP (1996) Testing for mixtures: a Bayesian entropic approach. In: Bayesian statistics, vol 5 (Alicante, 1994). Oxford Science Publications, Oxford University Press, New York, pp 255–276

Mukhopadhyay S, Gelfand A (1997) Dirichlet process mixed generalized linear models. J Am Stat Assoc 92:633–639

Müller P, Rosner G (1997) A Bayesian population model with hierarchical mixture priors applied to blood count data. J Am Stat Assoc 92:1279–1292

Müller P, Quintana FA, Rosner G (2004) A method for combining inference across related nonparametric Bayesian models. J R Stat Soc Ser B Stat Methodol 66(3):735–749

Müller P, Rosner GL, Iorio MD, MacEachern S (2005) A nonparametric Bayesian model for inference in related longitudinal studies. J R Stat Soc Ser C Appl Stat 54(3):611–626

Rodríguez A, Dunson DB, Gelfand AE (2008) The nested Dirichlet process, with discussion. J Am Stat Assoc 103:1131–1144

Roeder K, Wasserman L (1997) Practical Bayesian density estimation using mixtures of normals. J Am Stat Assoc 92(439):894–902

Rosner G, Müller P (1997) Bayesian population pharmacokinetic and pharmacodynamic analyses using mixture models. J Pharmacokinet Biopharm 25:209–233

Schumitzky A (1993) The nonparametric maximum likelihood approach to pharmacokinetic population analysis. In: Western simulation multiconference—simulation in health care. Society for Computer Simulation, San Diego, pp 95–100

Teh YW, Jordan MI, Beal MJ, Blei DM (2006) Sharing clusters among related groups: hierarchical Dirichlet processes. J Am Stat Assoc 101:1566–1581

Wade S, Mongelluzzo S, Petrone S (2011) An enriched conjugate prior for Bayesian nonparametric inference. Bayesian Anal 6(3):359–385

Wakefield J, Smith A, Racine-Poon A, Gelfand A (1994) Bayesian analysis of linear and nonlinear population models using the gibbs sampler. Appl Stat 43:201–221

Wakefield J, Aarons L, Racine-Poon A (1999) The Bayesian approach to population pharmacokinetic/pharmacodynamic modelling. In: Carlin B, Carriquiry A, Gatsonis C, Gelman A, Kass R, Verdinelli I, West M (eds) Case studies in Bayesian statistics. Springer, New York

Walker S, Wakefield J (1998) Population models with a nonparametric random coefficient distribution. Sankhya Ser B 60:196–214

Wang Y, Taylor JM (2001) Jointly modeling longitudinal and event time data with applcation to acquired immunodeficiency syndrome. J Am Stat Assoc 96:895–903

Wood W, Budman D, Korzun A, Cooper M, Younger J, Hart R, Moore A, Ellerton J, Norton L, Ferree C, Ballow A, Ill E, Henderson I (1994) Dose and dose intensity of adjuvant chemotherapy for stage ii, node positive breast cancer. N Engl J Med 330:1253–1259

Yang Y, Müller P, Rosner G (2010) Semiparametric Bayesian inference for repeated fractional measurement data. Chil J Stat 1:59–74

Zeger SL, Karim MR (1991) Generalized linear models with random effects: a Gibbs sampling approach. J Am Stat Assoc 86:79–86

Zhao L, Hanson TE, Carlin BP (2009) Mixtures of Polya trees for flexible spatial frailty survival modelling. Biometrika 96(2):263–276

Zhou H, Hanson T, Jara A, Zhang J (2015) Modelling county level breast cancer survival data using a covariate-adjusted frailty proportional hazards model. Ann Appl Stat 9:43–68

Chapter 8
Clustering and Feature Allocation

Abstract An important byproduct of inference in discrete mixture models is an implied random partition of experimental units. In fact, such random partitions are the main inference targets for many recently published applications of nonparametric Bayesian discrete mixture models. In this chapter we systematically consider the use of nonparametric Bayesian priors for inference on such random partitions. Many scientific inference problems are formalized as the related, more general problem of feature allocation. That is, inference on possibly overlapping random subsets of experimental units. We introduce some examples from data analysis for bioinformatics data and introduce the Polya urn model, product partition models, model based clustering and the Indian buffet process prior.

8.1 Random Partitions and Feature Allocations

Clustering Many applications call for a partition of experimental units into more homogeneous subgroups. This is known as clustering and feature allocation. Let $[n] = \{1, \ldots, n\}$ denote a set of experimental units, for example patients in a clinical study. To simplify the discussion we will from now on refer to the experimental units as "subjects", keeping in mind that the described models could just as well describe arrangements of any other experimental units, like studies, genes, proteins, schools etc.

A cluster arrangement $\rho_n = \{S_1, \ldots, S_K\}$ of $[n]$ is a partition, i.e., a family of subsets S_j with $S_j \cap S_{j'} = \emptyset$ for $j \neq j'$ and $\bigcup_{j=1}^{K} S_j = [n]$. The size K of ρ_n is part of the partition. When we want to highlight the dependence of K on n we write K_n. Sometimes we will find it more convenient to equivalently describe a partition by cluster membership indicators. Let $s_i = j$ if $i \in S_j$ denote cluster membership indicators. We add the convention of labeling clusters by appearance. That is, $s_1 = 1$ by definition, and $s_i \leq K_{i-1} + 1$, where $K_i = \max\{s_\ell, \ell \leq i\}$. There is a one-to-one mapping between ρ_n and $(s_1, \ldots, s_n)$. A probability model $p(\rho_n)$ describes a random partition of the subjects. When n is understood from the context, we will drop the subindex and just write $p(\rho)$.

Feature Allocation In some problems it is more natural to introduce an overlapping and not necessarily exhaustive grouping. For example, when grouping consumers by preferences for different genres of movies, we might want to consider features like drama, documentaries, etc. A feature is then a subset $S \subseteq [n]$. A feature allocation is a multiset $F_n = \{S_1, \ldots, S_K\}$ of features S_j without the restriction to mutually exclusive and exhaustive subsets. Consumers might have preferences for multiple genres, and some consumers might not record any preferences. We add a technical constraint that any subject can only be member in finitely many features. A partition is a special case of a feature allocation. Similar to cluster membership indicators, feature allocations can be alternatively represented by feature membership sets, $Y_i = \{j : i \in S_j\}$. Yet another representation of feature allocations that is often convenient is as an $(n \times K)$ binary matrix $\mathbf{Z}$ with $Z_{ij} = 1$ if $i \in S_j$ and $Z_{ij} = 0$ otherwise.

Sampling Model When random partitions $p(\rho_n)$ or feature allocations $p(F_n)$ are used for statistical modeling, the model construction is usually continued with some sampling model that relates observed responses y_i to the subgroups. For example,

$$p(y \mid \rho_n, \theta^\star) = \prod_{j=1}^{K} \left\{ \prod_{i \in S_j} p(y_i \mid \theta_j^\star) \right\} = \prod_i p(y_i \mid \theta_j^\star, j = s_i). \tag{8.1}$$

Here $\theta_j^\star$ are cluster specific parameters. We discuss some examples below. In a feature allocation problem we might use

$$p(y \mid F_n, \theta^\star) = \prod_{i=1}^{n} p(y_i \mid \theta_j^\star, j \in Y_i), \tag{8.2}$$

using, for example, $p(y_i \mid \theta_j^\star, j \in Y_i) = \mathsf{N}(\mu_i, \sigma^2)$ with $\mu_i = \sum_{j \in Y_i} \theta_j^\star$.

Least Squares Clustering Any prior model $p(\rho)$, together with a sampling model such as (8.1) defines a posterior random partition $p(\rho \mid y)$, which formalizes posterior uncertainty about the unknown cluster arrangement ρ. The use of such inference for any application gives rise to the practical problem of how to summarize the posterior $p(\rho \mid y)$. There is no such thing as a posterior mean clustering, or posterior median. The posterior mode $\rho^\star = \arg\max_\rho \{p(\rho \mid y)\}$ is often not very informative or typical of the probability model $p(\rho \mid y)$. This is because, first, $p(\rho^\star \mid y)$ often is a very small probability only, and second, because the partition ρ with the second highest posterior probability might have only negligibly less posterior probability, but might look entirely different. One summary that is often reported are posterior co-clustering probabilities, that is $P_{ij} \equiv p(s_i = s_j \mid y)$, arranged as an $(n \times n)$ matrix. Alternatively, Dahl (2006) proposes the least squares partition ρ_{LS}. For any partition ρ, let P_ρ denote the $(n \times n)$ matrix of co-clustering indicators $P_{\rho,ij} = I(s_i = s_j)$. The least squares partition ρ_{LS} is the partition with the least posterior mean distance to P_ρ. That is,

$$\rho_{LS} = \arg\min_{\hat\rho}\left\{\int d(P_\rho, P_{\hat\rho})\, dp(\rho \mid y)\right\} \quad (8.3)$$

The integral is a sum over all possible partitions. The distance counts the number of distinct elements. A simple program to implement the evaluation of ρ_{LS} is available at http://dahl.byu.edu/. The required input is a posterior Monte Carlo sample of partitions ρ from $p(\rho \mid y)$. A similar summary, for more general utility (or loss) functions is discussed in Quintana and Iglesias (2003). A similar construction is possible for feature allocations, to summarize $p(F_n \mid y)$.

8.2 Polya Urn and Model Based Clustering

Random Partitions and Random Probability Measures A common way to define priors $p(\rho_n)$ on partitions is through an indirect definition by sampling from a discrete random probability measure. Consider a discrete distribution $G(\cdot) = \sum w_h \delta_{m_h}(\cdot)$ with probability masses w_h in locations m_h. A random sample $\theta_i \mid G \overset{\text{iid}}{\sim} G$, $i = 1,\ldots, n$, implicitly defines a partition ρ_n by the following construction. Sampling from a discrete distribution implies a positive probability for ties, i.e., $\theta_{i_1} = \theta_{i_2}$ for some $i_1 \ne i_2$. Let $\theta_j^\star, j = 1,\ldots, K$, denote the $K \le n$ unique values and define $S_j = \{i : \theta_i = \theta_j^\star\}$. Then $\{S_1,\ldots, S_K\}$ defines a random partition of $[n]$. In other words, i.i.d. sampling from G implies a random partition $p(\rho_n \mid G)$. If G is a random probability measure then $p(\rho_n)$ can be defined by marginalizing w.r.t. G. We have already seen this construction before, in Sect. 2.3, under sampling from a random distribution with DP prior.

This indirect way of defining $p(\rho_n)$ could be criticized for building up an unnecessarily general and large model. If G is not of interest, but only the implied model $p(\rho_n)$, then one should think about modeling $p(\rho_n)$ directly. There seems to be no need for the detour via the random probability measure G. However, there are at least three good reasons to model $p(\rho_n)$ via G. First, the indirect construction ensures that $p(\rho_n)$ arises from marginalizing $p(\rho_{n+1})$. The marginalization property is formally stated as

$$p(\rho_n) = \sum_{s_{n+1}=1}^{K_n+1} p(\rho_{n+1}). \quad (8.4)$$

Such coherence across sample sizes is desirable. It would be embarrassing if inference for ρ_n were to depend upon whether or not we will ever consider an $(n+1)$-st experimental unit. Another reason for the construction via G is that in the limit, for large sample size n, the relative cluster sizes are asymptotically equal to the weights of the point masses w_h in G. A related third reason is that any exchangeable sequence of random partitions $p(\rho_n)$ can be represented as arising from random sampling under a discrete random probability measure G. Here $p(\rho_n)$ is called exchangeable if it is invariant under permutations of the indices $\{1, \ldots, n\}$. The result is known as Kingman's representation theorem (Kingman 1978, 1982). See, for example, Lee et al. (2013c), for a recent review.

DP Random Partition (Pólya Urn) The perhaps most popular random partition model $p(\rho_n)$ is the random partition that is induced by random sampling from a DP random probability measure. In other words, the generative model is as follows. First we generate $G \mid M, G_0 \sim \text{DP}(MG_0)$ from a DP prior. Next generate an i.i.d. sample $\theta_i \mid G \overset{iid}{\sim} G, i = 1, \ldots, n$. Now record the configuration of ties to define clusters S_j. The implied prior $p(\rho_n)$ is known as the Polya urn. We already encountered the Polya urn before, in Sect. 2.3, when discussing properties of the DP. Recall

$$p(\rho_n) = \frac{M^{K-1} \prod_{j=1}^{K} (n_j - 1)!}{(M+1) \cdot \ldots \cdot (M+n-1)}, \tag{8.5}$$

where $n_j = |S_j|$ is the number of elements in cluster j, or simply, the jth cluster size. There is an important subtlety about the representation of the partition. If the partition is recorded as a multiset $\rho_n = \{S_1, \ldots, S_K\}$ or as cluster membership indicators $(s_1, \ldots, s_n)$ with cluster labels that are indexed by appearance then the stated probability is correct. If, however, the partition is recorded as cluster membership indicators without any restrictions on the cluster labels, then an additional factor $1/K!$ needs to be added to (8.5). This is because, for example, $s = (1, 1, 1, 2, 3, 2)$ and $s' = (2, 2, 2, 3, 1, 3)$ record the same partition. The additional factor accounts for the $K!$ different ways of coding the partition with cluster membership indicators. Usually, an additional convention is added, requiring labeling by order of appearance. In the last example, this would single out partition s only.

Model Based Clustering A similarly popular prior on random partitions is model based clustering (Dasgupta and Raftery 1998; Fraley and Raftery 2002). The basic idea is simple. Consider sampling from a mixture model $y_i \overset{iid}{\sim} \sum_{h=1}^{H} w_h f(y_i \mid \theta_h^\star)$, $i = 1, \ldots, H$, for example, a location mixture of normal distributions with $f(\cdot \mid \theta_h^\star) = N(\cdot \mid \theta_h^\star, \sigma^2)$ for known σ^2. Next we replace the mixture model with an equivalent hierarchical model by introducing latent variables $s_i \in \{1, \ldots, H\}$ with

$$y_i \mid s_i = h, \boldsymbol{\theta}^\star \overset{ind}{\sim} f(y_i \mid \theta_h^\star),$$
$$p(s_i = h) = w_h. \tag{8.6}$$

If we interpret $s = (s_1, \ldots, s_n)$ as cluster membership indicators, then (8.6) implicitly defines a prior $p(\rho_n)$. A minor detail is the labeling of clusters. If order of appearance labeling is desired, then the labels s_i might have to be re-arranged. Also, it is possible that only $K \leq H$ distinct labels are generated (this is why we

8.2 Polya Urn and Model Based Clustering

Table 8.1 Example 24. Reported number of responses y_i and number of patients m_i for each one of the sarcoma subtypes

Subtype	y_i	m_i
Leiomyosarcoma	6	28
Liposarcoma	7	29
MFH	3	29
Osteosarcoma	5	26
Synovial	3	20
Angiosarcoma	2	15
MPNST	1	5
Fibrosarcoma	1	12
Ewing's	0	13
Rhabdo	0	2

used H instead of K for the number of terms in the mixture model). There is a connection between model-based clustering and the DP random partitions (Green and Richardson 2001). Consider model based clustering with a Dirichlet prior $(w_1, \ldots, w_H) \sim \text{Dir}(\delta_H, \ldots, \delta_H)$ for the weights in (8.6) and $\theta_h^\star \mid G_0 \stackrel{\text{iid}}{\sim} G_0$. For fixed n consider now a limit with $H \to \infty$ and $\delta_H \to 0$, such that $H\delta_H \to \alpha > 0$. The limiting model on $(y_1, \ldots, y_n)$ is identical to a DP mixture model $y_i \mid G \stackrel{\text{iid}}{\sim} \int f(y_i \mid \theta) \, G(d\theta)$, with $G \mid \alpha, G_0 \sim \text{DP}(\alpha G_0)$.

Example 24 (Clustering Sarcoma Subtypes) Leon-Novelo et al. (2012) consider a clinical study of patients with up to 10 subtypes of sarcoma. Table 8.1 shows the number of patients in each sarcoma subtype (m_i) and the number of tumor responses (y_i). We model the sarcoma data using a binomial likelihood, $y_i \mid \theta_i \stackrel{\text{ind}}{\sim} \text{Bin}(m_i, \theta_i)$ for $i = 1, \ldots, n = 10$. Here θ_i represents the true (and unknown) tumor incidence probability. To account for groupings among disease subtypes, we used model (8.6) with a fixed value of H and

$$y_i \mid s_i = h, \theta_h^\star \stackrel{\text{ind}}{\sim} \text{Bin}(m_i, \theta_h^\star).$$

The prior in (8.6) in particular implies that disease subtypes are a priori independently assigned to cluster h with probability w_h for $h = 1, \ldots, H$. Model specification is completed by assuming

$$(w_1, \ldots, w_H) \sim \text{Dir}(\alpha), \quad \theta_1^\star, \ldots, \theta_H^\star \stackrel{\text{iid}}{\sim} \text{Be}(a, b),$$

independently, with α an H-dimensional vectors with all components equal to 1.

Rather than adopting a prior distribution for the number of mixture components, we fitted the above model for every $H \in \{1, \ldots, 7\}$ and computed the LPML (Geisser and Eddy 1979). The highest value was attained when $H = 3$. Figure 8.1a summarizes the posterior similarity matrix, with entries $p(s_i = s_j \mid y)$ for all $1 \leq i, j \leq n$. The figure suggests the presence of two clusters, a large one including at least the first eight disease subtypes, and a second, smaller one, including Ewing's

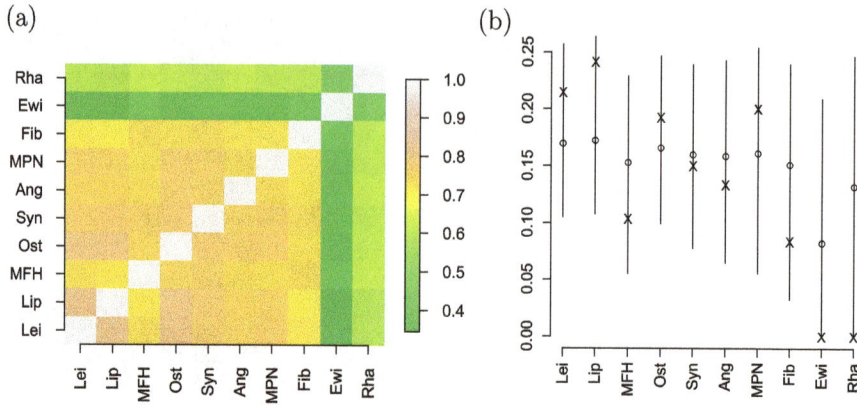

Fig. 8.1 Example 24. Panel (**a**) shows the posterior similarity matrix $p(s_i = s_j \mid \mathbf{y})$ for model (8.6) with $H = 3$. Panel (**b**) shows for each sarcoma the central 95 % credible interval for tumor response rates, with posterior means indicated as circles, obtained under model (8.6) with $H = 3$. For comparison, the empirical fraction $\hat{\theta}_i$, that is, the m.l.e.'s, are included as "×"

and possibly Rhabdo sarcomas. For comparison, least squared clustering (8.3) results in one large cluster including all subtypes except for Ewing's. Figure 8.1b shows inference for individual sarcoma subtypes. For each of the observed disease types we show the central 95 % credible interval for θ_i and the corresponding posterior mean, marked as a circle. For comparison, the empirical fractions of tumor responses, $\hat{\theta}_i$, that is, the maximum likelihood estimates, are marked by a cross. Except for the last two subtypes, for which no tumors were observed, all credible intervals include $\hat{\theta}_i$. The long intervals reflect the small sample sizes. Note also that with high posterior probability (32.6 %), the nine disease subtypes other than Ewing's are clustered together, which explains the closeness of the corresponding posterior means.

Software note: See the software appendix for this chapter for simple R code to implement model based clustering for this example.

8.3 Product Partition Models (PPMs)

8.3.1 Definition

Product partition models (PPMs) were introduced by Hartigan (1990) and Barry and Hartigan (1992). Their most characteristic feature is the so called *product distribution* for the random partition, which adopts the form of a product

$$p(\rho_n = \{S_1, \ldots, S_K\}) \propto \prod_{j=1}^{K} c(S_j), \tag{8.7}$$

8.3 Product Partition Models (PPMs)

where $c(S_j)$ is known as *cohesion* function of subset S_j, which represents how strongly we believe the elements in S_j are thought to be clustered together a priori. The normalization constant in (8.7) is $\sum_{\rho \in \mathcal{P}} \prod_{j=1}^{|\rho|} c(S_j)$, where $\mathcal{P}$ is the set of all possible partitions of $[n]$ into nonempty sets. The cohesion functions are restricted to be nonnegative functions of S_j, but in principle, any such function is valid. If $c(S)$ is only a function of the size of S, then the resulting model for ρ_n is invariant under permutations of the labels of units in $[n]$. Naturally, in practice one may wish to avoid defining $c(S)$ for every one of the $2^n - 1$ nonempty subsets of $[n]$, and resort instead to a more structured definition. A popular choice is $c(S) = M \times (|S| - 1)!$, where $|S|$ is the number of elements in S. It follows (see, e.g., Quintana and Iglesias 2003) that the resulting probability model for ρ_n is exactly (8.5), which can be characterized as the arrangement of ties under independent sampling from a DP random measure.

However, not every PPM can be interpreted as the implied random partition under some discrete random probability measure. Relatedly, not every possible choice of cohesion function generates a coherent family of models, that is, a class of models for which $p(\rho_n)$ in (8.7) arises from $p(\rho_{n+1})$ by marginalization of the $(n+1)$st unit,

$$p(\rho_n) = \sum_{s_{n+1}=1}^{K_n+1} p(\rho_{n+1}).$$

Recall that $K_n = |\rho_n|$ denotes the size of the partition. One example that violates this marginalization property is $c(S) = M \times (|S|)^2$. For further discussion about this and related issues, see Lee et al. (2013b).

Assume now a corresponding set of responses $\mathbf{y} = (y_1, \ldots, y_n)$, and let $\mathbf{y}^\star_S$ denote the responses arranged by cluster, that is, $\mathbf{y}^\star_S = (y_i : i \in S)$ for any $S \subseteq [n]$. The PPM then assumes that the joint model for $\mathbf{y}$ can be described in terms of independent sub-models for the partitioned data subsets, independent across clusters,

$$p(\mathbf{y} \mid \rho_n = \{S_1, \ldots, S_K\}) = \prod_{j=1}^{K} p(\mathbf{y}^\star_{S_j}). \tag{8.8}$$

For later reference we summarize the definition of a PPM.

Definition 8 (Product Partition Model) Let $c(S) \geq 0$ define a cohesion function for subsets $S \subseteq \{1, \ldots, n\}$. A random partition $p(\rho_n = \{S_1, \ldots, S_K\}) \propto \prod_{j=1}^{K} c(S_j)$ together with independent sampling across clusters as in (8.8) defines a product partition model (PPM).

The posterior distribution of ρ_n under (8.8) and (8.7) is again a PPM of the form (8.7), with cohesion functions given by $c_{post}(S_j) = c(S_j) p_{S_j}(\mathbf{y}^\star_{S_j})$. Barry and Hartigan (1992) considered also the case where partitions are restricted to be of *contiguous* type or in blocks, that is, $\rho_n = \{\{1, \ldots, i_1\}, \{i_1+1, \ldots, i_2\}, \ldots, \{i_{K-1}+1, \ldots, n\}\}$, where $1 \leq i_1 < i_2 < \cdots < i_{K-1} < n$, which is a particularly suitable framework for change-point detection problems. In this context Yao (1984) proposed cohesion functions of the form

$$c(\{i+1,\ldots,j\}) = \begin{cases} p(1-p)^{j-i-1} & \text{if } j < n \\ (1-p)^{j-i-1} & \text{if } j = n, \end{cases}$$

for any $1 \leq i < j \leq n$. The definition implies that the sequence of change points form a discrete renewal process having i.i.d. occurrence times with geometric distribution. See also Barry and Hartigan (1993), Loschi and Cruz (2005) and references therein.

We now complete the PPM with specific assumptions for a sampling model (8.8). We assume that the sampling model is exchangeable within clusters, and can be written as independent sampling conditional on cluster-specific parameters θ_j^*. Recall that a partition can be equivalently defined in terms of the cluster membership indicators s_i introduced earlier, with $s_i = j$ if $i \in S_j$. We assume

$$y_i \mid \boldsymbol{\theta}^*, \rho_n \stackrel{\text{ind}}{\sim} p(y_i \mid \theta_{s_i}^*), \quad \theta_1^*, \ldots, \theta_{K_n}^* \stackrel{\text{iid}}{\sim} F_0, \quad p(\rho_n) \propto \prod_{i=1}^{K_n} c(S_i). \tag{8.9}$$

Such an approach is adopted, for example, in the case of normal means in Crowley (1997).

We already mentioned the connection between parametric PPMs like (8.9) and BNP models based on the DP. With $c(S) = M \times (|S|-1)!$, model (8.9) is equivalent to what is left of

$$y_i \mid \theta_i \stackrel{\text{ind}}{\sim} p(y_i \mid \theta_i), \quad \theta_1, \ldots, \theta_n \mid F \stackrel{\text{iid}}{\sim} F, \quad F \sim \text{DP}(M, F_0)$$

after marginalizing with respect to the random probability measure F. See further discussion in Sect. 2.3 and in Quintana and Iglesias (2003) and Quintana (2006).

8.3.2 Posterior Simulation

Posterior simulation for PPMs is quite similar to inference for DP-based models (Sect. 2.4). The main change is in the updating of cluster membership indicators s_i. Let K^- denote the number of clusters after removing the ith individual from the sample. Denote by $S_1^-, \ldots, S_{K^-}^-$ the corresponding clusters and similarly for s_{-i}. Then

$$p(s_i = j \mid s_{-i}) \propto \begin{cases} \dfrac{c(S_j^- \cup \{i\})}{c(S_j^-)} & \text{for } j = 1, \ldots, K^- \\ c(\{i\}) & \text{for } j = K^- + 1. \end{cases} \tag{8.10}$$

8.3 Product Partition Models (PPMs)

If, for instance, $c(S) = M \times (|S| - 1)!$ then, after normalization, (8.10) becomes the Polya urn (2.9). Another common example is $c(S) = M$ for all $S \subset [n]$, in which case (8.10) becomes $p(s_i = j \mid s_{-i}) = 1/(K^- + M)$ for $j = 1, \ldots, K^-$ and $p(s_i = K^- + 1 \mid s_{-i}) = K^-/(K^- + M)$. With $M = 1$, the latter distribution reduces to the uniform on $\{1, \ldots, K^- + 1\}$. We refer to it as the uniform cohesion function. It is easy to adapt posterior simulation schemes for DP mixtures to the case of general PPMs. For example, recall Algorithm 8 of Neal (2000) from Section 2.4.3. The key step of the algorithm is the introduction of additional auxiliary parameters that can be created and discarded at every iteration. This has the effect of carrying along empty clusters, thus avoiding the need to perform analytical integrations that may or may not be available. Recall from Sect. 2.4.3 that m represents the number of extra clusters, to be carried along MCMC iterations. Equation (2.19) in Sect. 2.4.4 is replaced, after appropriate relabeling of the clusters, by

$$p(s_i = j \mid s_{-i}, y, \theta^*) \propto \begin{cases} p(y_i \mid \theta_j^*) \frac{c(S_j^- \cup \{i\})}{c(S_j^-)} & \text{for } j = 1, \ldots, K^- \\ p(y_i \mid \theta_j^*) \frac{c(\{i\})}{m} & \text{for } j = K^- + 1, \ldots, K^- + m. \end{cases}$$
(8.11)

Example 24 (ctd.) We consider again the sarcoma data of Table 8.1. This time, we adopt (8.7) as prior $p(\rho_n)$ for the partitions, again with a binomial sampling model with cluster-specific response rates θ_j^*,

$$y_i \mid \theta_{s_i}^*, \rho_n \stackrel{\text{ind}}{\sim} \text{Bin}(m_i, \theta_{s_i}^*), \quad \theta_1^*, \ldots, \theta_k^* \mid a, b \stackrel{\text{iid}}{\sim} \text{Be}(a, b), \text{ and } p(\rho_n) \propto \prod_{j=1}^{k} c(S_j),$$
(8.12)

We fit the model using Algorithm 8 of Neal (2000) modified as in (8.11).

Software note: R code to implement the model is provided in the on-line software page for this chapter.

Figure 8.2a shows the posterior similarity matrix under model (8.12), with $c(S) = M \times (|S| - 1)!$ and $M = 1$. The induced prior mean and variance of the number of clusters are $E(K) = 2.929$ and $\text{Var}(K) = 1.379$. Fixing the prior mean at $E(K) \approx 3$ makes inference comparable with the earlier analysis under model-based clustering with fixed $H = 3$. Compare with Fig. 8.1. The summaries are very similar, the main difference being a more marked separation between Ewing's and Rhabdo subtypes. In fact, the least squares clustering method of Dahl (2006) reports the same partition as before as posterior summary, namely, one singleton containing Ewing's, and a big cluster containing everything else. This is also supported by the fact that the posterior mode, mean and variance for K were 2, 2.032 and 0.768, respectively. The complete posterior distribution $p(K \mid y)$ is shown in Table 8.2.

We repeat the analysis using the uniform cohesion functions, for which the prior mean and variance of the number of clusters are $E(K) = 4.851$ and $\text{Var}(K) = 1.098$. The posterior similarity matrix under this analysis is shown in Fig. 8.2b. It

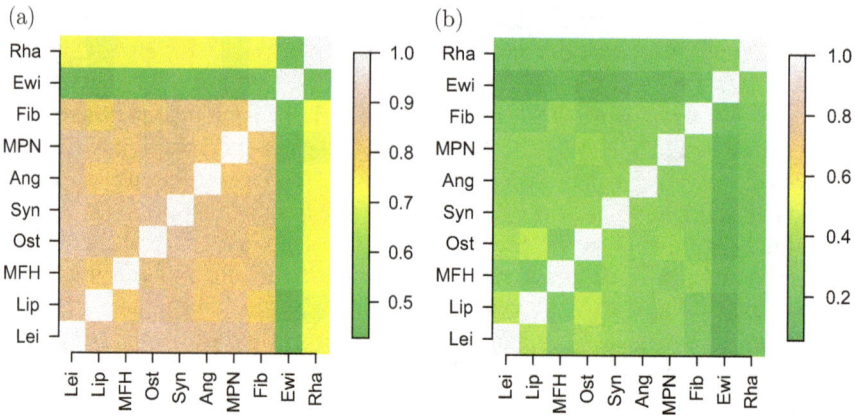

Fig. 8.2 Example 24. Posterior inference under the PPM (8.12). The graph shows the posterior similarity matrix $p(s_i = s_j \mid y)$ when using DP-style cohesion functions (*left panel*) (**a**) and when using uniform cohesion functions (*right panel*) (**b**)

Table 8.2 Example 24, inference under the PPM (8.12)

Posterior distribution of number of clusters							
$c(S)$	1	2	3	4	5	6	7
$M \times (\lvert S \rvert - 1)!$	0.293	0.448	0.201	0.051	0.006	0.001	0
M	0.001	0.022	0.252	0.435	0.223	0.060	0.007

The table shows the posterior probability distribution of the number of clusters under each of the displayed cohesion functions. Both distributions have theoretical support on $[n]$, but the estimation suggests a negligible probability mass after 6 and 7 clusters for DP and uniform cohesion functions, respectively

is quite different from the DP case and the inference under model based clustering. The median value of the co-clustering probabilities $p(s_i = s_j \mid y)$ is 0.2875. The low estimated similarity of the subtypes is also reflected in the least squares partition, which contains 7 clusters: one formed by Leiomyosarcoma and Liposarcoma, another formed by MFH, Synovial and Angiosarcoma, and all the other disease subtypes forming singletons. The posterior distribution $p(K \mid y)$ has mean, mode and variance 4, 4.065 and 0.872, respectively. See Table 8.2. By spreading its probability mass uniformly across all ρ, the prior with uniform cohesion functions implicitly favors small clusters relative to large ones. There is no preference for large coherent clusters.

Finally, we estimated the tumor response probabilities for all ten disease subtypes, under both choices of cohesion function discussed above. Figure 8.3 summarizes posterior inference as posterior means and central 95 % credible intervals, with circles and dashed lines for $c(S) = M \times (\lvert S \rvert - 1)!$ and triangles and dotted lines for $c(S) = M$. Empirical frequencies $\hat{\theta}_i$, that is, m.l.e. estimates, are marked by a cross. Compare with Fig. 8.1b. The posterior means under the PPM with DP-style cohesion functions are very close to those under model (8.6), but different

Fig. 8.3 Example 24. Inference under the PPM (8.12). For each sarcoma subtype we show the central 95 % credible interval for individual tumor incidence probabilities, with *dashed lines* and posterior means indicated as *circles* (DP-style cohesion functions) and *dotted lines* and *triangles* (uniform cohesion functions). For comparison, the empirical fraction of observed tumors are included as "X"

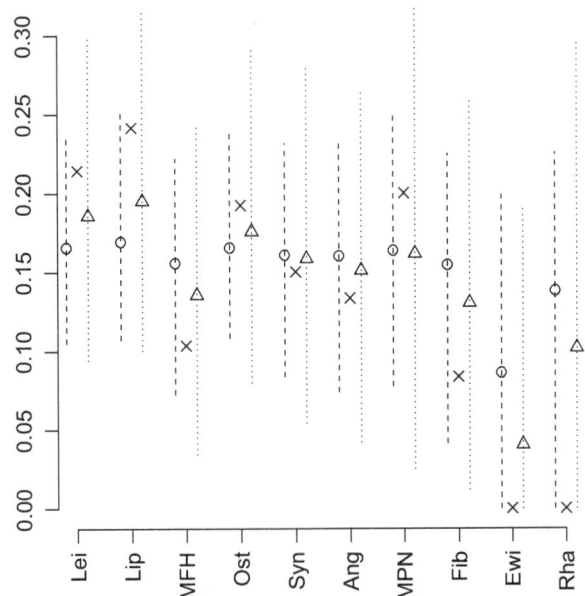

from those under the uniform cohesion functions. The posterior credible intervals are generally a bit shorter under the PPM with DP-style cohesion functions than for model based clustering, and generally longer for uniform cohesion functions. In the former case, the posterior means for sarcoma cases other than Ewing's are similar, because the model is borrowing strength across these subtypes. In turn, for $c(S) = M$, there is little borrowing strength, which explains the longer credible intervals and also the fact that the posterior means $E(\theta_i \mid y)$ are closer to $\hat{\theta}_i$. In summary, the choice of cohesion function can have substantial impact on the posterior inference, especially in problems with little data.

8.4 Clustering and Regression

8.4.1 The PPMx Model

We now add dependence on covariates to the PPM model (8.7). Consider, for example, a problem that involves clustering of patients into subpopulations. We would want to include a feature in the prior to favor clustering of patients with comparable baseline characteristics. Patients with similar prior treatment history, similar biomarkers, et cetera, should be more likely to cluster together in the same subpopulation. In other words, we want to introduce a regression on patient-specific covariates x_i in the random partition. Let $X = (x_1, \ldots, x_n)$ denote subject-specific covariates. We want to generalize the PPM prior $p(\rho_n)$ to a model $p(\rho_n \mid X)$. Müller et al. (2011) implement the desired regression on x_i by modifying the cohesion function $c(S)$ to include an extra factor that depends on covariates. Assume a q-dimensional covariate vector $x_i = (x_{i1}, \ldots, x_{iq})$, possibly including continuous, ordinal and categorical variables. Denote by $x_j^* = \{x_i : i \in S_j\}$ the set of covariate arranged by cluster. We introduce a *similarity function* as any nonnegative function g of the covariate values x_j^* such that high values of $g(x_j^*)$ indicate homogeneous covariate vectors, i.e. a cluster S_j of experimental units with covariates x_i that are judged to be similar.

Definition 9 (PPMx.) A PPMx model with similarity function $g(x_j^*)$, $g(\cdot) \geq 0$ is a random partition

$$p(\rho_n = \{S_1, \ldots, S_K\} \mid X) \propto \prod_{j=1}^{K} c(S_j) g(x_j^*), \qquad (8.13)$$

with normalization constant $\sum_{\rho \in \mathcal{P}} \prod_{\ell=1}^{|\rho|} c(S_\ell) g(x_\ell^*)$.

Equation (8.13) includes a slight abuse of notation. The covariates x_i need not be random variables. They could include selected dose levels or treatment choices. We put them in the conditioning set to indicate that the random partition model is indexed by x. The key component of (8.13) is the similarity function.

Defining the Similarity Function Formally, any nonnegative function g is a valid similarity function. In practice, though, ease of computation in the evaluation of $g(x^\star_j)$ is important. Müller et al. (2011) considered generic forms to construct similarity functions. A natural and easy way to compute $g(x^\star_j)$ is by introducing an auxiliary probability model that is used only to get an easy expression for the similarity function. The idea is to think of x_j^* as if x_i, $i \in S_j$, were randomly sampled from a hypothetical probability model with $q(x_i \mid \xi_j^\star)$ and prior $q(\xi_j^\star)$. Then

$$g(x_j^*) = \int \prod_{i \in S_j} q(x_i \mid \xi_j^\star) q(\xi_j^\star) \, d\xi_j^\star, \qquad (8.14)$$

which can be analytically evaluated when the distributions are chosen as conjugate pair. In summary, we use the marginal model under $q(\cdot)$ to define $g(x_j^*)$. Under most models the marginal is highest for sets of covariate values $x^\star_j$ that would be considered to be similar. Importantly, $q(\cdot)$ is only introduced for easy and efficient computation, without any notion of modeling a distribution of covariates x_i. Using candidate's formula, that is, Bayes theorem for the marginal model on $x^\star_j$ in (8.14), we get

$$g(x_j^*) = \frac{\prod_{i \in S_j} q(x_i \mid \tilde{\xi}_j^\star) q(\tilde{\xi}_j^\star)}{q(\tilde{\xi}_j^\star \mid x^\star_j)}, \qquad (8.15)$$

8.4 Clustering and Regression

where $\tilde{\xi}_j^*$ is *any* fixed value of ξ_j^*. Note that this expression can be readily evaluated and the dimension of $\tilde{\xi}_j^*$ does not depend on the cluster size. Some specific choices for particular data formats are as follows, assuming first, for simplicity, that the covariate x_i is univariate.

Continuous x_i: Define $\xi_j^* = (m_j, v_j)$. Let $q(x_i \mid \xi_j^*) = \mathsf{N}(x_i \mid m_j, v_j)$, and $q(m_j, v_j)$ be the conjugate normal-inverse chi-square (or gamma) prior distribution (see, for example, Gelman et al. 2004). Then (8.15) is easily evaluated. In this case, $g(x_j^*)$ is a scaled and correlated n_j-dimensional multivariate t density. Here $n_j = |S_j|$ is the size of the j-th cluster. Equation (8.15) avoids the explicit evaluation of this potentially high-dimensional density.

Categorical x_i: Consider a categorical covariate with c levels, $x_i \in \{1, \ldots, c\}$. Let $\xi_j^* = (\pi_1, \ldots, \pi_c)$ where $0 \leq \pi_r$ for all $r = 1, \ldots, c$ and $\sum_{r=1}^{c} \pi_r = 1$. Then use $q(x_i \mid \xi_j^*) \equiv \mathsf{Multin}(x_i \mid 1, \xi_j^*)$ and $q(\xi_j^*) \equiv \mathsf{Dir}(\xi_j^* \mid \alpha)$ for some suitable choice of α. In this case, $q(\xi_j^* \mid x_j^*)$ is again a multinomial distribution, and $g(x_j^*)$ is a Dirichlet-multinomial distribution. In the particular binary case ($c = 2$) we get the beta-binomial distribution.

Count covariates x_i: Assume $\xi_j^* > 0$. For $q(x_i \mid \xi_j^*)$ we assume a Poisson distribution with rate ξ^*, and for $q(\xi^*)$ we assume a gamma distribution. Then, $q(\xi_j^* \mid x_j^*)$ is again a gamma distribution and $g(x_j^*)$ reduces to the Poisson-gamma distribution.

Ordinal covariates x_i: we use the following construction. Assume an ordinal covariate with c categories. Johnson and Albert (1999) define an auxiliary probability model for x by introducing a latent variable z and a set of cutoffs $-\infty = \gamma_0 < \gamma_1 < \cdots < \gamma_{c-1} < \gamma_c = \infty$ and then set $x = r$ if $\gamma_{r-1} < z \leq \gamma_r$. For simplicity we fix the cutoffs as $\gamma_r = r - 1$ for $r = 1, \ldots, c$. As in the continuous case, let $\xi_j^* = (m_j, v_j)$. We use $q(z \mid \xi_j^*) = \mathsf{N}(z \mid m_j, v_j)$ and a normal-inverse chi-square (or gamma) distribution $q(\xi_j^*)$. Then $q(x_i = r \mid \xi_j^*) = q(\gamma_{r-1} < z \leq \gamma_r \mid \xi_j^*)$. Let $n_{jr} = \sum_{i \in S_j} I\{x_i = r\}$ count the number of covariates with value r in cluster j. The similarity function becomes

$$g(x_j^*) = \int_{\mathbb{R} \times \mathbb{R}^+} \prod_{r=1}^{c} \{\Phi_{m_j, v_j}(\gamma_r) - \Phi_{m_j, v_j}(\gamma_{r-1})\}^{n_{jr}} q(\xi_j^*) \, d\xi_j^*,$$

where $\Phi_{m,v}(\cdot)$ is the $\mathsf{N}(m, v)$ c.d.f.

Two more important details, about multiple covariates, of the same type, and of mixed types. First, the above procedures can be extended to the case of multivariate covariates of the same type by appropriately adjusting the auxiliary probability models. For instance, if x_i is a d-dimensional vector, then we may take $\xi_j^* = (m_j, v_j)$, $q(x_i \mid \xi_j^*) \equiv \mathsf{N}(x \mid m_j, v_j)$, and $q(\xi_j^*)$ to be a normal-Inverse Wishart distribution. Candidate's formula (8.15) can be used to evaluate the similarity function.

Second, to define a joint similarity function when x is a q-dimensional vector of mixed types of covariates, use

$$g(x_j^*) = \prod_{\ell=1}^{q} g^\ell(x_{j\ell}^*), \qquad (8.16)$$

where ℓ indexes covariates (or covariate types) and $g^\ell(\cdot)$ is the similarity function for the ℓ-th covariate (type).

Similar to the PPM model the PPMx prior (8.13) is usually used to define a statistical inference model together with a sampling model of the form (8.9).

Posterior Simulation A useful feature of a similarity function of the form (8.14) with DP-style cohesion functions is that the resulting joint model for data, parameters and random partition becomes formally equal to that obtained after marginalizing the random probability measure in a hypothetical DP mixture model for an augmented response vector $\tilde{y}_i = (y_i, x_i)$ with kernel $p(\tilde{y}_i \mid \theta_j^*, \xi_j^*) = p(y_i \mid \theta_j^*) q(x_i \mid \xi_j^*)$ and centering distribution in the DP prior $F_0(\theta^*, \xi^*) = p(\theta^*) q(\xi^*)$. This observation is useful for implementing posterior simulation.

The proposed choices of similarity functions $g(x_j^*)$ were driven by computational convenience. There are many other reasonable and valid alternatives (Figs. 8.4 and 8.5). For example, for categorical covariates one may use $g(x_j^*) = \exp\left(-\sum_{r=1}^{c} \hat{f}_{jr} \log(\hat{f}_{jr})\right)$, where $\hat{f}_{jr}$ is the proportion of covariate values equal to r in cluster j, and where we interpret $0 \times \log(0) = 0$.

8.4.2 PPMx with Variable Selection

In problems with a large number of covariates it is plausible that meaningful clusters might be characterized by just a subset of the covariates. We achieve this by introducing binary indicators $\gamma_{j\ell}$ for the jth cluster and ℓth covariate and assuming

$$p(\rho_n \mid \boldsymbol{\gamma}, X) \propto \prod_{j=1}^{K_n} \left\{ c(S_j) \times \left[\prod_{\ell=1}^{q} g(x_{j\ell}^\star)^{\gamma_{j\ell}} \right] \right\}. \qquad (8.17)$$

Model (8.17) defines a prior distribution on partitions, indexed by covariates with cluster-specific sets of covariates. Covariates can be active ($\gamma_{j\ell} = 1$) or inactive ($\gamma_{j\ell} = 0$). The model retains the product form. The model is completed with a prior model $p(\boldsymbol{\gamma})$ for the indicators. In Quintana et al. (2013) we use a normal hierarchical prior on logits. Let $z_{j\ell} = \text{logit } p(\gamma_{j\ell} = 1)$ denote the logit of the inclusion probability for covariate ℓ in cluster j on a logit scale. We assume a normal hierarchial model on $z_{j\ell}$.

8.4 Clustering and Regression

Adding covariate selection in the similarity function requires that the similarity function be calibrated such that $g(x^\star_j) > 1$ for a set of covariates $x^\star_j$ that are judged to be similar. A prior model with $g(x^\star_j) < 1$ for all $x^\star_j$ would a priori always favor no covariate selection and fail to formalize any prior preference for homogeneous clusters. We therefore use

$$\tilde{g}(x^\star_j) = \frac{g(x^\star_j)}{\prod_{i \in S_j} q(x_i \mid \tilde{\xi})}, \qquad (8.18)$$

for some conveniently chosen value of $\tilde{\xi}$ such as the m.l.e. of ξ given the complete set of covariate values X under the auxiliary model $q(X \mid \xi)$. Posterior simulation is greatly facilitated by the choice of (8.18), which has an important computational advantage. Candidate's formula (8.15) reduces to

$$\tilde{g}(x^\star_j) = \frac{q(\tilde{\xi})}{q(\tilde{\xi} \mid x^\star_j)}. \qquad (8.19)$$

The equality is true for any $\tilde{\xi}$ on the right hand side. The important advantage over direct evaluation of the marginal is that the dimension of ξ does not vary with cluster size.

Example 25 (ICU Readmission Rates) Quintana et al. (2013) discuss inference for readmission rates to a ICU (intensive care unit) in Portugal. Data from $n = 996$ patients include 17 variables: 12 physiology variables (heart rate, systolic blood pressure, body temperature, the ratio Pao2/Fio2 for ventilated patients, urinary output, serum urea level, WBC count, serum potassium, serum sodium level, serum bicarbonate level, bilirubin level and Glasgow coma score), age, type of admission (scheduled surgical, unscheduled surgical or medical) and three underlying disease variables (acquired immunodeficiency syndrome, metastatic cancer and hematologic malignancy). Covariates include a variety of different data formats. Covariates 1–12 are of continuous type, 13–14 are categorical, with 3 levels each, and 15–17 are binary. All variables are recorded in a vector of $p = 17$ covariates $x_i = (x_{i1}, \ldots, x_{ip})$, $i = 1, \ldots, n$.

Let y_i denote a binary indicator of death for the ith patient admitted to the ICU, $i = 1, \ldots, n$, with $y_i = 1$ if the patient died, and $y_i = 0$ otherwise. The proposed joint probability model for cluster-specific variable selection includes a sampling model expressed as a logistic regression for mortality with cluster-specific parameters. We recode each categorical covariate using two binary indicators, and add an extra intercept term, so that the resulting design vector $\tilde{x}_i$ has dimension 20. Given a partition ρ_n, represented as $(k, s_1, \ldots, s_n)$, we assume

$$\text{logit}\{p(y_i = 1 \mid s_i = j, \boldsymbol{\beta}^\star_j)\} = \boldsymbol{\beta}^{\star}_j \tilde{x}_i. \qquad (8.20)$$

We use similarity function (8.16) with a double-dipping similarity function g^ℓ which is defined as

$$g(x^\star_j) = \int \prod_{i \in S_j} q(x_i \mid \xi^\star_j) \, q(\xi^\star_j \mid x^\star_j) \, d\xi^\star_j.$$

with $q(\xi^\star_j \mid x^\star_j) \propto \prod_{i \in S_j} q(x_i \mid \xi^\star_j) q(\xi^\star_j)$ for conjugate pairs $q(x_i \mid \xi^\star_j)$ and $q(\xi^\star_j)$. It is important to point out here that $g(\cdot)$ need not be a probability model. There is no notion of modeling a distribution of covariates. As a probability model $g(x^\star_j)$ would be inappropriate due to the double use of the observed covariates.

The model is completed with a hierarchical prior on the regression coefficients $\beta^\star_j$. Figure 8.6 shows a summary of the inference.

8.4.3 Example 26: A PPMx Model for Outlier Detection

We discuss in more detail an application of the PPMx model to inference with possible outliers. We use the example to illustrate the impact of different choices of cohesion and similarity functions. Quintana and Iglesias (2003) considered estimating the slope or *systematic risk* in a normal Sharp model (Elton and Gruber 1995) for data on stock returns for Concha y Toro, one of the principal Chilean wine producers. The model is

$$y_i \mid \alpha, \beta, \sigma^2 \stackrel{ind}{\sim} N(\alpha + \beta x_i, \sigma^2), \qquad (8.21)$$

where observations $\{y_i\}$ are the monthly Concha y Toro stock returns, and covariates $\{x_i\}$ are the corresponding *Índice de Precio Selectivo de Acciones* (IPSA) values (the Chilean version of Dow-Jones index). It has been argued (Fama 1965; Blattberg and Gonedes 1974) that monthly stock returns data tend to exhibit little serial correlation. This is why such models usually include no serial correlation.

The example motivates a model for outlier detection. Without loss of generality we consider a regression as in (8.21). Quintana and Iglesias (2003) considered a PPM model for outlier detection and accurate estimation of the common parameter β. The proposed model considered observation-specific intercept parameters to capture atypical and possibly influential observations. We adopt here a PPMx version of that model, and assume

$$y_i \mid \theta^\star, \beta, \sigma^2 \stackrel{ind}{\sim} N(\theta^\star_{s_i} + \beta x_i, \sigma^2), \quad \text{and} \quad \theta^\star_j \mid \sigma^2 \stackrel{ind}{\sim} N(a, \tau_0^2 \sigma^2), \qquad (8.22)$$

with a hierarchical structure completed by assuming $\beta \mid \sigma^2 \sim N(b, \gamma_0^2 \sigma^2)$, $\sigma^2 \sim$ IGamma(ν_0, λ_0) and a PPMx random partition model (8.13).

8.4 Clustering and Regression

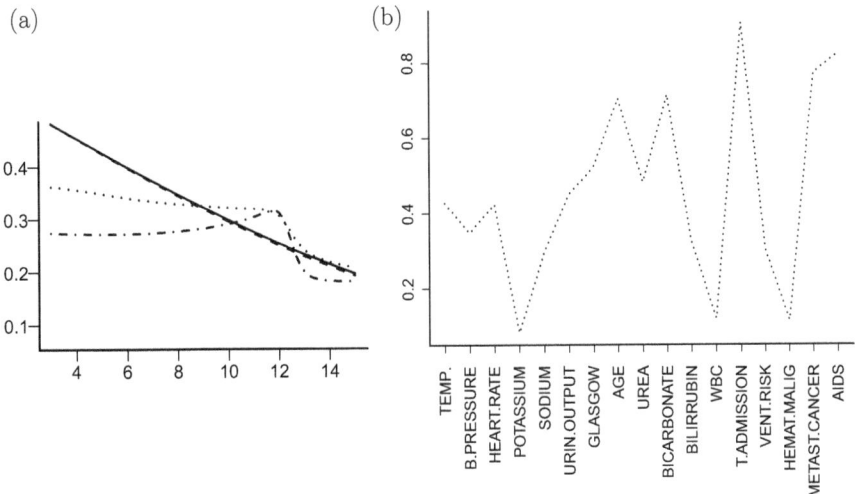

Fig. 8.4 Example 26. (**a**) The panels show the posterior distributions of β for prior 1 (*left*) and (**b**) prior 2 (*right*) under three versions of the PPMx model. One uses $g(x_j^*) = 1$ (g_1), another $g(x_j^*) = \exp(-\text{Var}(x_j^*))$ (g_2) and a third one (g_3) uses (8.14) with a normal-inverse gamma auxiliary model

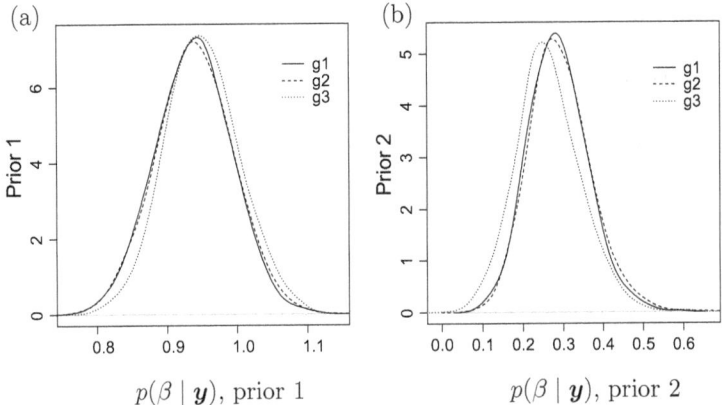

Fig. 8.5 Example 26. The *left panel* shows the raw data with IPSA values in the horizontal axis and Concha y Toro stock returns in the vertical axis. Outlying observations 43, 58, 98, 105, 106, and 111 are marked with *special characters*. The *right panel* shows the estimated posterior similarity matrix under Prior 1 and similarity function g_2. Observations have been relabeled so that the six outlying observations are in the last six positions

Prior Quintana and Iglesias (2003) chose the following hyper-parameter values: $a = 0$, $b = 1$, $\tau_0^2 = 1/3$, $\gamma_0^2 = 1/4$, $\nu_0 = 2.01$ and $\lambda_0 = 0.0101$. They were selected to express an informative prior under which only few observations are to be deemed as outliers. In particular, it follows that $E(\sigma^2) = 0.01$ and $\text{Var}(\sigma^2) =$

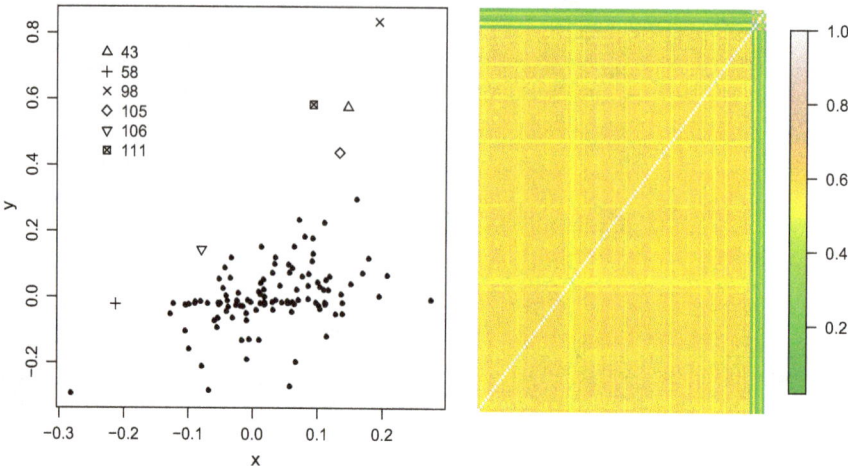

Fig. 8.6 Example 25. Panel (**a**) plots posterior estimated mortality against Glasgow score (keeping all other variables fixed). The *solid line* shows the prediction for the proposed model. The other lines show alternative models. Panel (**b**) shows posterior marginal variable inclusion probabilities. The averages are weighted with respect to the cluster sizes, that is $E(\sum_j \gamma_{j\ell} n_j/n \mid \text{data})$, plotted by covariate

0.01, with corresponding induced prior for β and baseline distributions being tightly concentrated around 1 and 0, respectively. Alternatively we also consider a different, vague prior with $\tau_0^2 = \gamma_0^2 = 100$. In the sequel we refer to the former as Prior 1 and to the latter as Prior 2.

Similarity Function We are interested in the effect of the similarity function on posterior inference and compare three alternative choices. Recall that $|S_j|$ is the size of the j-th cluster. The three similarity functions are: (1) $g_1(x_j^*) = 1$, which reduces the model to a regular PPM; (2) a function of the empirical variance, $g_2(x_j^*) = \exp\left(-\text{Var}(x_j^*)\right)$, where $\text{Var}(x_j^*) = |S_j|^{-1} \sum_{i \in S_j} (x_i - \bar{x}_j^*)$, and $\bar{x}_j^* = |S_j|^{-1} \sum_{i \in S_j} x_i$; and (3) a version of (8.14), which we refer to as g_3, with $\xi = v$, $q(x \mid v) \equiv N(x \mid 0, v)$ and $q(v) \equiv \text{IGamma}(v \mid r_0, r_1)$ with $r_0 = 2.0938$ and $r_1 = 0.02956$, which are determined so as to match the empirical mean and variance of the observed covariate values.

Results Figure 8.4 shows the resulting inference on the systematic risk. The left panel shows the posterior distribution of β for each of the three similarity functions for the informative Prior 1, while the right panel shows results under the vague Prior 2. The choice of similarity function, g_1, g_2 or g_3, has little effect under either prior. However, there is a striking difference on the support of $p(\beta \mid y)$ under one versus the other prior. This is because under Prior 1 the α_i are much more concentrated around their prior mean, in this case, $a = 0$. In contrast, under Prior 2 the α_i coefficients are free to adjust to the responses, leading to a considerable reduction in the slope β.

8.4 Clustering and Regression

Similarity functions g_1 and g_2: Applying the least squares algorithm of Dahl (2006) we find interesting results. Under the PPM model without covariates, that is g_1, and Prior 1 the selected partition has two clusters: one containing the subset $\{43, 98, 105, 106, 111\}$ and the other all the remaining observations. To a large extent, this agrees with the results in Quintana and Iglesias (2003), where the same subset of outlying points was detected, although grouped into two clusters rather than one. When using g_2 the result was again one large and one small cluster, the small one given by subset $\{43, 58, 98, 105, 106, 111\}$ and the large one with all the rest. Comparing these two, g_2 finds one more outlying observation, namely 58. These observations, together with a graphical representation of the posterior similarity matrix under Prior 1 and similarity function g_2 can be found in Figure 8.5. In the posterior similarity matrix under g_2, observations were relabeled so that the six potential outliers become the last six ones, placed together, and in the order stated above. For observation 58, all of the co-clustering probabilities in the similarity matrix lie below 50 %, which gives some support to its interpretation as an outlier.

While the previous results under Prior 1 using g_1 and g_2 are quite similar, under Prior 2 we find many more outliers. They can be grouped into 5 and 6 clusters under g_1 and g_2, respectively. The explanation is again the much less restrictive nature of the prior on the α_i coefficients. From the viewpoint of detecting outliers, Prior 2 is thus of little help as the main idea is to identify a few outliers, and not to declare a large portion of the sample as outlying observations.

Similarity functions g_3: Under either prior choice, that is Prior 1 or 2, when using g_3 the least squares algorithm gives over 50 clusters in both cases. The posterior similarity matrix in these two last cases has very small entries, with 99 % percentiles of 0.06 and 0.18. This means that g_3 induces many more clusters a posteriori than g_1 and g_2. However, when computing the LPML for each of the six models considered here, we find that Prior 2 with similarity function g_3 provides the best fit (Table 8.3).

Finally, Fig. 8.7 shows posterior predictive distributions under all combinations of Prior 1 and 2 and similarity functions g_1, g_2 or g_3. The predictions are for observations 1, 34, and 66, which represent, respectively, the minimum, median, and maximum observed values of x. We can see the shift in all these distributions as x increases. Prior 1 produces unimodal posteriors in all cases. Only Prior 2 and g_1 or g_2 lead to multimodal posteriors.

In summary, Prior 1, in particular in combination with g_1 or g_2, allows for reasonable outlier detection, but Prior 2, in particular with g_3, yields a better fit to the data, as seen from the LPML values.

Table 8.3 Example 26. The table shows the LPML values for each of Priors 1 and 2 and similarity functions g_1, g_2 and g_3, as defined in the text

Prior	Similarity function		
	g_1	g_2	g_3
1	76.74	76.51	71.34
2	133.85	136.80	186.04

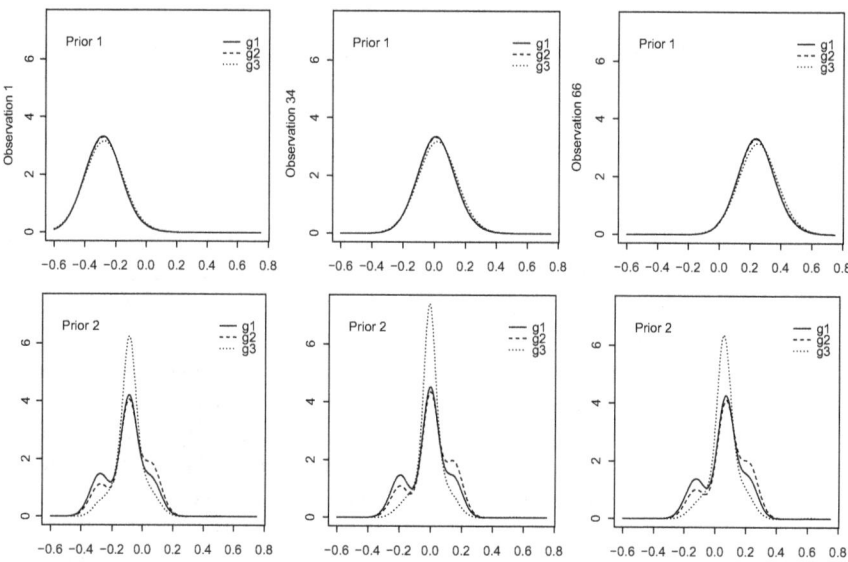

Fig. 8.7 Example 26. Posterior predictive distributions for stock returns example under Prior 1 (*top row*) and under Prior 2 (*bottom row*)

8.5 Feature Allocation Models

8.5.1 Feature Allocation

So far we discussed partitions of $[n] = \{1,\ldots,n\}$ into mutually exclusive and exhaustive subsets. We now extend the notion of partitions to *feature allocations*, that is, a family of subsets $\{S_1,\ldots,S_K\}$ which need not be mutually exclusive. Following Broderick et al. (2013), a feature is a subset $S \subset [n]$ and a feature allocation is a multiset $F_n = \{S_1,\ldots,S_K\}$ of features S_j, also called *blocks*, such that each index i can belong to any finite number of blocks. It follows that not every feature allocation is a partition, but every partition is a feature allocation. Recall the brief discussion of feature allocation models in Sect. 8.1. In particular, recall the $(n \times K)$ binary matrix $Z = [Z_{ik}]$ with feature membership indicators Z_{ik}. A feature allocation model is a prior $p(Z)$. If Z is directly observed, as it might be the case in the earlier example with recording movie preferences when the observed data are indicators Z_{ij} for customer i liking movies of type j, then the only inference of interest might be inference on hyper-parameters that index $p(Z)$ or posterior predictive inference for future experimental units, $i > n + 1$, and not much is left to do. In many applications, however, the feature allocation Z is latent and only linked to the observed data through some sampling model. For example we might only observe movie choices rather than preferences for different movie genres. Let y_i denote the observed movie choices for the i-th customer. We would add an assumed sampling model $p(y_i \mid Z, \boldsymbol{\theta}^\star)$ conditional on latent unobserved preferences Z. Here $\boldsymbol{\theta}^\star$ could be additional feature-specific parameters. Below, in Example 27 we will discuss an inference problem where Z represents the unknown latent composition of a tumor sample as a mixture of K cell subtypes. The observed data $\mathbf{y}$ are related to Z by an assumed sampling model. In general, let $\mathbf{y} = (y_i, i = 1, \ldots, n)$ denote the observed outcomes, and assume that the sampling model makes use of feature-specific parameters $\theta_j^\star$ and some additional common parameters η. Also, we assume conditional independence across i conditional on $Z, \boldsymbol{\theta}^\star, \eta$. This is the case in the later example. In summary,

$$y_i \stackrel{\text{ind}}{\sim} p(y_i \mid Z, \boldsymbol{\theta}^\star, \eta), \qquad (8.23)$$

$i = 1, \ldots, n$. The specific nature of $p(y_i \mid Z, \boldsymbol{\theta}^\star, \eta)$ depends on the problem. In most applications the sampling model for y_i might depend on Z only through the i-th row of Z.

8.5.2 Indian Buffet Process

The most popular prior model $p(Z)$ in feature allocation problems is the *Indian Buffet Process* (IBP), proposed in Griffiths and Ghahramani (2006). The name arises as follows. Consider n customers entering a restaurant one after another. Imagine a buffet with an unlimited number of dishes. The dishes will become the features in the IBP, that is, the dishes correspond to the columns of Z and the customers correspond to the rows of Z. The first customer selects a number of dishes, $K_1^+ \mid \alpha \sim \text{Poi}(\alpha)$. Without loss of generality we assume that the customer chooses the first K_1^+ dishes in the buffet. Thus $Z_{1j} = 1, j = 1, \ldots, K_1^+$. Now consider the i-th customer entering the restaurant. Let $K_{i-1} = \sum_{\ell=1}^{i-1} K_\ell^+$ denote the total number of dishes selected by the first $i-1$ customers and let Z_{i-1} denote the $(i-1) \times K_{i-1}$ binary matrix for the first $i-1$ customers and let $m_{i-1,j} = \sum_{\ell=1}^{i-1} Z_{\ell j}$ denote the number of customer so far who selected dish $j, j = 1, \ldots, K_{i-1}$. The ith customer takes a serving from each of the earlier selected dishes, $j = 1, \ldots, K_{i-1}$ with probability

$$p(Z_{ij} = 1 \mid Z_{i-1}) = \frac{m_{i-1,j}}{i}, \qquad (8.24)$$

i.e. with probability proportional to the popularity of this dish. After reaching the end of all previously selected dishes, the i-th customer then tries

$$K_i^+ \mid \alpha \sim \text{Poi}(\alpha/i) \qquad (8.25)$$

new dishes. The new dishes are indexed $j = K_{i-1} + 1, \ldots, K_i \equiv K_{i-1} + K_i^+$, we add K_i^+ new columns to Z, and set $Z_{ij} = 1$ and $Z_{\ell j} = 0$ for earlier customers $\ell = 1, \ldots, i-1$. It is possible that a customer goes hungry, with $\sum_j Z_{ij} = 0$. After the last, n-th customer has selected dishes we are left with $K = K_n$ dishes. This provides a constructive definition of a $(n \times K)$ random binary matrix Z. Note that the number of columns, K, is random. Letting $h_n = \sum_{i=1}^{n} 1/i$,

$$K_n \mid \alpha \sim \text{Poi}(\alpha h_n).$$

Implicit in the construction is a restriction of Z to indexing features by appearance. For reference we summarize the definition. Let $m_j = m_{n,j}$ denote the total number of customers who chose dish j.

Definition 10 (IBP) A random $(n \times K)$ binary matrix Z is said to follow an Indian buffet process (IBP) if

$$p(Z) = \frac{\alpha^K}{\prod_{i=1}^{n} K_i^+!} e^{-\alpha h_n} \prod_{j=1}^{K} \frac{(n-m_j)!(m_j-1)!}{n!}.$$

The model includes a random number of columns K and Z is constrained to indexing features by appearance.

It is sometimes convenient to use a slightly stricter restriction to so called *left ordered form*. Let $z_j = (Z_{1j}, \ldots, Z_{nj})$ denote the j-th column and interpret z_j as dyadic integer with Z_{1j} being the most significant digit. In left ordered form the columns are sorted by z_j. See Griffiths and Ghahramani (2006) for $p(Z)$ under constraint to left order form.

Similar to the DP prior, the IBP can be obtained as the limit of a finite feature allocation construction (Teh et al. 2007). For $k = 1, \ldots, K$ and $i = 1, \ldots, n$ let

$$w_k \mid \alpha, K \stackrel{\text{ind}}{\sim} \text{Be}(\alpha/K, 1) \quad \text{and} \quad Z_{ik} \mid w_k \stackrel{\text{ind}}{\sim} \text{Ber}(w_k), \tag{8.26}$$

be independent Bernoulli random variables. Taking the limit as $K \to \infty$, and dropping columns with all zeros we get the IBP prior $p(Z)$, except for the rearrangement into left ordered form (or ordering by appearance).

The construction (8.26) is symmetric in i. This is important for posterior simulation under the IBP. Consider a statistical inference problem with a sampling model of the form (8.23) under an IBP prior on the feature allocation Z. Assume that the model is completed with a prior probability model on the remaining parameters. Posterior inference is best implemented as posterior MCMC simulation. Let Z_{-i} denote the feature allocation without the i-th experimental unit, that is Z after removing the i-th row and any column that remains all zeroes after removing the i-th row. In setting up the MCMC transition probabilities we need the conditional prior probabilities $p(Z_{ij} \mid Z_{-i})$. The symmetry in the construction implies that the IBP prior is exchangeable across rows i. We can therefore assume without loss of generality that $i = n$ and use (8.24) and (8.25) to evaluate $p(Z_{ij} \mid Z_{-i})$.

8.5 Feature Allocation Models

Another, useful and instructive stick-breaking representation is given by Teh et al. (2007):

$$Z_{ik} \mid w_k \stackrel{\text{ind}}{\sim} \text{Ber}(w_k), \quad w_k = \prod_{j=1}^{k} v_j, \quad v_j \mid \alpha \stackrel{\text{iid}}{\sim} \text{Beta}(\alpha, 1), \qquad (8.27)$$

$k = 1, 2, \ldots$. The binary matrix Z is obtained after removing all columns that contain only zeros, which leaves us with a random $n \times K_n$ matrix with a random number of columns K_n. If desired, the columns could be re-arranged to restrict Z to left ordered form.

Example 27 (Tumor Heterogeneity) Lee et al. (2013a) and Xu et al. (2015) use an IBP prior to study tumor heterogeneity. The data are counts of point mutations in different samples. The underlying biological hypothesis is that a tumor is composed of different subpopulations of cells. We use the presence ($Z_{ij} = 1$) or absence ($Z_{ij} = 0$) of point mutations to characterize latent subpopulations. The data are counts from a next generation sequencing experiment. For each point mutation i, $i = 1, \ldots, n$, and each sample t, $t = 1, \ldots, T$ we count the number of reads that are mapped to the locus of that mutation (N_{ti}) and the number of reads out of those N_{ti} reads that actually carry the mutation (y_{ti}). We assume binomial sampling,

$$y_{ti} \mid p_{ti} \stackrel{\text{ind}}{\sim} \text{Bin}(N_{ti}, p_{ti}). \qquad (8.28)$$

The key assumption is that p_{ti} is due to the sample being composed of a small number of cell subpopulations, $j = 1, \ldots, K$, which include ($Z_{ij} = 1$) or not ($Z_{ij} = 0$) a particular mutation. The indicators Z_{ij} are combined into a $(n \times K)$ binary matrix $Z = [Z_{ij}]$. In this description, the columns z_j of Z represent the latent cell types. They are not directly observed, only indirectly by trying to explain the observed y_{ti} by representing sample t as being composed of these cell types. Let $\theta_{tj}^\star, j = 1, \ldots, K$ denote the fraction of cell type j in sample t. We assume

$$p_{ti} = \sum_{j=1}^{K} \theta_{tj}^\star Z_{ij} + \theta_{t0}^\star p_0, \qquad (8.29)$$

where the final term is added to allow for model mis-specification, measurement error and for subtypes that are too rare to be detected. We assume a Dirichlet prior on $\boldsymbol{\theta}_t^\star = (\theta_{t0}^\star, \theta_{t1}^\star, \ldots, \theta_{tK}^\star)$.

The key model element is the prior $p(Z)$. This is where we use the IBP prior,

$$Z \sim \text{IBP}(\alpha).$$

Figure 8.8 summarizes the estimated Z matrix. This formalizes the desired description of tumor heterogeneity. In this discussion we simplified the description. For diploid organisms, like humans, cell subtypes are characterized by pairs of

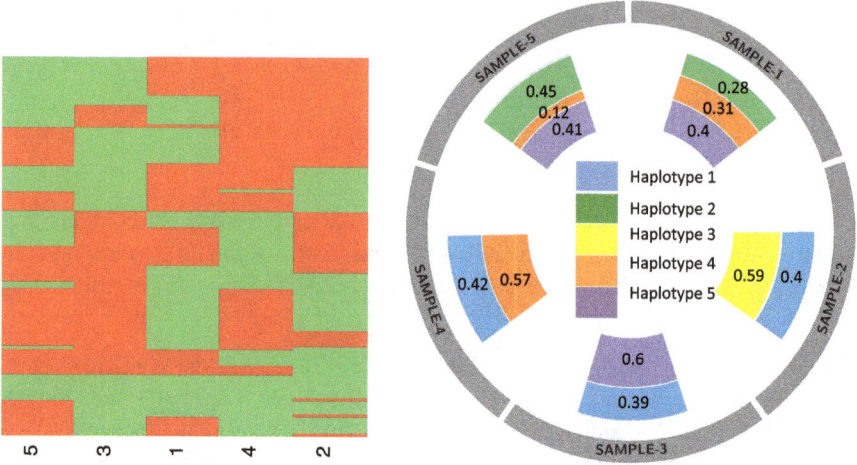

Fig. 8.8 Example 27. The *left panel* shows the estimated tumor heterogeneity characterized by the feature allocation matrix Z. The *columns* are the cell types, $j = 1, \ldots, 5$. The *rows* are the SNV's, $i = 1, \ldots, S$. The *right panel* shows the corresponding posterior estimated weights w_{tj} arranged by sample t in the *circle*

haplotypes. In that case the columns of Z should be interpreted as defining possible haplotypes, with $K > 2$ indicating tumor heterogeneity. See Lee et al. (2013a) for more discussion.

Finally we owe an explanation for the edges connecting the IBP with other models in Fig. 1 in the Preface. Thibaux and Jordan (2007) discuss an alternative definition of the IBP using a construction based on the Beta process (BP) and the Bernoulli process (BeP).

8.5.3 Approximate Posterior Inference with MAD Bayes

For large n and/or specific sampling models posterior inference with MCMC simulation becomes impractical due to slow mixing of the implemented Markov chain. This is the case in Example 27. The sampling model (8.28) introduces high posterior correlation of the $\theta_t^\star$ and Z, making it difficult to implement efficient posterior MCMC. Posterior simulation requires a transdimensional MCMC with reversible jump (RJ) transition probabilities that add or delete features. It is difficult to define RJ moves with practicable acceptance probabilities. This is not a critical problem in Example 27. A priori plausible numbers of distinct subclones are small, say between 1 and 10. Lee et al. (2013a) propose model selection to implement inference across K as an alternative to a more complicated transdimensional MCMC.

8.5 Feature Allocation Models

Alternatively, Broderick et al. (2013) introduce a clever scheme for approximate posterior inference that exploits an asymptotic similarity of the log posterior with a criterion function in a k-means clustering algorithm. The k-means algorithm is a fast popular rule-based clustering method (Hartigan and Wong 1979). The approximation is known as MAP-based asymptotic derivation (MAD) Bayes. The method is suitable for problems with a normal sampling model (8.23). The asymptotics are small-variance asymptotics for small variance in the normal sampling model. A similar asymptotic argument can be constructed with binomial sampling as in (8.28) and (8.29).

MAD Bayes Posterior Maximization

For reference we state the complete statistical inference model. We assume a sampling model

$$p(y \mid Z, \boldsymbol{\theta}^\star) \tag{8.30}$$

together with an IBP prior for Z and a prior for feature specific parameters $\boldsymbol{\theta}^\star = (\boldsymbol{\theta}^\star_1, \ldots, \boldsymbol{\theta}^\star_K)$:

$$p(Z \mid \alpha) \sim \text{IBP}(\alpha) \quad \text{and} \quad p(\boldsymbol{\theta}^\star_1, \ldots, \boldsymbol{\theta}^\star_K).$$

For example, the sampling model could be the binomial sampling $p(y \mid Z, \boldsymbol{\theta}^\star)$ of (8.28), noting that $p_{it} = p_{it}(Z, \boldsymbol{\theta}^\star)$ is determined by (8.29). The prior $p(\boldsymbol{\theta}^\star)$ could be the independent Dirichlet priors for the row vectors $\boldsymbol{\theta}^\star_t = (\theta^\star_{t0}, \theta^\star_{t1}, \ldots, \theta^\star_{tK})$ in Example 27. Note that in the example, we use $\boldsymbol{\theta}^\star_t$ to indicate the rows of the $(n \times K)$ matrix $\boldsymbol{\theta}^\star$ (rather than the feature-specific columns). The simple reason is the constraint to the row sums of 1.0, and the independence across rows. Also, we included the additional weight $\theta^\star_{t0}$.

The idea of MAD Bayes is to rescale $\log p(y \mid Z, \boldsymbol{\theta}^\star)$ by a factor β and take the limit as $\beta \to \infty$. At the same time, we reduce the parameter of the IBP prior as $\alpha = \exp(-\beta \lambda^2) \to 0$, for a fixed constant λ^2. The decreasing α avoids overfitting that would otherwise occur by maximizing the rescaled log likelihood function. In a moment we will recognize λ^2 as a penalty parameter for introducing additional features. For large β we get (Broderick et al. 2013; Xu et al. 2015)

$$-\frac{1}{\beta} \log p(Z, \boldsymbol{\theta}^\star \mid y) = c - \log p(y \mid Z, \boldsymbol{\theta}^\star) + K\lambda^2 \equiv Q(Z, \boldsymbol{\theta}^\star). \tag{8.31}$$

Here c is a constant (in $Z, \boldsymbol{\theta}^\star$). The last term is all that is left of the log IBP prior after taking the limit $\beta \to 0$. We recognize it as a penalty for the number of columns in Z, that is, for introducing additional features.

We are now ready to state the MAD Bayes algorithm to minimize the criterion function $Q(Z, \boldsymbol{\theta}^\star)$. We state it in the version of Xu et al. (2015), who adapt the

MAD Bayes algorithm of Broderick et al. (2013) for inference in Example 27. The algorithm is a variation of k-means. In the algorithm $\boldsymbol{\theta}_t^\star = (\theta_{t1}^\star, \ldots, \theta_{tK}^\star)$ denotes the t-th row of the $(T \times K)$ matrix $\boldsymbol{\theta}^\star$, rather than the feature-specific columns, simply because it makes it easier to impose the constraint to unit row sums. Similarly, row $z_i = (Z_{i1}, \ldots, Z_{iK})$ denotes the i-th row of the $(n \times K)$ binary matrix Z. Also, let $\boldsymbol{\theta}_{-t}^\star$ denote $\boldsymbol{\theta}^\star$ with the t-th row removed. Similarly for Z_{-i}.

Algorithm 10: *MAD-Bayes.*

1. $K = 1$ and $p(Z_{i1} = 1) = 0.5$, $i = 1, \ldots, n$ *(initialize Z)*
2. $\boldsymbol{\theta}_t^\star \sim \text{Dir}(1, 1, \ldots, 1)$ *for $t = 1, \ldots, T$ (initialize $\boldsymbol{\theta}^\star$).*
3. Repeat

   3.1 *for $i = 1, \ldots, n$: fixing $\boldsymbol{\theta}^\star$, Z_{-i} and K find*
   $z_i = \arg\min_{z_i} Q(Z, \boldsymbol{\theta}^\star)$,
   3.2 *for $t = 1, \ldots, T$: fixing Z (and thus K) and $\boldsymbol{\theta}_{-t}^\star$ find*
   $\boldsymbol{\theta}_t^\star = \arg\min_{\boldsymbol{\theta}_t^\star} Q(Z, \boldsymbol{\theta}^\star)$, subject to $\sum_{c=1}^K \theta_{tc} = 1$,
   3.3 Let Z' equal Z but with one new feature (labeled $K + 1$) with $Z_{i,K+1} = 1$ for one randomly selected index i.
   3.4 Find $\boldsymbol{\theta}^{\star\prime}$ that minimizes the objective given Z'.
   3.5 if $(Q(Z', \boldsymbol{\theta}^{\star\prime}) < Q(Z, \boldsymbol{\theta}^\star))$ then
   $(Z, \boldsymbol{\theta}^\star) := (Z', \boldsymbol{\theta}^{\star\prime})$

   until *(no changes made)*

8.6 Nested Clustering Models

Some applications call for clustering in more than one direction.

Example 28 (RPPA Data) Lee et al. (2013b) consider the following problem. Figure 8.9 shows levels of protein activation for $G = 55$ proteins in samples from $n = 256$ breast cancer patients. The data come from a reverse phase protein array (RPPA) experiment that allows to record protein activation for a large number of samples and proteins simultaneously. The idea is to identify sets of proteins that give rise to a clinically meaningful clustering of patients. The eventual goal is to exploit these subgroups for the development of optimal adaptive treatment allocations. This goal is in the far future.

The immediate goal is to identify subsets of proteins that are characterized by a common partition of patients. That is, two proteins g_1 and g_2 are in the same cluster if observed protein activation in the patient samples move in tandem for g_1 and g_2 and give rise to the same (nested) clustering of patients. In other words, we represent how different biologic processes give rise to different clusterings of the patient population by using that feature to define clusters of proteins. An important detail is that two proteins g_1 and g_2 can give rise to the same clustering of patients even if protein g_1 is always de-activated whenever g_2 is activated and vice versa. That is, sharing the same nested clustering of patients is more general than sharing a common parameter in a sampling model for protein activation.

8.6 Nested Clustering Models

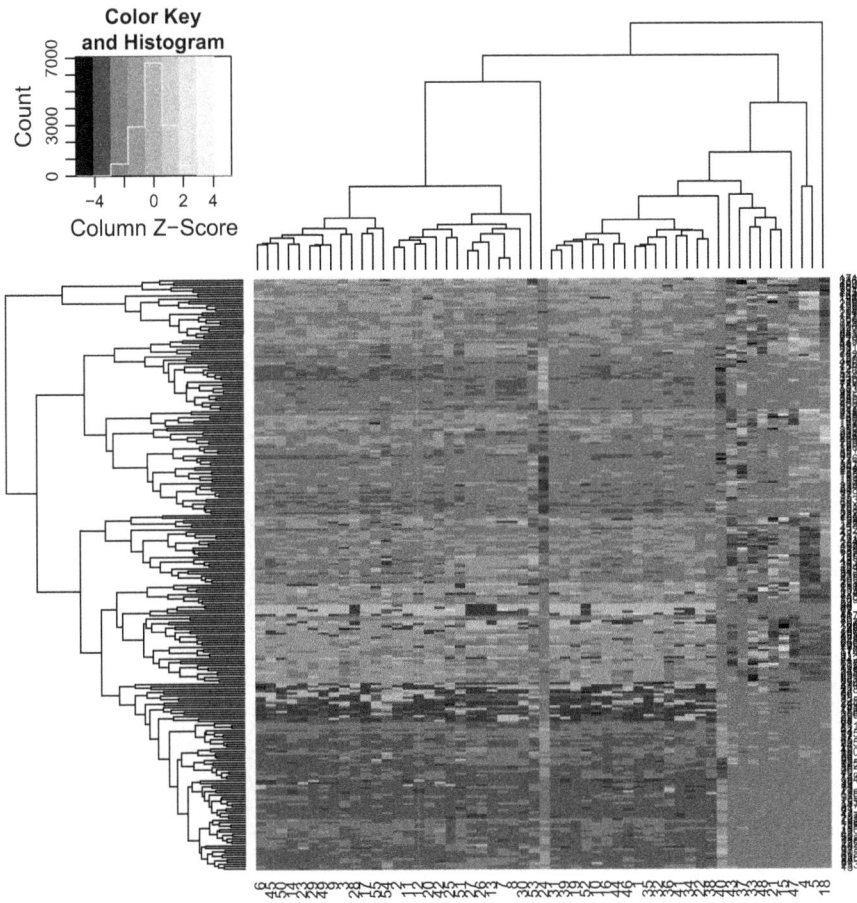

Fig. 8.9 Example 28. Protein activation for $n = 256$ patients (*rows*) and $G = 55$ proteins (*columns*). The dendrograms are estimated using hierarchical clustering

Let w_g denote cluster membership indicators to index a partition of proteins into $\{S_j;\ j = 0, \ldots, K\}$. For each subset S_j we define a protein-set specific partition of patients with respect to that protein set. Let c_{ji} denote cluster membership indicators for the partition of patients $i = 1, \ldots, n$ with respect to protein set j. In other words, we seek to identify a partition of proteins, $\boldsymbol{w} = (w_1, \ldots, w_G)$, and a nested partition of patients, $\boldsymbol{c}_j = (c_{j1}, \ldots, c_{jn})$, nested within each protein set. Figure 8.10 indicates protein clusters by vertical white lines, and the nested patient clusters by horizontal lines. There are two more important details. We allow for some proteins to be unrelated to any biologic process of interest, i.e., they do not give rise to a nested partition of patients. We collect these proteins in a special cluster $w_g = 0$ and define nested patient partitions only for clusters $j = 1, \ldots, K$. Similarly, we allow for the fact that some patients might not meaningfully fall into clusters with

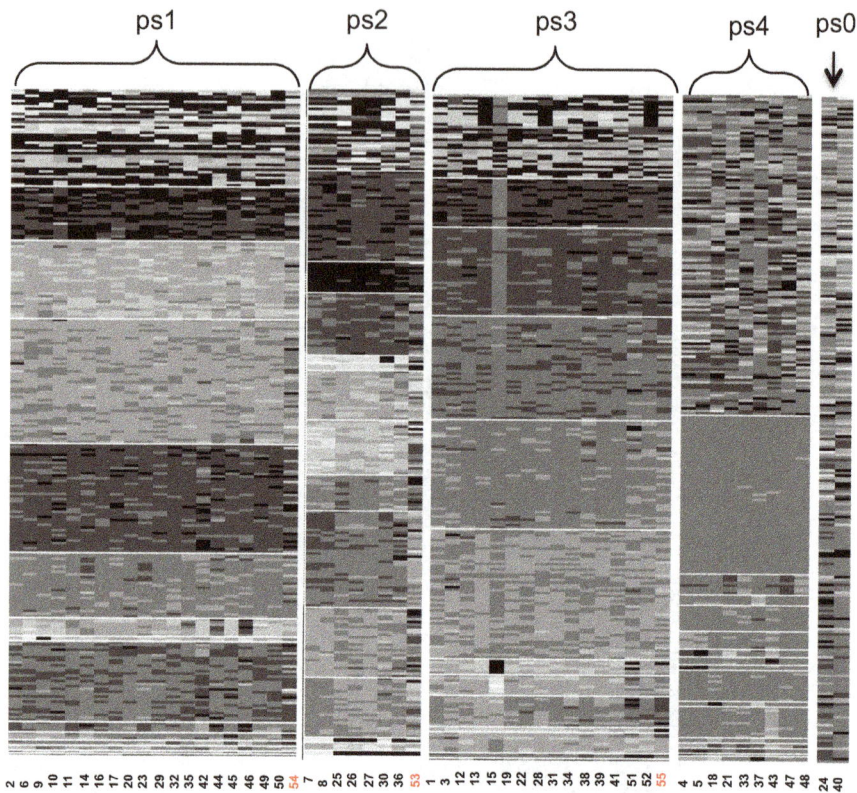

Fig. 8.10 Example 28. The image shows protein activation by patient (*rows*) and proteins (*columns*). The vertical white lines separate subsets S_j of proteins that give rise to different partitions of patients. Partitions of patients are indicated by *horizontal white lines*

respect to a particular protein set. We combine these patients in the special patient cluster $c_{ji} = 0$.

Lee et al. (2013b) define a prior model $p(w)$ for protein clusters, and conditional on w a prior $p(c \mid w) = \prod_{j=1}^{K} p(c_j)$ on random patient clusters with respect to each of the protein sets. Specifically, let $m_j = |S_j|$ denote the size of the j–th protein cluster.

$$p(w) = \pi_0^{m_0}(1-\pi_0)^{G-m_0} \frac{M^{K-1} \prod_{j=1}^{K}(m_j - 1)!}{(M+1)\cdot \ldots \cdot (M+G-m_0-1)} \qquad (8.32)$$

and similarly let $n_{jk} = |\{i : c_{ji} = k\}|$ denote the size of the k-th patient cluster with respect to the j-th protein set. We define

$$p(c_j \mid w) = \pi_1^{n_{j0}}(1-\pi_1)^{n-n_{j0}} \frac{\alpha^{K_j - 1} \prod_{k=1}^{K_j}(n_{jk} - 1)!}{(\alpha+1)\cdot \ldots \cdot (\alpha+n-n_{j0}-1)}. \qquad (8.33)$$

The prior $p(w)$ can be characterized as a zero-inflated Polya urn. Each protein is in cluster S_0 with probability π_0. The proteins that are not in S_0 form clusters $S_1, \ldots, S_K$ using the Polya urn defined in (8.5), with total mass parameter M. Similarly, $p(c_j \mid w)$ is another zero-inflated Polya urn, with probability π_1 for the zero cluster and a Polya urn with total mass parameter α for the remaining patients.

The prior model for the nested clusters on columns and rows is completed to a full inference model by defining a sampling model for observed data y_{gi}. We use a normal sampling model with protein and patient cluster specific parameters $\theta_{ig} = \theta_{kg}^{\star}$ for all i in the k-th cluster with respect to the protein set S_j that contains g, i.e.

$$y_{ig} \stackrel{\text{ind}}{\sim} N(\theta_{kg}^{\star}, \sigma_{\ell}^2), \quad \text{for } w_g = j \text{ and } c_{ji} = k \qquad (8.34)$$

and $y_{ig} \stackrel{\text{ind}}{\sim} N(m, \sigma_2^2)$ for $w_g = j$ and $c_{ji} = 0$, and $y_{ig} \stackrel{\text{ind}}{\sim} N(m, \sigma_3^2)$ for $w_g = 0$. The model is completed with conjugate priors on $\theta_{kg}^{\star}$, m and σ_{ℓ}^2, $\ell = 1, 2, 3$.

An important detail is that $\theta_{kg}^{\star}$ can vary across proteins $g \in S_j$ in the same protein set. The only feature that characterizes S_j is the shared nested clustering c_j, not any shared parameters.

Example 28 (RPPA Data, Ctd.) We implement inference on the desired nested clustering of patients with respect to different protein sets using the prior model (8.32) and (8.33), together with the sampling model in (8.34). The posterior distribution $p(w \mid y)$ and $p(c_j, j = 1, \ldots, K \mid w, y)$ is a probability model on a partition of patients nested within protein sets. Protein sets are formed to give rise to meaningful patient clusters. Figure 8.10 shows a summary of the posterior distribution on the random partitions. The displayed partition is found by the algorithm proposed in Dahl (2006).

References

Barry D, Hartigan JA (1992) Product partition models for change point problems. Ann Stat 20:260–279
Barry D, Hartigan JA (1993) A Bayesian analysis for change point problems. J Am Stat Assoc 88:309–319
Blattberg RC, Gonedes NJ (1974) A comparison of stable and student distribution as statistical models for stock prices. J Bus 47:244–280
Broderick T, Jordan MI, Pitman J (2013) Cluster and feature modeling from combinatorial stochastic processes. Stat Sci 28(3):289–312
Broderick T, Kulis B, Jordan MI (2013) MAD-Bayes: MAP-based asymptotic derivations from Bayes. In: Dasgupta S, McAllester D (eds) Proceedings of the 30th international conference on machine learning (ICML), 2013
Crowley EM (1997) Product partition models for normal means. J Am Stat Assoc 92:192–198
Dahl DB (2006) Model-based clustering for expression data via a Dirichlet process mixture model. In: Vannucci M, Do KA, Müller P (eds) Bayesian inference for gene expression and proteomics. Cambridge University Press, Cambridge

Dasgupta A, Raftery AE (1998) Detecting features in spatial point process with clutter via model-base clustering. J Am Stat Assoc 93:294–302

Elton EJ, Gruber MJ (1995) Modern portfolio theory and investment analysis, 5th edn. Wiley, New York

Fama E (1965) The behavior of stock market prices. J Bus 38:34–105

Fraley C, Raftery AE (2002) Model-based clustering, discriminant analysis, and density estimation. J Am Stat Assoc 97(458):611–631

Geisser S, Eddy W (1979) A predictive approach to model selection. J Am Stat Assoc 74:153–160

Gelman A, Carlin JB, Stern HS, Rubin DB (2004) Bayesian data analysis, 2nd edn. Texts in statistical science series. Chapman & Hall/CRC, Boca Raton, FL

Green PJ, Richardson S (2001) Modelling heterogeneity with and without the Dirichlet process. Scand J Stat 28(2):355–375

Griffiths TL, Ghahramani Z (2006) Infinite latent feature models and the Indian buffet process. In: Weiss Y, Schölkopf B, Platt J (eds) Advances in neural information processing systems, vol 18. MIT Press, Cambridge, MA, pp 475–482

Hartigan JA (1990) Partition models. Commun Stat Theory Meth 19:2745–2756

Hartigan JA, Wong MA (1979) Algorithm AS 136: A k-means clustering algorithm. J R Stat Soc Ser C: Appl Stat 28(1):100–108

Johnson VE, Albert JH (1999) Ordinal data modeling. Springer, New York

Kingman JFC (1978) The representation of partition structures. J Lond Math Soc 18(2):374–380. doi:10.1112/jlms/s2-18.2.374

Kingman JFC (1982) The coalescent. Stoch Process Appl 13(3):235–248. doi:10.1016/0304-4149(82)90011-4. http://dx.doi.org/10.1016/0304-4149(82)90011-4

Lee J, Müller P, Ji Y, Gulukota K (2015) A Bayesian feature allocation model for tumor heterogeneity. Annals of Applied Statistics: to appear

Lee J, Müller P, Zhu Y, Ji Y (2013b) A nonparametric Bayesian model for local clustering. J Amer Stat Ass 108:775–788

Lee J, Quintana FA, Müller P, Trippa L (2013c) Defining predictive probability functions for species sampling models. Stat Sci 28(2):209–222

Leon-Novelo LG, Bekele BN, Müller P, Quintana FA, Wathen K (2012) Borrowing strength with nonexchangeable priors over subpopulations. Biometrics 68(2):550–558

Loschi R, Cruz FRB (2005) Extension to the product partition model: computing the probability of a change. Comput Stat Data Anal 48:255–268

Müller P, Quintana FA, Rosner G (2011) A product partition model with regression on covariates. J Comput Graph Stat 20:260–278

Neal RM (2000) Markov Chain Sampling Methods for Dirichlet Process Mixture Models. J Comput Graph Stat 9:249–265

Quintana FA, Müller P, Papoila A (2015) cluster-specific variable selection for product partition models. Scandinavian J Stat to appear

Report, Pontificia Universidad Catolica de Chile, Department of Statistics, 2013

Quintana FA (2006) A predictive view of Bayesian clustering. J Stat Plann Inference 136(8):2407–2429

Quintana FA, Iglesias PL (2003) Bayesian clustering and product partition models. J R Stat Soc Ser B 65:557–574

Teh YW, Görür D, Ghahramani Z (2007) Stick-breaking construction for the Indian buffet process. In: Proceedings of the 11th conference on artificial intelligence and statistics, 2007

Thibaux R, Jordan M (2007) Hierarchical beta processes and the indian buffet process. In: Proceedings of the 11th conference on artificial intelligence and statistics (AISTAT), Puerto Rico, 2007

Xu Y, Müller P, Yuan Y, Gulukota K, Ji Y (2015) MAD Bayes for tumor – heterogeneity feature allocation with non-normal sampling. J Am Stat Ass (to appear)

Yao YC (1984) Estimation of a noisy discrete-time step function: Bayes and empirical Bayes approaches. Ann Stat 12:1434–1447

Chapter 9
Other Inference Problems and Conclusion

Abstract In this final chapter we briefly discuss some more specialized applications of nonparametric Bayesian inference, including the analysis of spatio-temporal data, model validation and causal inference. These themes are introduced to show by example the nature of the many application areas of nonparametric Bayesian inference that we did not include in earlier chapter.

We have discussed BNP approaches for some of the most common statistical inference problems, without any claim of an exhaustive discussion. We excluded several important problems, including, for example, inference for time-series data, spatio-temporal data, model validation, and causal inference. We briefly list some relevant references.

Spatio-Temporal Data Spatial data are measurements $\{Y(s_i) : i = 1, \ldots, n\}$ made at coordinates $s_1, \ldots, s_n \in \mathcal{D}$ for some set $\mathcal{D} \subset \mathbb{R}^d$. In *point-referenced data*, the coordinates may vary continuously over the fixed set $\mathcal{D}$. The case of *areal data* arises when $\mathcal{D}$ is partitioned into a finite number of smaller (areal) units. Finally, the case of *point-pattern data* follows when $\mathcal{D}$ is itself random (Banerjee et al. 2004). *Spatio-temporal data* includes additional indexing by time.

One of the earliest nonparametric models for spatial data appears in Gelfand et al. (2005). They considered replicated point-referenced data. Let $y = (Y(s_1), \ldots, Y(s_n))$ generically denote the complete responses for a given replicate, and let $y_1, \ldots, y_T$ denote the entire dataset. Assuming also the availability of a replicate-specific covariate vector x_t, their model assumes

$$y_t \mid \theta_t, \beta, \tau^2 \stackrel{ind}{\sim} \mathsf{N}(x_t'\beta + \theta_t, \tau^2 I), \quad \theta_t \mid G \stackrel{iid}{\sim} G, \quad G \sim \mathsf{DP}(M, G_0), \quad (9.1)$$

where G_0 is a zero-mean Gaussian process (compare Sect. 4.3.3) with covariance function $\sigma^2 H_\psi(\cdot, \cdot)$. The model is completed with conjugate hyper priors for β, τ^2, σ^2, and a gamma prior for M. Here H_ϕ is, for example, an exponential function of the form $H_\phi(s_j, s_i) = \exp(-\phi\|s_j - s_i\|)$, in which case ϕ is assigned a uniform prior on $(0, b_\phi]$.

Model (9.1) introduces spatial correlation through the random effects vectors θ_t, which are in turn assumed to originate from a DP model. This describes the sampling model as a countable location mixture of normals. Thus, given the collection of surfaces, any realization of the process selects a single sampled surface. Duan et al. (2007) extend the model to the generalized spatial DP which allows for different surface selection at different sites. The model involves a multivariate stick-breaking construction, where weights may be allowed to depend on spatial coordinates.

Reich and Fuentes (2007) introduced the spatial stick-breaking prior. The model introduces the spatial dependence in the construction of the weights. They use

$$Y(s) = \mu(s) + x(s)'\beta + \epsilon(s),$$

where $s = (s_1, s_2)$, $\mu(s) \sim F_s$ and F_s is a (potentially infinite) mixture of point masses with weights carrying the dependence on spatial coordinates s. Specifically, they considered $F_s(\cdot) = \sum_{i=1}^m p_i(s)\delta_{\theta_i}(\cdot)$ with a spatially varying stick breaking construction,

$$p_i(s) = V_i(s)\prod_{j<i}(1 - V_j(s)) \quad \text{with} \quad V_i(s) = w_i(s)V_i,$$

starting with $p_1(s) = V_1(s)$, and $\theta_i \stackrel{iid}{\sim} N(0, \tau^2)$, independent of the weights. Spatial dependence in the weights is introduced via the kernel functions $w_i(s)$. Here, $w_i(s)$ is centered at a knot $\psi_i = (\psi_{i1}, \psi_{i2})$ and the spread is controlled by a bandwidth parameter $\varepsilon_i = (\varepsilon_{i1}, \varepsilon_{i2})$. Reich and Fuentes (2007) considered several examples of kernel functions, for example, $w_i(s) = \prod_{j=1}^2 I(|s_j - \psi_{ji}| < \varepsilon_{ji}/2)$, with suitable hyper priors on ψ_i and ε_i. Another option is a square-exponential kernel of the form $w_i(s) = \prod_{j=1}^2 \exp(-(s_j - \psi_{ji})^2/\varepsilon_{ji}^2)$.

An alternative approach involving PPMs for disease mapping was developed by Hegarty and Barry (2008). Their goal is to identify areas of unusually high or low risk. The model involves a definition of cohesion functions for sets of areas. Cohesion of any subset S of areas is defined as $c(S) = \beta^{\ell(S)}$, where $\ell(S) = \sum_{A_i \in S} \ell_S(A_i)$ and $\ell_S(A_i)$ is the number of neighbors of A_i not in S. With this definition, they discourage maps with a large number of fragmented components. The model includes a Poisson-style likelihood function. See further details such as posterior simulation and applications in Hegarty and Barry (2008).

Model Comparison and Model Validation Many BNP priors can be naturally centered around a parametric model. This feature can be exploited to construct model validation of a parametric model by comparison with an encompassing non-parametric model. Carota et al. (1996) discuss the pitfalls of trying to implement such inference with a DP prior. Comparing $y_i \mid G \sim G$ and $G \sim \text{DP}(M, G_{0,\eta})$ versus an alternative parametric model $y_i \sim G_{0,\eta}$ fails. This is because the random probability measure G is a.s. discrete. The presence (or absence) of ties among the y_i would decide any model comparison. Berger and Guglielmi (2001) propose model validation of a parametric model by comparison with a BNP model based on a PT prior. The Bayes factor is evaluated using Eq. (3.5) (in Sect. 3.1.3). Alternatively the problems related to the discrete nature of the DP prior could be avoided by using model comparison with a DPM model. Basu and Chib (2003) discuss an elegant and computationally efficient strategy to evaluate the marginal probability under the DPM model, and thus the Bayes factor.

Besides using BNP models to validate a parametric model, a related problem is the comparison of alternative BNP models. Throughout the text we used log pseudo marginal likelihood (LPML) to compare competing models (Geisser and Eddy 1979), which only requires the evaluation of conditional predictive ordinates (CPO). Without loss of generality, assume that the model includes independent sampling conditional on some unknown parameters, $y_i \sim p(y_i \mid \boldsymbol{\theta})$, i.i.d., $i = 1, \ldots, n$, and let $\boldsymbol{y}_{-i} = (y_j, \ j \neq i)$. This is the case, for example, for DPM models (2.6). Then $\text{CPO}_i = p(y_i \mid \boldsymbol{y}_{-i}) = \int p(y_i \mid \boldsymbol{\theta}) \, dp(\boldsymbol{\theta} \mid \boldsymbol{y}_{-i})$ and $\text{LPML} = \sum_{i=1}^{n} \log(\text{CPO}_i)$.

An interesting use of BNP in model comparison arises in approaches for massive multiple comparisons. Guindani et al. (2009) use a DPM prior to interpret and generalize the optimal discovery procedure of Storey (2007).

Causal Inference A typical applications of causal inference is to clinical trials without randomization. Consider a stylized clinical study with two treatment arms, experimental therapy (E) versus control (C), a set of patient-specific baseline covariates (x_i), indicators $z_i \in \{C, E\}$ for treatment allocation and an outcome y_i. If treatment allocation is randomized then any difference in outcomes across the two treatment arms can be attributed to the treatment. Such randomized clinical trials are the gold standard of clinical research. However, in many cases such randomization is not possible. Inference that aims to compensate for the lack of randomization and report a causal treatment effect is known as causal inference. BNP methods have recently been proposed for such inference by Hill (2011) and Karabatsos and Walker (2012). Hill (2011) focused on modeling outcomes flexibly using Bayesian additive regression trees (BART). Karabatsos and Walker (2012) use a nonparametric mixture model with a stick-breaking prior for the probability of treatment assignment to provide a more accurately estimated propensity score in the inverse probability of treatment weighting (IPTW) method. Xu et al. (2013) use a DDP model to provide causal inference in dynamic treatment regimens by evaluating an average treatment effect as posterior inference on the difference of possible outcomes under competing treatments.

And we could continue the discussion with a long list of more applications of BNP methods to important, but perhaps also increasingly more specialized applications. In the selection of inference problems that we discussed at length earlier we tried to focus on generic and basic inference problems, recognizing that this categorization of BNP models does injustice to many important but more specialized applications. Many interesting applications appear in recent biostatistics literature. A good review of more sophisticated models for inference in biostatistics and bioinformatics appears in Dunson (2010).

Finally, the focus on data analysis problems lead us to not discuss any asymptotic properties of the proposed approaches. A major part of BNP research over the past years is concerned with such results. We refer interested readers to recent discussions in Ghosh and Ramamoorthi (2003), Phadia (2013) and the forthcoming book by Ghoshal and van der Vaart (2015).

References

Banerjee S, Carlin BP, Gelfand AE (2004) Hierarchical modeling and analysis for spatial data. Chapman & Hall/CRC, Boca Raton, FL
Basu S, Chib S (2003) Marginal likelihood and Bayes factors for Dirichlet process mixture models. J Am Stat Assoc 98:224–235
Berger J, Guglielmi A (2001) Bayesian testing of a parametric model versus nonparametric alternatives. J Am Stat Assoc 96:174–184
Carota C, Parmigiani G, Polson NG (1996) Diagnostic measures for model criticism. J Am Stat Assoc 91:753–762
Duan JA, Guindani M, Gelfand AE (2007) Generalized spatial Dirichlet process models. Biometrika 94:809–825
Dunson D (2010) Nonparametric Bayes applications to biostatistics. Cambridge University Press, Cambridge, pp 223–273
Geisser S, Eddy W (1979) A predictive approach to model selection. J Am Stat Assoc 74:153–160
Gelfand AE, Kottas A, MacEachern SN (2005) Bayesian nonparametric spatial modeling with Dirichlet process mixing. J Am Stat Assoc 100:1021–1035
Ghosh JK, Ramamoorthi RV (2003) Bayesian nonparametrics. Springer, New York
Ghoshal S, van der Vaart A (2015) Fundamentals of nonparametric Bayesian inference. Cambridge University Press, Cambridge
Guindani M, Müller P, Zhang S (2009) A Bayesian discovery procedure. J R Stat Soc. Ser B (Stat Methodol) 71(5):905–925
Hegarty A, Barry D (2008) Bayesian disease mapping using product partition models. Stat Med 27(19):3868–3893
Hill JL (2011) Bayesian nonparametric modeling for causal inference. J Comput Graph Stat 20(1):217–240
Karabatsos G, Walker SG (2012) A Bayesian nonparametric causal model. J Stat Plann Inference 142(4):925–934
Phadia EG (2013) Prior processes and their applications. Springer, Berlin
Reich BJ, Fuentes M (2007) A multivariate semiparametric Bayesian spatial modeling framework for hurricane surface wind fields. Ann Appl Stat 1(1):249–264
Storey JD (2007) The optimal discovery procedure: a new approach to simultaneous significance testing. J R Stat Soc Ser B (Stat Methodol) 69(3):347–368
Xu Y, Müller P, Wahed AS, Thall PF (2013) Bayesian nonparametric estimation for dynamic treatment regimes with sequential transition times. ArXiv e-prints 1405.2656

Appendix A
DPpackage

While BNP models are extremely powerful and have a wide range of applicability, they are not as widely used as one might expect. One reason for this has been the gap between the type of software that many users would like to have for fitting models and the software that is currently available. The most general programs currently available for Bayesian inference are BUGS (see, e.g., Gilks et al. 1994), OpenBugs (Thomas et al. 2006), and JAGS (Plummer 2003). BUGS can be accessed from the publicly available R program (R Development Core Team 2014), using the R2WinBUGS package (Strurtz et al. 2005). OpenBugs can run on Windows and Linux, as well as from inside R. JAGS can also run on Windows and Linux, and from R using the rjags package. In addition, various R packages exist that directly fit particular Bayesian models. We refer to Appendix C in Carlin and Louis (2008), for an extensive list of software for Bayesian modeling. Although the number of fully Bayesian programs continues to burgeon, with many available at little or no cost, they generally do not include semiparametric models. Two exceptions to this rule are the R package bayesm (Rossi et al. 2005; Rossi and McCulloch 2008), including functions for some models based on DP priors (Ferguson 1973), and the Bayesian regression software by Karabatsos (2014), which includes a wide variety of BNP regression problems in a menu-driven package. However, the range of different BNP models is huge. It is practically impossible to build flexible and efficient software for the full generality of such models.

Here we provide a brief introduction to a publicly available R package that is designed to bridge the previously mentioned gap, the DPpackage, originally presented in Jara (2007) and Jara et al. (2011). Although the name of the package is due to the DP, the package now includes many other priors on function spaces. Currently, DPpackage includes models based on the DP (Sect. 2.1), mixtures of DP (MDP, Sect. 2.2) DPM models (DPM, Sect. 2.2), linear dependent DP (LDDP, Sect. 4.4.2), linear dependent Poisson-Dirichlet processes (LDPD, Jara et al. 2010), weight dependent DP (WDDP, Sect. 4.4.4), finite mixture of DPM of normals (HDPM, Sect. 7.3.1), centrally standardized DP (CSDP, Sect. 5.2.1), PTs (Sect. 3.1),

© Springer International Publishing Switzerland 2015
P. Mueller et al., *Bayesian Nonparametric Data Analysis*, Springer Series in Statistics, DOI 10.1007/978-3-319-18968-0

mixtures of PTs (MPT, Sect. 3.2.1), mixtures of triangular distributions (Perron and Mengersen 2001), random Bernstein polynomials (Petrone 1999a,b; Petrone and Wasserman 2002) and dependent Bernstein polynomials (Barrientos et al. 2011). The package also includes models based on penalized B-splines (Sect. 4.3.2). The package is available from the Comprehensive R Archive Network at http://CRAN. R-project.org/package=DPpackage.

A.1 Overview

The design philosophy behind DPpackage is quite different from most comparable general purpose languages. The most important design goal has been the implementation of model-specific MCMC algorithms. A direct benefit of this approach is that the sampling algorithms can be made dramatically more efficient than in a general purpose function based on black-box algorithms.

Fitting a model in DPpackage begins with a call to an R function, for instance, DPmodel, or PTmodel. Here "model" is a descriptive name for the model being fitted, for example DPcdensity. Typically, the model function will take a number of arguments that control the MCMC sampling strategy. In addition, the model(s) formula(s), data, and prior parameters are passed to the model function as arguments. The common arguments in every model function are listed next.

(i) prior: A list with values for the prior hyper-parameters.
(ii) mcmc: A list which must include the integers nburn giving the number of initial burn-in scans, nskip giving the thinning interval, nsave giving the total number of scans to be saved, and ndisplay giving the number of saved scans to be displayed on the screen, that is, the function reports on the screen when every ndisplay iterations have been carried out and returns the process runtime in seconds. For some specific models, one or more tuning parameters for Metropolis steps may be needed and must be included in this list. The names of these tuning parameters are explained in each specific model description in the associated help files.
(iii) state: An object list giving the current value of the parameters, when the analysis is the continuation of a previous MCMC simulation, or giving the starting values for a new Markov chain. The latter is useful to run multiple chains starting from different points.
(iv) status: A logical variable indicating whether it is a new run (TRUE) or the continuation of a previous analysis (FALSE). In the latter case, the current value of the parameters must be specified in the object state.

Inside the R function the inputs are organized in a more useable form, MCMC simulation is implemented in a shared library that is written in a compiled language, and the posterior Monte Carlo sample is summarized, labeled, assigned into an output list, and returned. The output list includes,

(i) `state`: A list containing the current value of the parameters.
(ii) `save.state`: An object list containing the MCMC samples for the parameters. This list contains two matrices `randsave` and `thetasave`, which contain the MCMC samples of the variables with random distribution (errors, random effects, etc.) and the parametric part of the model, respectively.

As an example of the extraction of the output elements, consider the generic model fit:

```
fit <- DPmodel(..., prior, mcmc, state, status, ....)
```

The lists can be extracted using the following code:

```
fit$state
fit$save.state$randsave
fit$save.state$thetasave
```

Based on these output objects, it is possible to use, for instance, the boa (Smith 2007) or the coda (Plummer et al. 2009) R packages to evaluate convergence diagnostics. For illustration, we consider the coda package here. It requires a matrix of posterior draws for relevant parameters to be saved as a mcmc object. Assume that we have obtained fit1, fit2, and fit3, by running a model function three times, specifying different starting values for each run. To compute the Gelman-Rubin convergence diagnostic statistic for the first parameter stored in the thetasave object, the following commands may be used:

```
library("coda")
coda.obj <- mcmc.list(
   chain1 = mcmc(fit1$save.state$thetasave[,1]),
   chain2 = mcmc(fit2$save.state$thetasave[,1]),
   chain3 = mcmc(fit3$save.state$thetasave[,1]))
gelman.diag(coda.obj, transform = TRUE)
```

The second command line saves the results as a mcmc.list object class and the third command line computes the Gelman-Rubin statistic from these three chains.

Generic R functions such as print, plot, summary and anova have methods to display the results of a DPpackage model fit. The function print displays the posterior means of the hyper-parameters in the model, and summary displays posterior summary statistics (mean, median, standard deviation, naive standard errors, and credibility intervals). By default, the function summary computes the 95 % highest posterior density (HPD) intervals using the Monte Carlo method proposed by Chen and Shao (1999). Alternatively the user can display the order statistic estimator of the 95 % credible interval by using the following code:

```
summary(fit, hpd = FALSE)
```

The plot function displays the trace plots and a kernel-based estimate of the posterior distribution for the parameters of the model. Similarly to summary, the plot function displays the 95 % HPD regions in the density plot and the posterior mean. The same plot but considering the 95 % credible region can be obtained by using the following code:

```
plot(fit, hpd = FALSE)
```

The anova function computes simultaneous credible regions for a vector of parameters from the MCMC sample using the method described by Besag et al. (1995). The output of the anova function is an anova-like table containing the pseudo-contour probabilities for each of the factors included in the linear part of the model.

A.2 An Example

We show how model fitting functions in DPpackage are implemented in the context of density regression. Conditional density estimation (Sect. 4.4.4) is the fully nonparametric version of traditional regression problems for data $\{(x_i, y_i)\}_{i=1}^n$, where $x_i \in \mathcal{X} \subset \mathbb{R}^p$ is a set of predictors, and $y_i \in \mathbb{R}$ is the response variable. Rather than assuming a functional form for the mean function and/or a common error distribution the problem is cast as inference for a family of conditional distributions

$$\{G_x : x \in \mathcal{X} \subset \mathbb{R}^p\},$$

where $y_i \mid x_i \overset{ind.}{\sim} G_{x_i}$. The current version of DPpackage considers several BNP models for related random probability distributions including particular implementations of the DDP model proposed in MacEachern (1999, 2000), a natural generalization of the approach discussed by Müller et al. (1996) for nonparametric regression to the context of conditional density estimation. In this section we show how to perform conditional density estimation using BNP models for related probability distributions, also referred to as Bayesian density regression, using the DPcdensity and LDDPdensity functions. See the discussion in Sects. 4.4.4 and 4.4.2, Eq. (4.12) for a discussion of the models. We briefly review these models below.

A.2.1 The Models

The LDDP Model In Sects. 4.4.1 and 4.4.2 we reviewed the DDP model as an approach to define a prior model for an uncountable set of random measures indexed by a single continuous covariate, say x, $\{G_x : x \in \mathcal{X} \subset \mathbb{R}\}$. We will use the version of the model defined in (4.12) as the linear dependent DP (LDDP). We augment β_h to (β_h, σ_h), to include the kernel variance in the mixture of (4.12). Inference in

A.2 An Example

this model is implemented in the `LDDPdensity` function. In summary, we fit the following model to the regression data $(y_i, \boldsymbol{x}_i)$, $i = 1, \ldots, n$:

$$y_i \mid G \stackrel{ind.}{\sim} \int \mathsf{N}\left(y_i \mid \boldsymbol{x}_i' \boldsymbol{\beta}, \sigma^2\right) dG(\boldsymbol{\beta}, \sigma^2),$$

and $G \mid \alpha, G_0 \sim DP(\alpha G_0)$, where $G_0 \equiv \mathsf{N}(\boldsymbol{\beta} \mid \boldsymbol{\mu}_b, \boldsymbol{S}_b) \, \mathsf{Ga}\left(\sigma^{-2} \mid \tau_1/2, \tau_2/2\right)$. The LDDP model specification is completed with the following hyper-priors:

$$\alpha \mid a_0, b_0 \sim \mathsf{Ga}(a_0, b_0), \quad \tau_2 \mid \tau_{s_1}, \tau_{s_2} \sim \mathsf{Ga}(\tau_{s_1}/2, \tau_{s_2}/2),$$
$$\boldsymbol{\mu}_b \mid \boldsymbol{m}_0, \boldsymbol{S}_0 \sim \mathsf{N}(\boldsymbol{m}_0, \boldsymbol{S}_0) \quad \text{and} \quad \boldsymbol{S}_b \mid \nu, \boldsymbol{\Psi} \sim \mathsf{IWis}(\nu, \boldsymbol{\Psi}).$$

The WDDP Model Alternatively we will implement conditional regression as in Sect. 4.4.4. Let $\boldsymbol{x}_i$ denote a p-dimensional vector of continuous predictors. We fit a DPM of multivariate Gaussian distributions to an augmented response vector $\tilde{\boldsymbol{y}}_i = (y_i, \boldsymbol{x}_i)'$, $i = 1, \ldots, n$. The implied conditional distribution (4.14) takes the form

$$f_z(y_i) = \sum_{l=1}^{\infty} \omega_l(\boldsymbol{x}_i) \mathsf{N}(y_i \mid \beta_{0l} + \boldsymbol{x}_i' \boldsymbol{\beta}_l, \sigma_l^2). \tag{A.1}$$

This is (4.14) under a DPM model for $\tilde{\boldsymbol{y}}$ before marginalizing w.r.t. G. Recall from Sect. 4.4.4 that we refer to this model as weight dependent Dirichlet process (WDDP). A similar density regression is proposed in Dunson et al. (2007).

Inference under the WDDP is implemented in the `DPpackage` function `DPcdensity`. In summary, the model is

$$\tilde{\boldsymbol{y}}_i \mid G \stackrel{iid}{\sim} \int \mathsf{N}(\tilde{\boldsymbol{y}}_i \mid \boldsymbol{\mu}, \boldsymbol{\Sigma}) dG(\boldsymbol{\mu}, \boldsymbol{\Sigma}), \quad \text{and} \quad G \mid \alpha, G_0 \sim DP(\alpha G_0). \tag{A.2}$$

The baseline distribution G_0 is the conjugate normal-inverted-Wishart (IW) distribution $G_0 \equiv \mathsf{N}\left(\boldsymbol{\mu} \mid \boldsymbol{m}_1, \kappa_0^{-1} \boldsymbol{\Sigma}\right) \mathsf{IWis}(\boldsymbol{\Sigma} \mid \nu_1, \boldsymbol{\Psi}_1)$. The model is completed with the hyper-priors $\alpha \mid a_0, b_0 \sim \mathsf{Ga}(a_0, b_0)$, $\boldsymbol{m}_1 \mid \boldsymbol{m}_2, \boldsymbol{S}_2 \sim \mathsf{N}(\boldsymbol{m}_2, \boldsymbol{S}_2)$, $\kappa_0 \mid \tau_1, \tau_2 \sim \mathsf{Ga}(\tau_1/2, \tau_2/2)$, and $\boldsymbol{\Psi}_1 \mid \nu_2, \boldsymbol{\Psi}_2 \sim \mathsf{IWis}(\nu_2, \boldsymbol{\Psi}_2)$. The model implies a weight dependent mixture model, as in expression (A.1), with

$$\omega_l(z) = \frac{\omega_l \mathsf{N}(z \mid \boldsymbol{\mu}_{2l}, \boldsymbol{\Sigma}_{22l})}{\sum_{j=1}^{\infty} \omega_j \mathsf{N}(z \mid \boldsymbol{\mu}_{2j}, \boldsymbol{\Sigma}_{22j})}, \quad \beta_{0l} = \mu_{1l} - \boldsymbol{\Sigma}_{12l} \boldsymbol{\Sigma}_{22l}^{-1} \boldsymbol{\mu}_{2l}, \quad \boldsymbol{\beta}_l = \boldsymbol{\Sigma}_{12l} \boldsymbol{\Sigma}_{22l}^{-1},$$

and

$$\sigma_l^2 = \sigma_{11l}^2 - \boldsymbol{\Sigma}_{12l} \boldsymbol{\Sigma}_{22l}^{-1} \boldsymbol{\Sigma}_{21l},$$

where the weights ω_l follow a DP stick-breaking construction and the remaining elements arise from the standard partition of the vectors of means and (co)variance matrices given by

$$\boldsymbol{\mu}_l = \begin{pmatrix} \mu_{1l} \\ \mu_{2l} \end{pmatrix} \text{ and } \boldsymbol{\Sigma}_l = \begin{pmatrix} \sigma^2_{11l} & \boldsymbol{\Sigma}_{12l} \\ \boldsymbol{\Sigma}_{21l} & \boldsymbol{\Sigma}_{22l} \end{pmatrix},$$

respectively.

The DPcdensity function fits a marginalized version of the model, where the random probability measure G is integrated out. Full inference on the conditional density at covariate level z is obtained by using the ϵ-DP approximation proposed by Muliere and Tardella (1998), with $\epsilon = 0.01$.

A.2.2 Example 29: Simulated Data

Data We replicate the results reported by Dunson et al. (2007), where a different approach is proposed. Following Dunson et al. (2007), we simulate $n = 500$ observations from a mixture of two normal linear regression models, with the mixture weights depending on the predictor, different error variances and a non-linear mean function for the second component,

$$y_i \mid x_i \overset{ind.}{\sim} \exp\{-2x_i\}N(y_i|x_i, 0.01) + (1 - \exp\{-2x_i\})\, N(y_i|x_i^4, 0.04), \quad i = 1, \ldots, n.$$

The predictor values x_i are simulated from a uniform distribution, $x_i \overset{iid}{\sim} U(0,1)$. The following code is useful to plot the true conditional densities and the mean function:

```
R> dtrue <- function(grid, x) {
+     exp(-2 * x) * dnorm(grid, mean = x, sd = sqrt(0.01)) +
+     (1 - exp(-2 * x)) * dnorm(grid, mean = x^4, sd = sqrt(0.04))
+ }
R> mtrue <- function(x) exp(-2 * x) * x + (1 - exp(-2 * x)) * x^4
```

The data were simulated using the following code:

```
R> set.seed(0)
R> nrec <- 500
R> x <- runif(nrec)
R> y1 <- x + rnorm(nrec, 0, sqrt(0.01))
R> y2 <- x^4 + rnorm(nrec, 0, sqrt(0.04))
R> u <- runif(nrec)
R> prob <- exp(-2 * x)
R> y <- ifelse(u < prob, y1, y2)
```

Fit Using DPcdensity Inference under model (A.2) is implemented in the DPpackage function DPcdensity. We fit the model using the hyper-parameters $a_0 = 10$, $b_0 = 1$, $\nu_1 = \nu_2 = 4$, $\boldsymbol{m}_2 = (\bar{y}, \bar{x})'$, $\tau_1 = 6.01$, $\tau_2 = 3.01$ and

A.2 An Example

$S_2 = \Psi_2^{-1} = 0.5S$, where S is the sample covariance matrix for the response and predictor. The following code illustrates how the hyper-parameters are specified:

```
R> w <- cbind(y, x)
R> wbar <- apply(w, 2, mean)
R> wcov <- var(w)
R> prior <- list(a0 = 10, b0 = 1, nu1 = 4, nu2 = 4, s2 = 0.5 * wcov,
+      m2 = wbar, psiinv2 = 2 * solve(wcov), tau1 = 6.01, tau2 = 3.01)
```

A total number of 25,000 scans of the Markov chain cycle implemented in the DPcdensity function were completed. A burn-in period of 5000 samples was discarded and the chain was then subsampled at every fourth iterate to get a final Monte Carlo sample size of 5000. The following code implements this MCMC specification:

```
R> mcmc <- list(nburn = 5000, nsave = 5000, nskip = 3, ndisplay = 1000)
```

The following commands were used to fit the model, where the conditional density estimates were evaluated on a grid of 100 points on the range of the response:

```
R> fitWDDP <- DPcdensity(y = y, x = x, xpred = seq(0, 1, 0.02),
+      ngrid = 100, compute.band = TRUE, type.band = "HPD",
+      prior = prior, mcmc = mcmc, state = NULL, status = TRUE)
```

Fit Using LDDPdensity Using the same MCMC specification, we also fitted the LDDP model to the same data. We used the function LDDPdensity to fit a mixture of B-splines models with $x'\beta = \beta_0 + \sum_{j=1}^{6} \psi_j(x)\beta_j$, where $\psi_k(x)$ corresponds to the kth B-spline basis function evaluated at x, as implemented in the bs function of the splines R package. The LDDP model was fitted using Zellner's g-prior (Zellner 1983), with $g = 10^3$. The following values for the hyper-parameters were considered: $a_0 = 10$, $b_0 = 1$, $m_0 = (X'X)^{-1} X'y$, $S_0 = g(X'X)^{-1}$, $\tau_1 = 6.01$, $\tau_{s1} = 6.01$, $\tau_{s2} = 2.01$, $\nu = 9$, and $\Psi^{-1} = S_0$. The following code shows the prior specification:

```
R> library("splines")
R> W <- cbind(rep(1, nrec), bs(x, df = 6, Boundary.knots = c(0, 1)))
R> S0 <- 1000 * solve(t(W) %*% W)
R> m0 <- solve(t(W) %*% W) %*% t(W) %*% y
R> prior <- list(a0 = 10, b0 = 1, m0 = m0, S0 = S0, tau1 = 6.01,
+      taus1 = 6.01, taus2 = 2.01, nu = 9, psiinv = solve(S0))
```

The following commands were used to fit the model, where the conditional density estimates were evaluated on a grid of 100 points on the range of the response,

```
R> xpred <- seq(0, 1, 0.02)
R> Wpred <- cbind(rep(1, length(xpred)),
+      predict(bs(x, df = 6, Boundary.knots = c(0, 1)), xpred))
R> fitLDDP <- LDDPdensity(formula = y ~ W - 1, zpred = Wpred, ngrid = 100,
+      compute.band = TRUE, type.band = "HPD", prior = prior, mcmc = mcmc,
+      state = NULL, status = TRUE)
```

Results Figures A.1 and A.2 show the true density, the estimated density and pointwise 95 % HPD intervals for a range of values of the predictor for the WDDP and LDDP model, respectively. The estimates correspond approximately to the true densities in each case. The figures also display the plot of the data along with the estimated mean function, which is very close to the true one under both models.

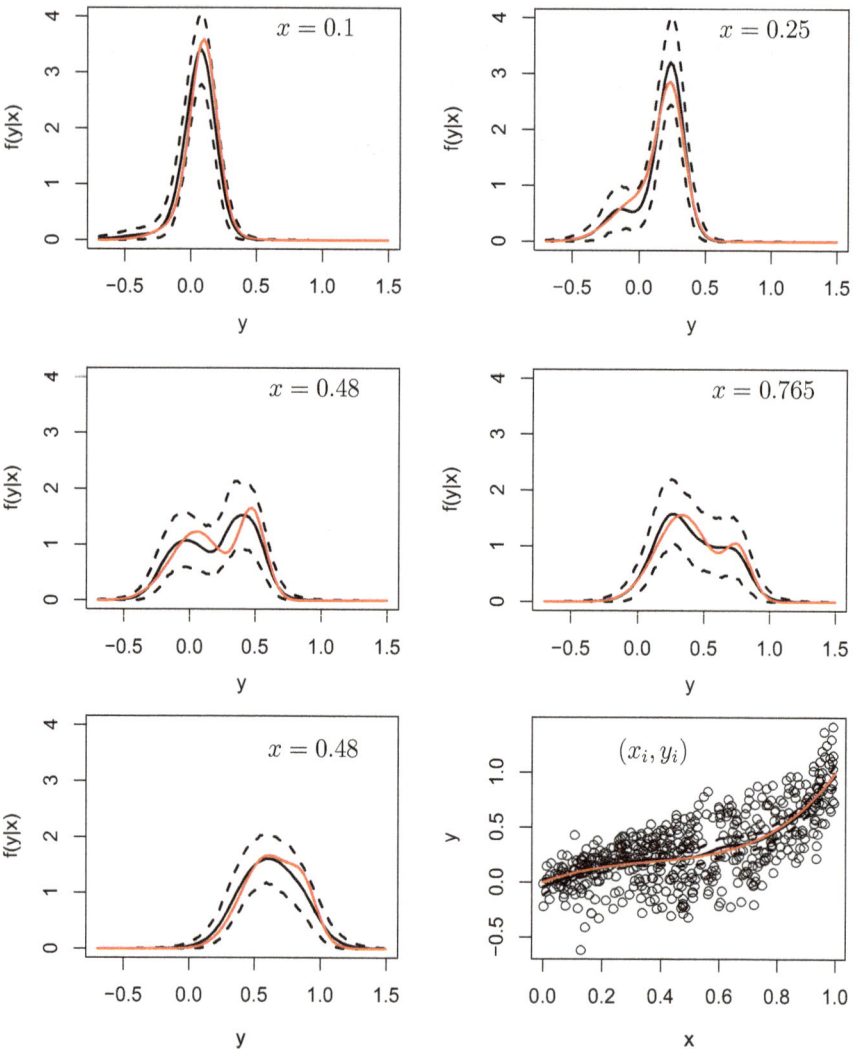

Fig. A.1 Example 29. WDDP model: True conditional densities of $y \mid x$ (*in red*), posterior mean estimates (*black continuous line*) and pointwise 95 % HPD intervals (*black dashed lines*) for x as indicated in the first five panels. The last panel shows the data, along with the true and estimated mean regression curves

A.2 An Example

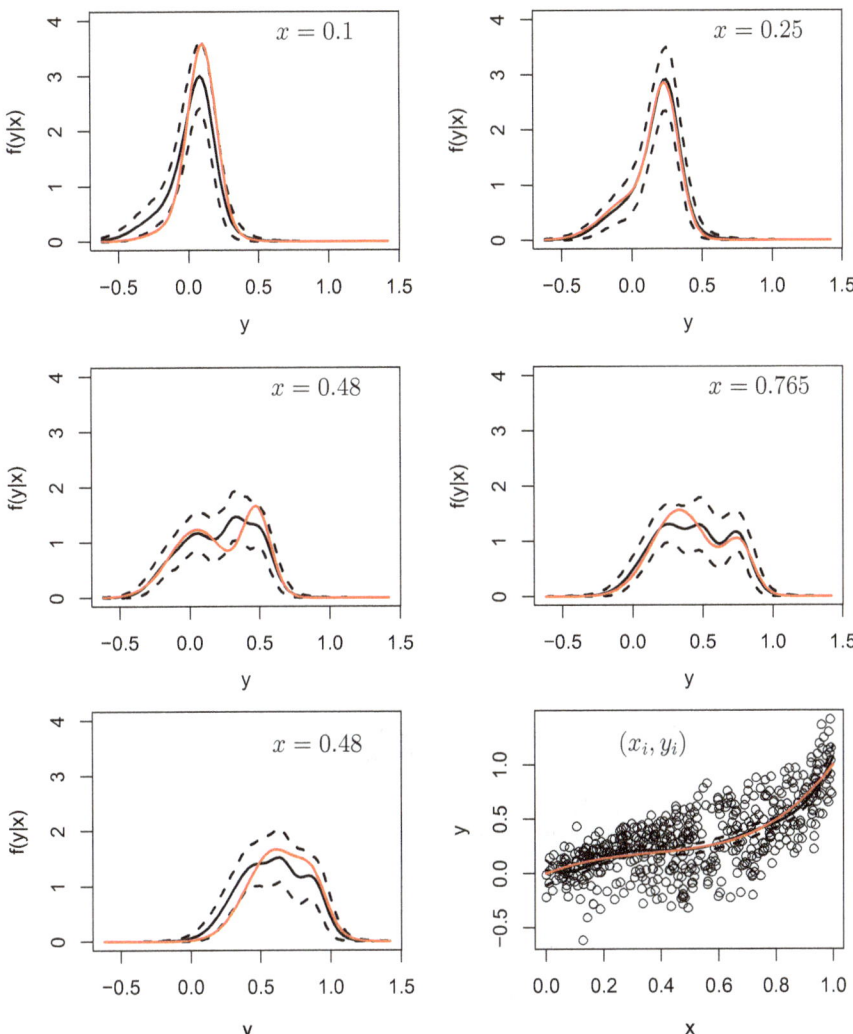

Fig. A.2 Example 29. LDDP model: True conditional densities of $y \mid x$ (*in red*), posterior mean estimates (*black continuous line*) and pointwise 95 % HPD intervals (*black dashed lines*) for x as indicated in the first five panels. The last panel shows the data, along with the true and estimated mean regression curves

In both functions, the posterior mean estimates and the limits of pointwise 95 % HPD intervals for the conditional density for each value of the predictors are stored in the model objects densp.m, and densp.l and densp.h, respectively. The following code illustrates how these objects can be used in order to get the posterior estimates for $x = 0.1$ in the LDDP model. This code was used to draw the plots displayed in Figs. A.1 and A.2.

```
R> par(cex = 1.5, mar = c(4.1, 4.1, 1, 1))
R> plot(fitLDDP$grid, fitLDDP$densp.h[6,], lwd = 3, type = "l", lty = 2,
+    main = "", xlab = "y", ylab = "f(y|x)", ylim = c(0, 4))
R> lines(fitLDDP$grid, fitLDDP$densp.l[6,], lwd = 3, type = "l", lty = 2)
R> lines(fitLDDP$grid, fitLDDP$densp.m[6,], lwd = 3, type = "l", lty = 1)
R> lines(fitLDDP$grid, dtrue(fitLDDP$grid, xpred[6]), lwd = 3,
+    type = "l", lty = 1, col = "red")
```

Finally, both functions return the posterior mean estimates and the limits of pointwise 95 % HPD intervals for the mean function in the model objects meanfp.m, and meanfp.l and meanfp.h, respectively. The following code was used to obtain the estimated mean function under the LDDP model, along with the true function.

```
R> par(cex = 1.5, mar = c(4.1, 4.1, 1, 1))
R> plot(x, y, xlab = "x", ylab = "y", main = "")
R> lines(xpred, fitLDDP$meanfp.m, type = "l", lwd = 3, lty = 1)
R> lines(xpred, fitLDDP$meanfp.l, type = "l", lwd = 3, lty = 2)
R> lines(xpred, fitLDDP$meanfp.h, type = "l", lwd = 3, lty = 2)
R> lines(xpred, mtrue(xpred), col = "red", lwd = 3)
```

References

Barrientos F, Jara A, Quintana FA (2011) Dependent Bernstein polynomials for bounded density regression. Techical Report, Department of Statistics, Pontificia Universidad Católica de Chile

Besag J, Green P, Higdon D, Mengersen K (1995) Bayesian computation and stochastic systems (with discussion). Stat Sci 10:3–66

Carlin BP, Louis TA (2008) Bayesian methods for data analysis, 3rd edn. Chapman and Hall/CRC, New York

Chen MH, Shao QM (1999) Monte Carlo estimation of Bayesian credible and HPD intervals. J Comput Graph Stat 8(1):69–92

Dunson DB, Pillai N, Park JH (2007) Bayesian density regression. J R Stat Soc B 69:163–183

Ferguson TS (1973) A Bayesian analysis of some nonparametric problems. Ann Stat 1:209–230

Gilks WR, Thomas A, Spiegelhalter DJ (1994) A language and program for complex Bayesian modelling. Statistician 43:169–178

Jara A (2007) Applied Bayesian non- and semi-parametric inference using DPpackage. Rnews 7:17–26

Jara A, Lesaffre E, De Iorio M, Quintana FA (2010) Bayesian semiparametric inference for multivariate doubly-interval-censored data. Ann Appl Stat 4:2126–2149

Jara A, Hanson TE, Quintana FA, Müller P, Rosner GL (2011) DPpackage: Bayesian semi- and nonparametric modeling in R. J Stat Softw 40(5):1–30

Karabatsos G (2014) Software user's manual for Bayesian regression: nonparametric and parametric models. Techical Report, University of Illinois-Chicago. http://www.uic.edu/~georgek/HomePage/BayesSoftware.html

MacEachern S (1999) Dependent nonparametric processes. In: ASA proceedings of the section on Bayesian statistical science. American Statistical Association, Alexandria

MacEachern SN (2000) Dependent Dirichlet processes. Techical Report, Department of Statistics, The Ohio State University

Muliere P, Tardella L (1998) Approximating distributions of random functionals of Ferguson-Dirichlet priors. Can J Stat 26:283–297

Müller P, Erkanli A, West M (1996) Bayesian curve fitting using multivariate normal mixtures. Biometrika 83:67–79

Perron F, Mengersen K (2001) Bayesian nonparametric modeling using mixtures of triangular distributions. Biometrics 57:518–528

Petrone S (1999a) Bayesian density estimation using Bernstein polynomials. Can J Stat 27:105–126

Petrone S (1999b) Random bernstein polynomials. Scand J Stat 26:373–393

Petrone S, Wasserman L (2002) Consistency of Bernstein polynomial posterior. J R Stat Soc B 64:79–100

Plummer M (2003) JAGS: A program for analysis of Bayesian graphical models using Gibbs sampling. In: Proceedings of the 3rd international workshop on distributed statistical computing (DSC 2003)

Plummer M, Best N, Cowles K, Vines K (2009) CODA: output analysis and diagnostics for MCMC. R package version 0.13-4

R Development Core Team (2014) R: A language and environment for statistical computing. R Foundation for Statistical Computing, Vienna. http://www.R-project.org. ISBN 3-900051-07-0

Rossi P, McCulloch R (2008) Bayesm: Bayesian inference for marketing/micro-econometrics. http://faculty.chicagogsb.edu/peter.rossi/research/bsm.html. R package version 2.2-2

Rossi P, Allenby G, McCulloch R (2005) Bayesian statistics and marketing. Wiley, New York

Smith BJ (2007) Boa: An r package for mcmc output convergence assessment and posterior inference. J Stat Softw 21:1–37

Strurtz S, Ligges U, Gelman A (2005) R2WinBUGS: a package for running WinBUGS from R. J Stat Softw 12:1–16

Thomas A, O'Hara B, Ligges U, Sibylle S (2006) Making BUGS open. Rnews 6:12–17

Zellner A (1983) Applications of Bayesian analysis in econometrics. Statistician 32:23–34

List of Examples

Some examples appear in multiple places when we use the same data to illustrate different methods. Below is a list of all examples, with the section numbers.

1. Density estimation: Chap. 1
2. Oral cancer: Chap. 1, Sects. 6.1, 6.2.1, 6.2.2, 6.2.3
3. T-cell receptors: Sects. 2.1.2, 2.2
4. Gene expression: Sects. 2.2, 3.1.3
5. Old Faithful geyser: Sects. 4.2, 4.3.1, 4.3.2, 4.3.3, 4.4.1, 4.4.2, 4.4.3
6. Doppler function: Sect. 4.3.1
7. Nitrogen oxide: Sect. 4.3.2
8. Breast cancer: Sects. 4.4.1, 6.4
9. Baseball: Sect. 5.1.1
10. Jane Austen: Sect. 5.1.2
11. Teacher evaluation: Sect. 5.1.3
12. Unemployment data: Sects. 5.2.1, 5.2.2
13. Epilepsy trial: Sect. 5.2.3
14. Mexican DWI Sect. 5.2.4
15. Sperm deformity: Sect. 5.3
16. Columbian children mortality: Sect. 6.3.2

17. Breast retraction: Sect. 6.4
18. Lung cancer: Sect. 6.4.
19. Mammogram usage: Sect. 7.1
20. Population PD—CALGB 8881: Sect. 7.2
21. Two related studies—CALGB 8881 and 9160: Sect. 7.3.1
22. Multiple studies—CALGB 8881, 9160 and 8541: Sect. 7.3.2
23. Pregnancies: Sect. 7.3.3
24. Sarcoma: Sects. 8.2, 8.3
25. ICU readmission: Sect. 8.4.2
26. Concha y Toro: Sect. 8.4.3
27. Tumor heterogeneity: Sect. 8.5.2
28. RPPA data: Sect. 8.6
29. Simulated data: Appendix

Index

accelerated failure time (AFT) model, **107**, 109
    ANOVA DDP, 111
    Dirichlet process, 52
    LDTF process, 114
accelerated hazards (AH) model, 109
additive hazards model, 109
additive model, 61
    generalized, 90
AFT. *See* accelerated failure time (AFT) model
AH. *See* accelerated hazards (AH) model
asymptotic properties, 178

BART. *See* Bayesian additive regression tree (BART)
Bayes factor, 81
Bayesian additive regression tree (BART), **64**, 177
bayesm, 179
bayesSurv
    bayessurvreg2, 107
BayesX, 61, 90, 105, 110
beta process, 103
binomial response, 77
BNPdensity, 49
boa, 181
B-spline, 4, **60**, 61, 106, 107, 180, 185
BUGS, 179
    R2WinBUGS, 179

CART. *See* classification and regression tree (CART)
catdata, 88

categorical response, 80
    regression, 86
causal inference, 177
centrally standardized Dirichlet process (CSDP), 87, 88, 91
classification, 96, 138
classification and regression tree (CART), 63
clustering. *See* partition
    model based (*see* model based clustering)
coda, 181
cohesion function, 150
    uniform, 153
completely random measure (CRM), 48
conditional regression, 72, 183
contingency table, 80, 83
cosine expansion, 59
covariance function, 62, 175
CRM. *See* completely random measure (CRM)
CSDP. *See* centrally standardized Dirichlet process (CSDP)

DDP. *See* dependent Dirichlet process (DDP)
density regression. *See* conditional regression
dependent Dirichlet process (DDP), **65**, 136, 177
    ANOVA, **67**, 67, 70, 136
    linear, 185
    posterior simulation, 67
dependent increments models, 103
Dirichlet-multinomial process, 27
Dirichlet process (DP), **8**, 27, 34, 48, 65, 78, 127, 177, 180
    centrally standardized, **87**, 91, 180

© Springer International Publishing Switzerland 2015
P. Mueller et al., *Bayesian Nonparametric Data Analysis*, Springer Series in Statistics, DOI 10.1007/978-3-319-18968-0

enriched, 141
ϵ-, 184
finite (*see* finite Dirichlet process)
generalized (*see* generalized Dirichlet process)
hierarchical, 140
linear dependent (*see* linear dependent Dirichlet process)
marginal distribution, 11
mean, 93
mixture of, 15
nested, 140
partition, 15, **148**, 152
posterior updating, 9
weight dependent, 73, 183
Dirichlet process mixture (DPM), **12**, 72, 78, 84, 98, 127, 180, 183
ANOVA, 70
clustering, **15**
finite mixture of (*see* finite mixture of DPM)
hierarchical (*see* hierarchical DPM)
posterior distribution, 12
posterior simulation, **18**, 20–22
discrete wavelet transform, 55
DP. *See* Dirichlet process (DP)
DPM. *See* Dirichlet process mixture (DPM)
DPpackage
CSDPbinary, 88
DPcdensity, 73, 183, 184
DPdensity, 46
DPglmm, 94
DProc, 98
FPTFbinary, 91
gam, 90
HDPMdensity, 134
LDDP, 68, 137
LDDPdensity, 99, 183, 185
LDDProc, 99
LDDPsurvival, 111, 114
LDTFPdensity, 70
LDTFPglmm, 129
LDTFPsurvival, 114
PSgam, 61
PTdensity, 40
PTglmm, 127

feature allocation, 145, **164**
finite Dirichlet process, **25**, 53
posterior simulation, 26
finite mixture of DPM, 180
finite mixture of random probability measures, 132

finite Polya tree (FPT), 41
posterior simulation, 42, 45
FPT. *See* finite Polya tree (FPT)
frailty, 109
functional mixed effects model, 58

gamma process, 70
Gaussian process, **62**, 65, 66, 175
generalized additive models, 63
treed, 63
generalized Dirichlet process, 28
generalized linear mixed model (GLMM), 92, 127
generalized linear model (GLM), 86
semiparametric, 87
GLM. *See* generalized linear model (GLM)
GLMM. *See* generalized linear mixed model (GLMM)
GP. *See* Gaussian process (GP)

hazard rate, 3
time-dependent covariates, 109
time-dependent regression, 109
HDPM. *See* hierarchical Dirichlet process mixture (HDPM)
hierarchical DPM, 134
homogeneity test, 80

IBP. *See* Indian buffet process (IBP)
Indian buffet process, 165

JAGS, 179
rjags, 179

k-means, 169

LDDP. *See* linear dependent Dirichlet process (LDDP)
LDTFP. *See* linear dependent tail-free process (LDTFP)
linear dependent Dirichlet process (LDDP), **68**, 99, 111, 114, 180, 183
linear dependent Poisson-Dirichlet, 180
linear dependent tail-free process (LDTFP), 70, **113**, 114, 127
locally weighted linear regression, 72
log pseudo marginal likelihood (LPML), 95, 108, 115, 149, **177**
LPML. *See* log pseudo marginal likelihood (LPML)

MAD Bayes. *See* MAP-based asymptotic derivation
MAP-based asymptotic derivation, 169
matrix stick breaking process, 141
mixed effects model, 126
mixture of beta, 90
mixture of Polya tree (MPT), **39**, 52, 98, 101, 108, 109, 180
  multivariate, 127
model based clustering, 148
model comparison, 176
model validation, 176
MPT. *See* mixture of Polya tree (MPT)

neural network, 58
neutral to the right (NTR), 102
nonparametric regression
  basis expansion, 54
  B-spline, 69
  Dirichlet process mixture, 52
  Dirichlet process residuals, 52
  Polya tree residuals, 52
normalized generalized gamma process, 48
normalized generalized Gaussian process, 49
normalized inverse Gaussian, 48
Normalized random measures with independent increments (NRMI), 48
NRMI
  mixture of, 49
NTR. *See* neutral to the right (NTR)

`OpenBugs`, 179
ordinal response
  multivariate, 83
  regression, 95

partition, 145
  least squares, 146
  nested, 170
PH. *See* proportional hazards (PH) model
pharmacodynamic models, 129
pharmacokinetic models, 129
Pitman Yor process, 28
Poisson Dirichlet process, 28
Polya tree (PT), **34**, 52, 70, 91, 101, 177
  dependent, 70
  marginal, 37
  mixture of (*see* mixture of Polya tree (MPT))
  partially specified (*see* finite Polya tree (FPT))
  posterior, 37

posterior simulation, 43
predictive distribution, 40
prior centering, 35
Polya urn, **15**, 78, **148**, 153
  zero-inflated, 173
population PK/PD models, 129
PPM. *See* product partition model (PPM)
PPMx model, 156
probit model
  multivariate, 84
product partition model (PPM), 150
  change-point problem, 152
  predictor dependent, 73
  spatial, 176
proportional hazards (PH) model, 2, **105**, 109, 127
proportional odds, 108, 109
pseudo contour probability, 117
PT. *See* Polya tree (PT)
PY. *See* Pitman Yor process
pyramid scheme, 55

`R2BayesX`, 4, 105, 109
  `bayesx`, 106
ROC curve, 96
  area under the curve, 96
  empirical, 98

similarity function, 156
slice sampler, 23
spatio-temporal data, 175
`spBayesSurv`, 109
species sampling model (SSM), 27
`splines`
  `bs`, 185
SSM. *See* species sampling model (SSM)
stick breaking construction, **8**, 28, 65, 176
  multivariate, 176
  spatial, 176

tail free (TF) process, 26, 34, 114
  linear dependent (*see* linear dependent tail free process)
TF. *See* tail free (TF) process
`tgp`, 63

wavelets, 54
WDDP. *See* weight dependent Dirichlet process (WDDP)
weight dependent Dirichlet process (WDDP), 180